UCLA Symposia on Molecular and Cellular Biology, New Series

Series Editor, C. Fred Fox

RECENT TITLES

Volume 77
Signal Transduction in Cytoplasmic Organization and Cell Motility, Peter Satir, John S. Condeelis, and Elias Lazarides, *Editors*

Volume 78
Tumor Progression and Metastasis, Garth L. Nicolson and Isaiah J. Fidler, *Editors*

Volume 79
Altered Glycosylation in Tumor Cells, Christopher L. Reading, Senitiroh Hakomori, and Donald M. Marcus, *Editors*

Volume 80
Protein Recognition of Immobilized Ligands, T.W. Hutchens, *Editor*

Volume 81
Biological and Molecular Aspects of Atrial Factors, Philip Needleman, *Editor*

Volume 82
Oxy-Radicals in Molecular Biology and Pathology, Peter A. Cerutti, Irwin Fridovich, and Joe M. McCord, *Editors*

Volume 83
Mechanisms and Consequences of DNA Damage Processing, Errol C. Friedberg and Philip C. Hanawalt, *Editors*

Volume 84
Technological Advances in Vaccine Development, Laurence Lasky, *Editor*

Volume 85
B Cell Development, Owen N. Witte, Norman R. Klinman, and Maureen C. Howard, *Editors*

Volume 86
Synthetic Peptides: Approaches to Biological Problems, James P. Tam and Emil Thomas Kaiser, *Editors*

Volume 87
Gene Transfer and Gene Therapy, I. Verma, R. Mulligan, and A. Beaudet, *Editors*

Volume 88
Molecular Biology of the Eye: Genes, Vision, and Ocular Disease, Joram Piatigorsky, Toshimichi Shinohara, and Peggy S. Zelenka, *Editors*

Volume 89
Liposomes in the Therapy of Infectious Diseases and Cancer, Gabriel Lopez-Berestein and Isaiah J. Fidler, *Editors*

Volume 90
Cell Biology of Virus Entry, Replication, and Pathogenesis, Richard W. Compans, Ari Helenius, and Michael B.A. Oldstone, *Editors*

Volume 91
Bone Marrow Transplantation: Current Controversies, Robert Peter Gale and Richard E. Champlin, *Editors*

Volume 92
The Molecular Basis of Plant Development, Robert Goldberg, *Editor*

Volume 93
Cellular and Molecular Biology of Muscle Development, Laurence H. Kedes and Frank E. Stockdale, *Editors*

Volume 94
Molecular Biology of RNA, Thomas R. Cech, *Editor*

Volume 95
DNA-Protein Interactions in Transcription, Jay D. Gralla, *Editor*

Volume 96
Stress-Induced Proteins, Mary Lou Pardue, James R. Feramisco, and Susan Lindquist, *Editors*

Volume 97
Molecular Biology of Stress, Shlomo Breznitz and Oren Zinder, *Editors*

Volume 98
Metal Ion Homeostasis: Molecular Biology and Chemistry, Dean H. Hamer and Dennis R. Winge, *Editors*

Volume 99
Human Tumor Antigens and Specific Tumor Therapy, Richard S. Metzgar and Malcolm S. Mitchell, *Editors*

Volume 100
Mechanisms of Action and Therapeutic Applications of Biologicals in Cancer and Immune Deficiency Disorders, J. Groopman, C. Evans, and D. Golde, *Editors*

Volume 101
Molecular Biology of Plant-Pathogen Interactions, Brian Staskawicz, Paul Ahlquist, and Olen Yoder, *Editors*

Please contact the publisher for information about previous titles in this series.

Molecular Biology of Plant-Pathogen Interactions

Molecular Biology of Plant-Pathogen Interactions

Proceedings of a UCLA Colloquium
Held at Steamboat Springs, Colorado
March 26–April 1, 1988

Editors

Brian Staskawicz
Department of Plant Pathology
University of California
Berkeley, California

Paul Ahlquist
Institute for Molecular Virology
Department of Plant Pathology
University of Wisconsin
Madison, Wisconsin

Olen Yoder
Department of Plant Pathology
Cornell University
Ithaca, New York

Alan R. Liss, Inc. • New York

Address all Inquiries to the Publisher
Alan R. Liss, Inc., 41 East 11th Street, New York, NY 10003

Printed in the United States of America

Library of Congress Cataloging-in-Publication Data

Molecular biology of plant-pathogen interactions.

(UCLA symposia on molecular and cellular biology ; new ser. v. 101)
Bibliography: p.
Includes index.
1. Plant-pathogen relationships—Molecular aspects—Congresses. I. Staskawicz, Brian John. II. Ahlquist, Paul. III. Yoder, Olen. IV. Series.
SB732.7.M65 1989 581.2′3 88-27205
ISBN 0-8451-4700-5

Contents

Contributors

Paul Ahlquist, Institute for Molecular Virology, and Department of Plant Pathology, University of Wisconsin, Madison, WI 53706 **[xv,105]**

Richard F. Allison, Institute for Molecular Virology, and Department of Plant Pathology, University of Wisconsin, Madison, WI 53706 **[105]**

David Baulcombe, Department of Molecular Genetics, Institute of Plant Science Research, Trumpington, Cambridge CB2 2LQ, England **[257]**

Roger N. Beachy, Department of Biology, Washington University, St. Louis, MO 63130 **[269]**

D.M. Bisaro, Department of Molecular Genetics, and Ohio State Biotechnology Center, Ohio State University, Columbus, OH 43210 **[199]**

John F. Bol, Department of Biochemistry, Leiden University, 2333 AL Leiden, The Netherlands **[247]**

J.M. Bonneville, Department of Plant Biology, Friedrich-Miescher-Institut, CH-4002 Basel, Switzerland **[153]**

L. Brand, Department of Plant Molecular Biology, Biological Sciences, Monsanto Company, St. Louis, MO 63198 **[199]**

Alan D. Brooks, Department of Botany and Center for Agricultural Biotechnology, University of Maryland, College Park, MD 20742 **[35]**

C. K. Browning, Department of Molecular Genetics, and Ohio State Biotechnology Center, Ohio State University, Columbus, OH 43210 **[199]**

P. Bubrick, Department of Plant Pathology, University of California, Riverside, CA 92521 **[117]**

Clifford D. Carpenter, Department of Plant Pathology, University of Massachusetts, Amherst, MA 01003 **[217]**

James C. Carrington, Department of Microbiology, Oregon State University, Corvallis, OR 97331 **[129]**

Susan M. Cary, Department of Microbiology, Oregon State University, Corvallis, OR 97331 **[129]**

Vitaly Citovsky, Department of Molecular Plant Biology, University of California Berkeley, Berkeley, CA 94720 **[3]**

Greg L. Cleveland, Department of Botany and Center for Agricultural Biotechnology, University of Maryland, College Park, MD 20742 **[35]**

The numbers in brackets are the opening page numbers of the contributors' articles.

Alan Collmer, Department of Botany and Center for Agricultural Biotechnology, University of Maryland, College Park, MD 20742 **[35]**

Ben J.C. Cornelissen, MOGEN International N.V., 2333 CB Leiden, The Netherlands **[247]**

Michael Dabrowski, Department of Biology, Indiana University, Bloomington, IN 47405 **[19]**

W.O. Dawson, Department of Plant Pathology, University of California, Riverside, CA 92521 **[117]**

Martine Devic, Department of Molecular Genetics, Institute of Plant Science Research, Trumpington, Cambridge CB2 2LQ, England **[257]**

M.D. Dickman, Ohio State Biotechnology Center, Ohio State University, Columbus, OH 43210; present address: Department of Plant Pathology, University of Nebraska, Lincoln, NE 68583-0722 **[87]**

William G. Dougherty, Department of Microbiology, Oregon State University, Corvallis, OR 97331 **[129]**

Rik Eggen, Department of Molecular Biology, Agricultural University, 6703 BC Wageningen, The Netherlands **[141]**

J.S. Elmer, Department of Plant Molecular Biology, Biological Sciences, Monsanto Company, St. Louis, MO 63198 **[199]**

Henk Engel, Department of Biology C-013, University of California San Diego, La Jolla, CA 92093; present address: Department of Biochemistry, University of Groningen, 9747 AG Groningen, The Netherlands **[217]**

J. Fütterer, Department of Plant Biology, Friedrich-Miescher-Institut, CH-4002 Basel, Switzerland **[153]**

R. Frederick, Department of Plant Pathology, University of California, Berkeley, CA 94720 **[49]**

W.E. Gardiner, Department of Molecular Genetics, and Ohio State Biotechnology Center, Ohio State University, Columbus, OH 43210 **[199]**

Stanton B. Gelvin, Department of Biological Sciences, Purdue University, West Lafayette, IN 47907 **[19]**

Rob Goldbach, Department of Virology, Agricultural University, 6709 PD Wageningen, The Netherlands **[141]**

K-B. Goldberg, Department of Plant Pathology, University of Kentucky, Lexington, KY 40546-0091 **[229]**

K. Gordon, Department of Plant Biology, Friedrich-Miescher-Institut, CH-4002 Basel, Switzerland **[153]**

S. Gowda, Department of Plant Pathology, University of Kentucky, Lexington, KY 40546-0091 **[229]**

C. Grimm, Institute of Molecular Biology and Biotechnology, Research Center of Crete, Heraklio, Greece; present address: Department of Plant Pathology, University of California, Berkeley, CA 94720 **[49]**

E.L. Halk, Agrigenetics Advanced Science Company, Madison, WI 53716 **[283]**

Bryan Harrison, Department of Virology, Scottish Crop Research Institute, Dundee DD2 5DA, Scotland **[257]**

Sheng Yang He, Department of Botany and Center for Agricultural Biotechnology, University of Maryland, College Park, MD 20742 **[35]**

K.K. Hill, Agrigenetics Advanced Science Company, Madison, WI 53716 **[283]**

Bradley I. Hillman, Department of Plant Pathology, University of California, Berkeley, CA 94720; present address: Department of Cell and Developmental Biology, Roche Institute of Molecular Biology, Roche Research Center, Nutley, NJ 07110 **[59,185]**

T. Hohn, Department of Plant Biology, Friedrich-Miescher-Institut, CH-4002 Basel, Switzerland **[153]**

Elizabeth Howard, Department of Molecular Plant Biology, University of California Berkeley, Berkeley, CA 94720 **[3]**

Stephen H. Howell, Department of Biology C-013, University of California San Diego, La Jolla, CA 92093 **[217]**

Martine Jaegle, Department of Molecular Genetics, Institute of Plant Science Research, Trumpington, Cambridge CB2 2LQ, England **[257]**

N.P. Jarvis, Agrigenetics Advanced Science Company, Madison, WI 53716 **[283]**

Joon M. Ji, Department of Biology, Indiana University, Bloomington, IN 47405 **[19]**

J. Jiricny, Department of Plant Biology, Friedrich-Miescher-Institut, CH-4002 Basel, Switzerland **[153]**

Howard S. Judelson, Department of Vegetable Crops, University of California, Davis, CA 95616 **[71]**

J. Kiernan, Department of Plant Pathology, University of Kentucky, Lexington, KY 40546-0091 **[229]**

P.E. Kolattukudy, Ohio State Biotechnology Center, Ohio State University, Columbus, OH 43210 **[87]**

K.J. Krahn, Agrigenetics Advanced Science Company, Madison, WI 53716 **[283]**

Sondra G. Lazarowitz, Department of Embryology, Carnegie Institution of Washington, Baltimore, MD 21210 **[167]**

L.W. Liao, Agrigenetics Advanced Science Company, Madison, WI 53716 **[283]**

P.B. Lindgren, Department of Plant Pathology, University of California, Berkeley, CA 94720; present address: Plant Biology Laboratory, The Salk Institute, La Jolla, CA 92037 **[49]**

L.S. Loesch-Fries, Agrigenetics Advanced Science Company, Madison, WI 53716 **[283]**

Asuncion Martinez, Department of Biology, Indiana University, Bloomington, IN 47405 **[19]**

D.J. Merlo, Agrigenetics Advanced Science Company, Madison, WI 53716 **[283]**

Richard W. Michelmore, Department of Vegetable Crops, University of California, Davis, CA 95616 **[71]**

M. Mindrinos, Department of Plant Pathology, University of California, Berkeley, CA 94720 **[49]**

T. Jack Morris, Department of Plant Pathology, University of California, Berkeley, CA 94720 **[185]**

Richard S. Nelson, Department of Biology, Washington University, St. Louis, MO 63130; present address: Division of Plant Biology, Noble Foundation, Ardmore, OK 73402 **[269]**

S.E. Nelson, Agrigenetics Advanced Science Company, Madison, MI 53716 **[283]**

Donald Nuss, Department of Cell and Developmental Biology, Roche Institute of Molecular Biology, Roche Research Center, Nutley, NJ 07110 **[59]**

N.J. Panopoulos, Department of Plant Pathology, University of California, Berkeley, CA 94720 **[49]**

T. Dawn Parks, Department of Microbiology, Oregon State University, Corvallis, OR 97331 **[129]**

Allison J. Pinder, Department of Embryology, Carnegie Institution of Washington, Baltimore, MD 21210 **[167]**

B. Pisan, Department of Plant Biology, Friedrich-Miescher-Institut, CH-4002 Basel, Switzerland **[153]**

G.K. Podila, Ohio State Biotechnology Center, Ohio State University, Columbus, OH 43210 **[87]**

Patricia A. Powell, Department of Biology, Washington University, St. Louis, MO 63130; present address: Department of Molecular Biology, Salk Institute, San Diego, CA 92138-9216 **[269]**

Brendan Rae, Department of Cell and Developmental Biology, Roche Institute of Molecular Biology, Roche Research Center, Nutley, NJ 07110 **[59]**

L. Rahme, Department of Plant Pathology, University of California, Berkeley, CA 94720 **[49]**

K.E. Rashka, Agrigenetics Advanced Science Company, Madison, WI 53716 **[283]**

Walt Ream, Department of Biology, Indiana University, Bloomington, IN 47405 **[19]**

James C. Register, III, Department of Biology, Washington University, St. Louis, MO 63130 **[269]**

R. Richins, Department of Plant Pathology, University of Kentucky, Lexington, KY 40546-0091 **[229]**

Jeffrey L. Ried, Department of Botany and Center for Agricultural Biotechnology, University of Maryland, College Park, MD 20742 **[35]**

E. Roberts, Ohio State Biotechnology Center, Ohio State University, Columbus, OH 43210; present address: Washington State University, Pullman, WA 99164 **[87]**

S.G. Rogers, Department of Plant Molecular Biology, Biological Sciences, Monsanto Company, St. Louis, MO 63198 **[199]**

H. Sanfaçon, Department of Plant Biology, Friedrich-Miescher-Institut, CH-4002 Basel, Switzerland **[153]**

J. Schoelz, Department of Plant Pathology, University of Kentucky, Lexington, KY 40546-0091; present address: Department of Plant Pathology, University of Missouri, Columbia, MO 65211 **[229]**

M. Schultze, Department of Plant Biology, Friedrich-Miescher-Institut, CH-4002 Basel, Switzerland **[153]**

R. Shepherd, Department of Plant Pathology, University of Kentucky, Lexington, KY 40546-0091 **[229]**

Anne E. Simon, Department of Biology C-013, University of California San Diego, La Jolla, CA 92093; present address: Department of Plant Pathology, University of Massachusetts, Amherst, MA 01002 **[217]**

Brian Staskawicz, Department of Plant Pathology, University of California, Berkeley, CA 94720 **[xv]**

G. Sunter, Department of Molecular Genetics, and Ohio State Biotechnology Center, Ohio State University, Columbus, OH 43210 **[199]**

James Tartaglia, Department of Cell and Developmental Biology, Roche Institute of Molecular Biology, Roche Research Center, Nutley, NJ 07110; present address: Department of Immunology, New York State Department of Health, Albany, NY 12201 **[59]**

Ab van Kammen, Department of Molecular Biology, Agricultural University, 6703 BC Wageningen, The Netherlands **[141]**

Jan A.L. van Kan, Department of Biochemistry, Leiden University, 2333 AL Leiden, The Netherlands **[247]**

K. Veluthambi, Department of Biological Sciences, Purdue University, West Lafayette, IN 47907 **[19]**

Jan Verver, Department of Molecular Biology, Agricultural University, 6703 BC Wageningen, The Netherlands **[141]**

Pieter Vos, Department of Molecular Biology, Agricultural University, 6703 BC Wageningen, The Netherlands **[141]**

Joan Wellink, Department of Molecular Biology, Agricultural University, 6703 BC Wageningen, The Netherlands **[141]**

Barbara Winsor, Department of Molecular Plant Biology, University of California Berkeley, Berkeley, CA 94720 **[3]**

Olen Yoder, Department of Plant Pathology, Cornell University, Ithaca, NY 14853-5908 **[xv]**

M. Young, Department of Plant Pathology, University of Kentucky, Lexington, KY 40546-0091; present address: Division of Plant Industry, CSIRO, Canberra, Australia **[229]**

Patricia Zambryski, Department of Molecular Plant Biology, University of California Berkeley, Berkeley, CA 94720 **[3]**

Preface

The UCLA Colloquium on **Molecular Biology of Plant–Pathogen Interactions** was held at Steamboat Springs, Colorado, from March 26 to April 1, 1988, with the principal aim of examining the molecular basis of plant disease from the perspective of both host and pathogen. This conference was the first international meeting dedicated to an integrated discussion of the molecular biology and host interactions of bacterial, fungal, and viral plant pathogens. The result was a series of timely and interactive sessions that examined the most recent advances throughout the field of molecular plant pathology. The conference was attended by over 250 scientists and was held concurrently with the UCLA Symposium on Molecular Biology of Plant Development, making these meetings a highlight of plant research communication in 1988.

Major advances in the identification and cloning of bacterial genes involved in pathogenesis, virulence, and host specificity have been accomplished in the last few years. This detailed knowledge has led to a closer molecular understanding of basic disease processes at the molecular level in several well-defined model plant-bacterial interactions.

The molecular basis of *Agrobacterium* transformation was examined in great detail, and the precise mechanism of plant transformation is beginning to be unravelled. A major advancement in this area is the discovery that certain genes in the *vir* region have been shown to be involved in coding proteins that facilitate T-DNA transfer. In addition, it has been established that the *vir* region contains two genetic loci, *virA* and *virG*, that are involved in controlling the induction of other *vir* genes and that are involved in the signal perception and signal transduction mediated by specific plant metabolites.

The molecular analysis of bacterial pathogenesis is being investigated in many laboratories around the world, and mutational analysis has revealed the occurrence of numerous genes that are necessary for pathogenicity and virulence. Many unresolved questions remain because the biochemical functions of many such genes have yet to be determined. In contrast, tremendous progress has been achieved in the cloning and analysis of genes encoding virulence functions such as phytohormone production and pectinolytic enzymes. Furthermore, genes controlling the induction of race-specific resistance have further strengthened the gene-for-gene hypothesis and have been cloned in several host-pathogen interactions. The question of whether the gene products of avirulence genes act directly or indirectly with the host to elicit a defense reaction remains unresolved.

The ability to introduce genes into phytopathogenic fungi by transformation has allowed researchers to approach the molecular analysis of fungal pathogenesis from a new perspective. During the meeting it became evident that most *Ascomycetes* can be transformed with existing vectors and that technology for other groups of fungi is rapidly developing. In addition to gene insertion, fungal transformation systems are being used to isolate genes from fungal genomes by functional complementation. For example, genes controlling fungal mating type have been isolated from several fungi, both *Ascomycetes* and *Basidiomycetes*, and characterized at the molecular level. Moreover, several laboratories have developed sufficient technology that they are poised to isolate genes that might be involved in fungal pathogenicity and virulence. Such genes may control synthesis of fungal products, including cellular and extracellular enzymes, low molecular weight toxins, and hormones, or they may encode products involved in race-specificity. Evaluation of the role of these genes in pathogenesis will be facilitated by the observation that site-specific gene disruptions and gene replacements occur in plant pathogenic fungi.

The considerable biological diversity of plant viruses was also well represented in this meeting. In addition to their intrinsic importance as pathogens, the relatively small genomes of viruses are well suited to global manipulation by present molecular genetic approaches, offering important opportunities for studying many facets of plant-pathogen interactions. In the varied systems discussed, significant advances were evident concerning both the processes of virus multiplication and the associated host interactions that govern resistant or pathogenic outcomes of infection.

In studies of RNA viruses, which constitute the majority of plant viruses, topics addressed included determinants of host specificity, as well as the mechanisms of viral protein processing and RNA replication. The extreme specificity of the latter processes for viral substrates has been explored in detailed characterization of recognition sites in both proteins and RNA templates, providing potential targets for further antiviral strategies. Also discussed were the biochemical properties and virulence determinants of a group of small pathogenic RNA molecules, including viroids, the simplest known independent pathogens, and the helper-dependent satellite RNAs of some viruses. Particularly elegant biochemical characterizations were presented on the autocatalytic RNA processing abilities of some satellite and viroid RNAs. Recent advances in plant DNA viruses include direct genetic mapping of host response and pathogenicity determinants in the reverse-transcribing, dsDNA caulimoviruses, as well as elucidation of novel translational mechanisms for gene expression and regulation. The unusual molecular biology and practical importance of ssDNA geminiviruses continue to attract growing research activity, which is reflected by important progress on viral DNA replication and gene expression and by initial work on the molecular basis of host range.

One of the most exciting recent developments in plant pathology has been the production of transgenic plants that possess effective resistance to specific viruses. Strategies already successfully pursued for engineered resistance include the expression of viral coat protein genes and the expression of cloned satellite RNAs. Presentations on engineered coat protein expression included demonstrations of protection in several new virus–host systems and further insight into the mechanisms underlying coat-mediated protection. In addition to the demonstrated use of complete satellite RNAs to inhibit replication of their natural helper viruses, a striking new possibility emerging from studies of viroids and some satellite RNAs is the engineering of new site specificities for their RNA-cleaving "ribozyme" properties. This approach should allow cleavage of specific sites in selected RNAs, either to destroy selected incoming viral genomes or to alter cellular gene expression posttranscriptionally.

On the challenging frontier of host responses to infection, prospects to use homologous or heterologous transposons to isolate plant resistance genes were discussed at length in several presentations. Impressive results were also presented on the "PR" proteins of tobacco, which are synthesized in response to necrosis-inducing infections and other stimuli, and whose appearance correlates with the onset of increased general resistance to a wide range of viruses, fungi, and bacteria. Virus-induced tobacco genes have been studied extensively: a number of PR protein genes have been cloned; the organization of their multigene families has been investigated; and specific antifungal functions (chitinase; 1,3-β-gluconase) has been associated with several PR gene products. There isolated PR genes promise significant further opportunities for elucidating the steps in plant gene induction in response to infection, as well as more opportunities to engineer pathogen resistance into plants.

The conference as a whole defined a dramatic advance, in just one or two years, in the conceptual state of plant pathology. Longstanding speculations are being replaced by specific observations, and much of the progress is attributable to new developments in molecular genetic manipulation of viruses and fungi, and to elegant applications of the established power of bacterial genetics. Major challenges remain, and foremost among them is the need to advance understanding of the host side of infection to approach the state of pathogen characterization. However, the growing ability to map and manipulate plant genomes and the current availability of several isolated plant genes with probable roles in defense responses provide specific tools with which to examine plant recognition and response to infection challenge.

The current momentum promises still more exciting prospects for definition of the primary components that interact in the confrontation of plants with pathogens, as well as the results of such interaction. As a summary of the conference, this book provides a picture of the current stage of advancement toward those goals.

Support for this meeting was provided by Unilever Research; Zoecon Research Institute, Sandoz Corporation; Protection Corporation; Ciba-Geigy Corporation, Biotechnology Research; Diatech, Ltd., London; Northrup King Company; Agracetus; DeKalb-Pfizer Genetics; and Pioneer HiBred International, Inc. Additional support was provided by The Director's Fund, established with gifts from Pfizer, Inc.; Amoco Technology Company, Biotechnology Division; Bio-Rad Laboratories; Bristol-Myers Company, Pharmaceutical Research and Development Division; Codon; DNAX Research Institute; Eastman Kodak Company; Genetics Institute, Inc.; American Hoechst Corporation; Immunex Corporation; Life Technologies, Inc.; Minnesota Mining & Manufacturing Company; New England Biolabs; Sandoz Research Institute; Ciba-Geigy Corporation, Pharmaceuticals Division; Wyeth Laboratories; and Warner Lambert/Parke-Davis; and by grant, 88-37234-3288 from the U.S. Department of Agriculture.

Brian Staskawicz
Paul Ahlquist
Olen Yoder

I. MECHANISM OF AGROBACTERIUM TRANSFORMATION

Molecular Biology of Plant–Pathogen Interactions, pages 3–18

PROTEINS THAT MEDIATE DNA TRANSFER BY AGROBACTERIUM TUMEFACIENS TO PLANT CELLS: SUMMARY AND PERSPECTIVES

Vitaly Citovsky, Elizabeth Howard, Barbara Winsor and Patricia Zambryski

Department of Molecular Plant Biology, University of California Berkeley, Berkeley, Ca. 94720

The genetic transformation of plant cells by *Agrobacterium tumefaciens* is a unique phenomenon of interkingdom DNA transfer, and it has been the focus of extensive research over the last ten years. As a result, the following sequence of events for the *Agrobacterium*-plant cell interaction has emerged (Figure 1). Wounded but otherwise metabolically active plant cells secrete phenolic compounds (for example, acetosyringone (AS) and alpha-hydroxy-acetosyringone for *Nicotiana tabacum* [1,2]) which are recognized by specific receptors on the bacterial membrane. The recognition involves positive chemotaxis towards the recipient plant cell (3), and results in the activation of a particular set of genes contained within the 35 kbp virulence (*vir*) region (1,2) of the Ti (tumor inducing) plasmid of the bacterium. Six virulence loci, *virA*, *virB*, *vir C*, *virD*, *virE*, and *virG* (4) are involved in the generation of a transferable DNA copy (T-DNA), which when mobilized from the Ti plasmid to the plant cell, induces tumor formation. Production of the T-DNA is initiated with recognition of 25 bp directly repeated sequences at each end of the element (5 and references therein), by a specific *vir* encoded endonuclease(6-10)to produce nicks between the 3rd and 4th base of the bottom strand of the 25 bp border repeats (11,12). Soon after border nicking single strand copies of the T-DNA region,

Figure 1

SEQUENCE OF EVENTS IN THE AGROBACTERIUM-PLANT CELL INTERACTION

recognition of the susceptible plant cell by *Agrobacterium*

a) secretion of phenolic compounds (*vir* signals) by wounded plant cell
b) positive chemotaxis towards wounded plant cell
c) attachment of *Agrobacterium* to plant cell surface (mediated by chromosomal virulence loci, *chvA*, *chvB*, *pscA* ?)

↓

binding of *vir* signals to bacterial membrane receptors (*vir* A)

↓

transmembrane signalling which induces *virG* mediated transcriptional activation of *vir* gene expression

↓

generation of a transferable T-DNA copy

a) VirD1/VirD2 endonuclease-induced nicks at bottom strand of T-DNA borders
b) unwinding of T-strand from right to left (facilitated by VirD1/VirD2 and VirE2 ?)

↓

assembly of transfer complex (VirD1/VirD2,VirE2, VirB polypeptides ?)

↓

transfer of T-strand complex through bacterial and plant cell membranes (*vir* products unknown)

↓

localization to plant nucleus

↓

integration into plant genome

designated T-strands (13), are detectable within _vir_ induced _Agrobacteria_ (8,13,14). T-strands are presumably unwound either prior to (or concommitant with) bottom strand replacement DNA synthesis and assembled into a complex with _vir_-specific proteins. Ultimately the T-strands are transferred into the recipient cell where they are integrated into the plant nuclear genome (15 and references therein). While molecular mechanisms leading to generation of the T-strands are emerging, later steps of the transfer process are still obscure.

The transfer process can be divided into three main stages: i) recognition of the recipient plant cell and induction of the virulence response; ii) production of T-strand, and iii) formation of the T-DNA transfer complex. For each of the steps in the T-DNA transfer process shown in Figure 1, we list the relevant bacterial proteins which have been assigned to carry out the reactions outlined (see also Table 1). In the following sections we review and evaluate the progress towards understanding the roles of particular proteins in mediating each of these steps. Finally, proteins known to be plant inducible but with no assigned function will be discussed.

PROTEINS MEDIATING BACTERIAL RECOGNITION OF AND RESPONSE TO RECIPIENT PLANT CELLS

Recognition of susceptible (wounded) plant cells by _Agrobacterium_ involves binding to the host cell and induction of virulence specific bacterial genes. The binding process was found to be mediated by the products of constituitively expressed chromosomal loci _chvA_, _chvB_ (16,17) and _pscA_ (18). The first two loci are located on a 15.5 kbp fragment of the bacterial chromosome. While the function of _chvA_ remains unknown, it has been shown that the 8kb _chvB_ locus encodes a protein of approximately 235 kDa that acts as an

Table 1

CHARACTERIZATION OF OCTOPINE VIRULENCE PROTEINS

Locus	Size (kb)	Forms tumors?	Size (kDa) Predicted	Size (kDa) Observed	Location	Assigned function(s)
<u>virA</u>	2.0	-	70	ND	M	AS sensor, kinase ?
<u>virG</u>	0.6	-	30	36	C?	activates <u>vir</u> expression
<u>virB</u>	9.5	-	26,12,11.7,22 66,23.5,32.5 9,26,73,38	33,80 25	M	transmembrane channel?
<u>virC</u>	1.8	+/-	26,23	ND	?	enhances virulence, host range
<u>virD</u>	4.5	-	16,47, 21,76	16,56	C?	border endonuclease, T-strand production, pilot protein?
<u>virE</u>	1.8	-/+	60	65	C/M	ssDNA binding protein

ND-not determined; M-membrane; C-cytoplasm. See text for references.

intermediate in the synthesis of cyclic beta-1,2-glucan(19,20). The pscA locus is approximately 3.0 kbp and is involved in the synthesis of the major neutral and acidic extracellular polysaccharides (18). Evidently, chvB and pscA (and possibly chvA) loci have major effects on the composition of the bacterial cell wall and potentially plasma membrane. It is not known, however, how the products of these loci enhance bacterial attachment to the plant cell nor whether they interact with plant cell wall components or directly with plasma membranes of the wounded cells. If these proteins do bind plasma membranes of the wounded cell directly, specificity for plant membranes rather than cell wall components could target the bacteria to breaks in the cell wall. Potentially such direct access to the recipient cell plasma membrane would facilitate subsequent DNA transfer.

Induction of vir expression by plant phenolics is mediated by the products of the virA and virG loci (21). Insertion mutations in these genes result in greatly attenuated (virA) or totally deficient (virG) induction of the other vir loci. The model for virA/virG activation of the vir loci is based on significant amino acid homology between the products of these loci and other pairs of bacterial proteins which act as sensor-regulators of gene expression in response to extracellular stimuli (21-23). For example, the envZ/ompR, ntrB/ntrC and phoR/phoB pairs of genes allow E.coli to respond to the changes in osmolarity or nitrogen and phosphate concentrations, respectively. The first gene in each pair encodes a membrane protein which directly senses the external signal. The protein product of the second member of the pair acts as a positive transcriptional activator. That virA functions as a sensor molecule in Agrobacterium derives from recent results indicating that the virA polypeptide localizes to the inner membrane (24). The mechanism of virA transmembrane signalling which results in virG induction is unknown. Nor has it been shown whether the virG polypeptide binds directly to other vir promotor regions or effects induction by interaction with the RNA polymerase or another protein factor.

PROTEINS RESPONSIBLE FOR T-STRAND PRODUCTION

Currently, only two vir proteins, namely the VirD1 and VirD2 polypeptides, are known to directly participate in the generation of T-strand molecules (8,12). Mutant analysis revealed that these proteins are responsible for the T-DNA border specific endonuclease activity (6-10). Resultant nicks at the right and left borders are presumably then used as initiation and termination sites for T-strand production. Other proteins essential to the generation of T-strands are thought to be constituitive chromosomal products. Transfer of the T-DNA is strictly polar, in a leftward direction from the right border (5,25). Polarity of the T-strand makes sense, since only the DNA to the left of the right T-DNA border is transferred. This raises the question of how the T-strand generating proteins distinguish between homologous right and left border repeats to effect polar transfer. One possibility is that since the Ti plasmid sequences surrounding right and left 25 bp border repeats are different, these adjacent regions influence the recognition and utilization of each border. If this is true, sequence context specific to each border, as well as protein complexes capable of recognizing and interacting with such sequences must be an integral part of the transfer process. In fact, in the simple case of the single T-DNA element of the nopaline Ti plasmid, sequences surrounding the right border of the T-DNA promote efficient transfer, whereas sequences surrounding the left border attenuate transfer relative to that obtained with isolated border sequences (26,27). Earlier work with the more the complex octopine Ti plasmid containing three adjacent T-DNA elements, described a 24 bp consensus sequence capable of promoting the T-DNA transfer. This sequence, designated _overdrive_, is found adjacent to the right borders of the octopine Ti plasmid (28). Recent data demonstrate that _overdrive_ acts an enhancer; it stimulates T-DNA transfer when placed in either orientation, on either side or at variable distance (up to 6 kbp) from the border repeat sequences (29, W. Ream unpublished results). The latter results explain how the octopine Ti plasmid can transfer three T-DNA elements using only two _overdrive_ sequences.

The mechanisms by which these sequences are utilized by _Agrobacterium_ proteins are still unknown. Our preliminary results indicate that the VirD2 product is tightly associated with the T-strand molecule (E.A. Howard, unpublished observations) following the nicking reaction at the right border. Since earlier work showed that the 3' end of the T-strand is available to exonuclease digestion (13), it is likely that the 5' end of the T-strand at the border nick site remains associated with the VirD2 product. These observations can be understood if there are two types of VirD1/VirD2 border interactions. One is a simple nicking reaction at the left border sequence. There are only two participants in this event - VirD endonuclease and the border repeat. The second type of interaction is more complex. The _overdrive_ region (or its unidentifed counterpart in the nopaline plasmid) is proposed (see also 30) to act as an assembly site for a putative processing complex. This complex includes VirD endonuclease, bacterial helicase and possibly other proteins such as DNA polymerase. The processing complex becomes associated with the sequences adjacent to the right border repeat. Three subsequent reactions will then take place at the right border: nicking, tight attachment of the VirD2 protein to the 5' end of the nick and unwinding of the bottom (T) strand leftwards from the right border.

PROTEINS OF THE T-DNA TRANSFER COMPLEX

All of the processes summarized above have evolved to produce a structure, the T-DNA transfer complex, capable of penetrating through bacterial and recipient plant cell plasma membranes and possibly cell walls to introduce new genetic information into the plant genome. Major functions which may be attributed to the proteins of the transfer complex include protection of the T-strand molecule, recognition of transmembrane routes from the bacterium to the recipient plant cell, targeting of the transfer complex to the plant nucleus, and efficient integration of the transferred DNA into the plant genome.

One protein characterized as a probable part of the transfer complex is the VirE2 polypeptide. The protein product of the *virE2* locus was shown to possess a single stranded (ss) DNA binding activity (31-33). Similar to other known bacterial ssDNA binding proteins, VirE2 protein binds ssDNA in a highly cooperative manner but without any apparent sequence specificity (V. Citovsky, M.L. Wong, and P. Zambryski, manuscript in preparation.). Electron microscopy studies show that VirE2-coated linear ssDNA molecules appear as fully unfolded rigid structures as opposed to collapsed DNA molecules observed in the absence of the protein (V. Citovsky, M.L. Wong, and P. Zambryski, *op. cit.*). The observation that the VirE2 protein is one of the most abundantly produced *vir* products (31,35) lends support to the idea that it has a structural and protective function in the transfer complex . For example, to completely coat a 20 kb nopaline T-strand molecule would require about 700 molecules (assuming a 30 nucleotide binding site)(34). The amount of VirE2 product observed in plant-induced *Agrobacterium* is consistent with this estimate (31,35).

The VirE2 ssDNA binding protein is one of the largest prokaryotic ssDNA binding proteins identified to date (reviewed in 36); potentially this protein has several functional domains that act at different steps of the T-DNA transfer process. In fact, the ssDNA binding activity may not be its major function. An unusual feature of the *virE2* locus is that mutants in its locus can be complemented to wild-type virulence if co-innoculated on plants with *Agrobacterium* carrying a complete wild-type *vir* region (37). The extracellular complementation of *virE* mutants indicates potentially that the product(s) of this locus can be translocated through the bacterial envelope. For example, the VirE2 protein may facilitate passage of the T-DNA complex through bacterial membranes and possibly through plant cell plasma and nuclear membranes. Transmembrane secretion of VirE2 (or VirE2-T-strand complexes) may be mediated by the products of the *virB* locus since proteins encoded by the N-terminal half of this locus were found to fractionate to the cell envelope (35). It is conceivable that *virB* polypeptides form membrane channels through which T-DNA transfer complexes are secreted. Finally, although existing data are tentative, it has been suggested that *virE* specific proteins also play a role in the integration of the T-DNA into the plant cell genome (38).

Another *vir* protein likely to be part of the transfer complex is a product of the *virD* locus. As mentioned above, the VirD2 protein was found tightly associated with the T-strand. This protein potentially serves as a plant cell and/or nuclear localization signal that together with the products of the *virE* locus facilitates translocation of the transfer complex through bacterial and plant membranes.

PROTEINS WITH NONASSIGNED FUNCTIONS

The biological function of most of the plant-induced Agrobacterium proteins have not yet been elucidated. For example, polypeptides of the 9.5 kbp virB locus are uncharacterized (except for their cell fractionation and relative abundance). The sequence of this locus predicts eleven open reading frames (ORFs)(39). However, only three virB polypeptides encoded by the N-terminus of the virB locus have been observed in vir induced Agrobacteria (35), and they do not correspond to any of the predicted ORFs. The C-terminal half of the virD locus contains sufficient information to encode two possible ORFs of 21 kDa and 76 kDa whose roles are unknown (40,41). The virC locus sequence predicts two polypeptides of 26 kDa and 23 kDa (42); again the functions of the virC products are unknown. The sequence of the virE locus of the octopine Ti plasmid predicts a second ORF of 7 kDa at the 5' end (43), and several possible small ORFs are also found at the 5' end of the nopaline virE locus (44). The significance of these small virE encoded polypeptides remains to be determined (see Table 1).

Moreover, there are at least five additional proteins, designated virulence related proteins (VRPs), which are induced in Agrobacterium by plant signal molecules (35). Production of VRPs is dependent on intact virA and virG loci, i.e. they are under the control of the vir regulatory system. One VRP of apparent molecular weight 45 kDa is encoded by pinF (plant inducible locus F)(4) which maps adjacent to the vir region. Another VRP of apparent molecular weight 27 kDa is encoded by an unknown region of the Ti plasmid, while other VRPs are likely to be chromosomally encoded (35). The existence of VRPs indicates another level of genetic and functional complexity in the T-DNA transfer process. While pinF seems to be nonessential (4), other VRPs may be involved in the T-DNA transfer either directly by specifying components of the transfer machinery, or indirectly by affecting the general metabolism of the bacterial cell during its interaction with the plant cell.

WHAT IS THE MECHANISM OF THE T-DNA TRANSFER?

We propose that the T-DNA transfer by *Agrobacterium* essentially combines two different mechanisms of DNA transfer, namely bacterial conjugation and viral infection. The first step includes induction of the mobilization of the T-DNA element using plant signals by a conjugation-like process with such characteristic features as site-specific nicking, generation of a single stranded transferable DNA molecule and 5' to 3' polarity of the DNA transfer (45). In strong support that a conjugative mechanism is operative for this process is the observation that the mobilization functions (*mob*) and the origin of transfer (*oriT*) of a bacterial plasmid (pRSF1010), when transformed into an *Agrobacterium* strain harboring the entire *vir* region (in the absence of the native Ti plasmid with its relevant T-DNA region), promoted transfer of RSF1010 into plants (46). Thus, a bacterial origin of transfer, in the presence of its particular mobilization proteins, was capable of exploiting *Agrobacterium*'s system for bacterial/plant DNA transfer to effect its own "conjugative" transfer. This observation suggests that the border sequences of the T-DNA are functionally analogous to plasmid *oriT's*. Thus, at least a subset of the virulence genes (such as *virD* and *virB*) must be analogous to the transfer genes of bacterial conjugation. Agrobacterium, then, may have adapted components of its (bacterial) conjugative system to allow for DNA transfer to plant cells.

A conjugation model is not sufficient to explain the entire process of Agrobacterium infection of plant cells since, unlike DNA transferred between bacteria during conjugation, T-DNA must be capable of penetrating the plant cell membrane, localizing to and penetrating the nuclear membrane and finally, integrating efficiently into the plant genome. These latter events are classical features of virus-cell interaction. It is tempting to speculate that once the T-DNA transfer complex is formed (by a conjugation-like mechanism), the Agrobacterium cell functions as a viral envelope which hosts an infectious deoxyribonucleoprotein complex. Envelope-like functions of the bacterial membrane would then facilitate (by formation of membrane pores, for example) passage of the transfer complex into the plant cell. All subsequent steps would be carried out by this complex in a virus-like manner. This model assumes an independent and self-sufficient role for the T-DNA complex. If this is true, *in vitro* reconstitution of the T-DNA transfer complex could be a useful tool for genetic modification of plants.

Acknowledgements: Current research is supported by NSF grant DMB-861772 to P.Z.

REFERENCES

1. Stachel, S.E., Messens, E., Van Montagu, M., Zambryski, P. (1985) Identification of the signal molecules produced by wounded plant cells that activate T-DNA transfer in *Agrobacterium tumefaciens*. Nature (London) 318, 624-629
2. Stachel, S.E., Nester, E.W., Zambryski, P. (1986) A plant cell factor induces *Agrobacterium tumefaciens vir* gene expression. Proc. Natl. Acad. Sci. USA 83, 379-383

3. Ashby, A.M., Watson, M.D., Shaw, C.H. (1987) A Ti-plasmid determined function is responsible for chemotaxis of A. tumefaciens towards the plant wound compound acetosyringone. FEMS Microbiol. Lett. 41, 189-192
4. Stachel, S.E., Nester, E.W. (1986) The genetic and transcriptional organization of the vir region of the A6 Ti-plasmid of Agrobacterium. EMBO J. 5, 1445-1454
5. Wang, K., Herrera-Estrella, L., Van Montagu, M., Zambryski, P. (1984) Right 25 bp terminus sequence of the nopaline T-DNA is essential for and determines direction of T-DNA transfer from Agrobacterium to the plant genome. Cell 38, 35-41
6. Alt-Moerbe, J., Rak, B., Schroeder, J. (1986) A 3.6 kbp segment from the vir region of Ti plasmids contains genes responsible for border sequence-directed production of T-region circles in E. coli. EMBO J. 5, 1129-1135
7. Yanofsky, M.F., Porter, S.G., Young, C., Albright, L.M., Gordon, M.P., Nester, E.W. (1986) The virD operon of Agrobacterium tumefaciens encodes a site-specific endonuclease. Cell 47, 471-477
8. Stachel, S.E., Timmerman, B., Zambryski, P. (1987) Activation of A. tumefaciens vir gene expression generates multiple single-stranded T-strand molecules from the pTiA6 T-region: requirement for 5' virD products. EMBO J. 6, 857-863
9. Veluthambi, K., Jayaswal, R.K., Gelvin, S.B. (1987) Virulence genes A, G, and D mediate the double stranded border cleavage of T-DNA from the Agrobacterium Ti-plasmid. Proc. Natl. Acad. Sci. USA 84, 1881-1885
10. Yamamoto, A., Iwahashi, M., Yanofsky, M.F., M.F., Nester, E.W., Takebe, I., Machida, Y. (1987) The proximal region in the virD locus of Agrobacterium tumefaciens is necessary for the plant inducible circularization of T-DNA. Molec. Gen. Genet. 206, 174-177
11. Wang, K., Stachel, S.E., Timmerman, B., Van Montagu, M., Zambryski, P. (1987) Site-specific nick occurs within the 25 bp transfer promoting border sequence following induction of vir gene expression in Agrobacterium tumefaciens. Science 235, 587-591

12. Albright, L.M., Yanofsky, M.F., Leroux, B., Ma, D., Nester, E.W. (1987) Processing of the T-DNA of A. tumefaciens generates border nicks and linear, single stranded T-DNA. J. Bacteriol. 169, 1046-1055
13. Stachel, S.E., Timmerman, B., Zambryski, P. (1986) Generation of single-stranded T-DNA molecules during the initial stages of T-DNA transfer from Agrobacterium tumefaciens to plant cells. Nature 322, 706-712
14. Veluthambi, K., Ream, W., Gelvin, S. (1988) Virulence genes, borders and overdrive generate single stranded T-DNA molecules from the A6 Ti-plasmid plasmid of Agrobacterium. J. Bacteriol., in press
15. Gheysen, G., Van Montagu, M., Zambryski, P. (1987) Integration of A. tumefaciens T-DNA involves rearrangements of target plant DNA sequences. Proc. Natl. Acad. Sci. USA 84, 6169-6173
16 Douglas, C.J., Halperin, W., Nester, E.W. (1982) Agrobacterium tumefaciens mutants affected in attachment to plant cells. J. Bacteriol. 152, 1265-1275
17 Douglas, C.J., Staneloni, R.J., Rubin, R.A., Nester, E.W. (1985) Identification and genetic analysis of an Agrobacterium tumefaciens chromosomal virulence region. J. Bacteriol. 161, 850-860
18. Thomashow, M.F., Karlinsey, J.E., Marks, J.R., Hurlbert, R.E. (1987) Identification of a new virulence locus in A. tumefaciens that affects polysaccharide composition and plant-cell attachment. J. Bacteriol. 169, 3209-3216
19. Zorreguieta, A., Geremia, R.A., Cavaignac, S., Cangelosi, G.A., Nester, E.W., Ugalde, R.A. (1988) A chromosomal virulence locus of Agrobacterium is the structural gene for an intermediate in -1,2-glucan synthesis. J. Bacteriol., in press
20. Puvanesarajah, V., Schell, F.M., Stacey, G., Douglas, C.J., Nester, E.W. (1985) Role for 2-linked beta-D-glucan in the virulence of A. tumefaciens. J. Bacteriol. 164, 102-106
21. Stachel, S.E., Zambryski, P. (1986) VirA and virG control the plant-induced activation of the T-DNA transfer process of Agrobacterium tumefaciens. Cell, 46, 325-333
22. Winans, S.C., Ebert, P.R., Stachel, S.E., Gordon, M.P., Nester, E.W. (1986) A gene essential for

Agrobacterium virulence is homologous to a family of positive regulatory loci. Proc. Natl. Acad. Sci. USA 83, 8278-8282

23. Ronson, C.W., Nixon, B.T., Ausubel, F.M. (1987) Conserved domains in bacterial regulatory proteins that respond to environmental stimuli. Cell 5, 579-581
24. Leroux, B., Yanofsky, M.F., Winans, S.C., Ward, J.E., Ziegler, S.F., Nester, E.W. (1987) Characterization of the virA locus of Agrobacterium tumefaciens: a transcriptional regulator and host range determinant. EMBO J. 6, 849-856.
25 Peralta, E.G., Ream, L.W. (1985) T-DNA border sequences required for crown gall tumorigenesis. Proc. Natl. Acad. Sci. USA 82, 5112-5116
26. Jen, G., Chilton, M.D. (1986) The right border region of pTiT37 T-DNA is intrinsically more active than the left border region in promoting T-DNA transformation. Proc. Natl. Acad. Sci. USA 83, 3895-3899
27. Wang, K., Genetello, C., Van Montagu, M., Zambryski, P. (1987) Sequence context of the T-DNA border repeat element determines its relative activity during T-DNA transfer to plant cells. Mol. Gen. Genet. 210, 338-346
28. Peralta, E.G., Hellmiss, R., Ream, T. (1986) Overdrive, a T-DNA transmission enhancer on the A. tumefaciens tumor-inducing plasmid. EMBO J. 5, 1137-1142
29. Van Haaren, M.J.J., Sedee, N.J.A., Schilperoort, R.A., Hooykaas, P.J.J. (1987) Overdrive is a T-region transfer enhancer which stimulates T-strand production in A. tumefaciens. Nucl. Acids Res. 15, 8983-8997
30. Zambryski, P. (1988) Basic processes underlying Agrobacterium mediated DNA transfer to plant cells. Ann. Rev. Genetics, in press
31. Citovsky, V., De Vos, G., Zambryski, P. (1988) Single stranded DNA binding protein encoded by the virE locus of Agrobacterium tumefaciens. Science 240, 501-504.
32. Das, A. (1988) The A. tumefaciens virE operon encodes a single stranded DNA binding protein. Proc. Natl. Acad. Sci. USA, in press
33. Christie, P.J., Ward, J.E., Winans, S., Nester, E.W. (1988) The Agrobacterium tumefaciens virE2 gene product is a single stranded DNA binding protein that associates with T-strands. J. Bacteriol., in press
34. Gietl, C., Koukolikova-Nicola, Z., Hohn, B. (1987) Mobilization of T-DNA from Agrobacterium to plant cells involves a protein that binds single stranded DNA. Proc. Natl. Acad. Sci. USA 84, 9006-9010

35. Engstrom, P., Zambryski, P., Van Montagu, M., Stachel, S.E. (1987) Characterization of A. tumefaciens virulence proteins induced by the plant factor acetosyringone. J. Mol. Biol., 197, 635-645
36. Chase, J.W., Williams, K.R. (1986) Single stranded DNA binding proteins required for DNA replication. Ann. Rev. Biochem. 55, 103-136
37. Otten, L., DeGreve, H., Leemans, J., Hain, R., Hooykass, P., Schell, F.M. (1984) Restoration of virulence of vir region mutants of A. tumefaciens strain B6S3 by coinfection with normal and mutant Agrobacterium strains. Mol. Gen. Genet. 195, 159-163
38. Gardener, R.C., Knauf, V. (1986) Transfer of Agrobacterium DNA to plants requires a T-DNA border but not the virE locus. Science 231, 725-727
39. Ward, J.E., Akiyoski, D., Regier, D., Datta, A., Gordon, M.P., Nester, E.W. (1988) Characterization of the virB operon from Agrobacterium tumefaciens Ti plasmid. J. Biol. Chem, in press
40. Porter, S.G., Yanofsky, M.F., Nester, E.W. (1987) Molecular characterization of the virD operon from A. tumefaciens. Nucl. Acids Res. 15, 7503-7517
41. Jayaswal, R.K., Veluthambi, K., Gelvin, S.B., Slightom, J.L. (1987) Double stranded T-DNA cleavage and the generation of single stranded T-DNA molecules in E. coli by a virD encoded border specific endonuclease from A. tumefaciens. J. Bacteriol. 169, 5035-5045
42. Yanofsky, M.F., Nester, E.W. (1986) Molecular characterization of a host-range determining locus from Agrobacterium tumefaciens. J. Bacteriol. 168, 244-250
43. Winans, S.C., Allenza, P., Stachel, S.E., McBride, K.E., Nester, E.W. (1987) Characterization of the virE operon of the Agrobacterium Ti-plasmid pTiA6. Nucl. Acids Res. 15, 825-837
44. Hirooka, T., Rogowsky, P.M., Kado, C.I. (1987) Characterization of the virE locus of A. tumefaciens plasmid pTiC58. J. Bacteriol. 169, 1529-1536
45. Stachel, S.E., Zambryski, P.C. (1986) Agrobacterium tumefaciens and the susceptible plant cell: a novel adaptation of extracellular recognition and DNA conjugation. Cell 47, 155-157
46. Buchanan-Wollaston, V., Passiatore, J.E., Cannon, F. (1987) The mob and oriT mobilization functions of a bacterial plasmid promote its transfer to plants. Nature 328, 172-175

Molecular Biology of Plant–Pathogen Interactions, pages 19–31

THE OVERDRIVE ENHANCER SEQUENCE STIMULATES PRODUCTION OF T-STRANDS FROM THE AGROBACTERIUM TUMEFACIENS TUMOR-INDUCING PLASMID[1]

Joon M. Ji[2], Asuncion Martinez[2], Michael Dabrowski[2], K. Veluthambi[3], Stanton B. Gelvin[3], and Walt Ream[2]

[2] Department of Biology, Indiana University, Bloomington, Indiana 47405

[3] Department of Biological Sciences, Purdue University, West Lafayette, Indiana 47907

ABSTRACT During crown gall tumorigenesis a specific segment of the *A. tumefaciens* tumor-inducing (Ti) plasmid, the T-DNA, integrates into plant nuclear DNA. Similar 23-base-pair (bp) direct repeats at each end of the T-region signal T-DNA borders, and efficient T-DNA transmission requires two discrete sequences: the right-hand border repeat and the 24 bp T-DNA transmission enhancer sequence called *overdrive*. T-DNA transmission apparently initiates when the *virD* endonuclease produces a site-specific nick in the bottom strand of the right-hand border repeat. Subsequent events generate T-strands, linear single-stranded DNA molecules containing the entire bottom strand of the T-region. A synthetic right border repeat in its wild-type orientation promotes T-DNA transmission (virulence) at a low frequency; a conserved Ti plasmid sequence (*overdrive*) which normally flanks the right border repeat greatly stimulates virulence. We investigated the influence of location on the ability of *overdrive* to stimulate right

[1] W.R. thanks the American Cancer Society for a Junior Faculty Research Award (JFRA-175), the National Science Foundation for grant PCM8316006, and the National Institutes of Health for Research Career Development Award K04 AI00838-01 and for grant R01 GM38294-01. A NSF Presidential Young Investigator Award (DMB8351152) with matching funds from Agrigenetics Research Associates supported S.B.G.

border function. The *overdrive* sequence normally lies either 15 bp or 16 bp to the right of two known right border repeats, but *overdrive* retained its activity when relocated, in either orientation, 75 bp to the left of the border repeat. The T-DNA transmission enhancer stimulated virulence significantly when moved 553 bp to the right of the border repeat, but distances greater than 3,000 bp diminished its activity. Upon cocultivation with tobacco protoplasts, strains carrying a functional *overdrive* accumulated substantially more T-strands than strains lacking the enhancer sequence. Introduction of a multicopy cosmid carrying the *virG*, *virC*, *virD*, and *virE* operons suppressed the phenotype of an *overdrive* deletion mutant, restoring wild-type levels of virulence and T-strand production. Mutations in the *virC* operon reduced virulence to the same extent as deletion of the *overdrive* sequence. Double mutants exhibited the same virulence as the single mutant parents suggesting that *virC*-encoded proteins function at *overdrive*.

INTRODUCTION

Crown gall tumors form on most dicotyledonous plants when virulent strains of *Agrobacterium tumefaciens*, containing a 190 kilobase-pair (kb) tumor inducing (Ti) plasmid, infect wounded plant tissue (1). A specific segment of the Ti plasmid, the T-DNA, transfers into plant cells and stably integrates into plant nuclear DNA (2,3). The T-DNA encodes enzymes for biosynthesis of auxin and cytokinin thereby causing transformed cells to grow as crown gall tumors (1).

T-DNA transmission (transfer and integration) involves specific DNA-protein interactions. Similar 23-base-pair (bp) direct repeats at each end of the T-region signal T-DNA borders (4-6), and efficient T-DNA transmission requires two discrete sequences: the right-hand border repeat (7-9) and the 24 bp T-DNA transmission enhancer sequence called *overdrive* (7,8,10,11). Virulence (*vir*) genes located outside of the T-region on the Ti plasmid also play an essential role (12). Wounded plant cells produce phenolic compounds (acetosyringone) which induce the expression of the *vir* genes (13). The first two genes in the *virD* operon encode an endonuclease activity which generates specific nicks and cuts within the border repeats (14-19). T-DNA transmission apparently initiates when the virD endonuclease produces a site-specific nick in the bottom strand of the right-hand border repeat (14,16,19). Subsequent events generate T-strands, linear single-stranded DNA molecules containing the entire bottom strand of the T-region (16). T- strands may represent intermediates in T-DNA transmission.

The right border repeat plays an essential role in virulence. A synthetic right border repeat in its wild-type orientation promotes T-DNA transmission (7-9) (virulence) at a low frequency; a conserved Ti plasmid sequence (overdrive) which normally flanks the right border repeat greatly stimulates virulence (7,8). Our previous work showed: overdrive functions fully in either orientation whereas the border repeat promotes T-DNA transmission best in one direction, and the exact spacing and sequence between a border repeat and overdrive can vary slightly without reducing border function (7).

In this study we: (1) investigated further the effects of location and distance on the ability of overdrive to promote T-DNA transmission, (2) identified molecular events stimulated by the overdrive enhancer sequence, and (3) used genetic experiments to identify proteins that act at overdrive. The overdrive sequence normally lies either 15 bp or 16 bp to the right of two known right border repeats (7), but overdrive retained its activity when relocated, in either orientation, 75 bp to the left of the border repeat. The T-DNA transmission enhancer stimulated virulence significantly when moved 553 bp to the right of the border repeat, but distances greater than 3,000 bp diminished its activity.

Overdrive stimulated molecular events which likely play a role in virulence. Upon cocultivation with tobacco protoplasts, strains carrying a functional overdrive accumulated substantially more T-strands than strains lacking the enhancer sequence. Introduction of a multicopy cosmid carrying the virG, virC, virD, and virE operons suppressed the phenotype of an overdrive deletion mutant, restoring wild-type levels of virulence and T-strand production. Apparently, extra copies of specific vir genes generated abnormally abundant amounts of vir proteins and rendered the overdrive sequence unnecessary. Thus, overdrive played a quantitative role in T-DNA transmission by stimulating early events in this process under conditions where the concentrations of specific vir proteins limited T-DNA transfer and virulence. This relationship of T-DNA right borders to overdrive resembles that of inverted repeats to recombinational enhancers in several site-specific inversion systems (20-24).

Genetic experiments identified a specific vir locus which encodes proteins that likely act at overdrive. Transposon insertions in the virC operon reduced virulence to the same extent as deletions removing the overdrive sequence. We constructed virC overdrive double mutants which exhibited the same virulence as the single mutant parents suggesting that virC-encoded proteins function at overdrive.

MATERIALS AND METHODS

We used methods and strains described earlier (7,8,25).

RESULTS

Position and Orientation Independence of Overdrive.

To determine whether the order of the border repeat and overdrive affects the efficiency of T-DNA transmission, we inserted the synthetic overdrive in each orientation 76 bp to the left of the pTiA6 TL right border repeat (WR1151 & WR1152; Fig. 1). Both strains exhibited the same virulence as a wild-type strain (WR1101), and these strains exhibited much greater virulence than the parental strain (WR1076) which lacked overdrive. Thus, overdrive stimulated T-DNA transmission greatly when placed, in either orientation, to the left of the border repeat, and overdrive retained its function when positioned 60 bp farther than normal from the border repeat.

Effect of Distance on Overdrive Activity.

To test whether overdrive could act over a substantial distance to stimulate T-DNA transmission, we increased the distance between overdrive and the TL right border repeat. Using a synthetic linker oligonucleotide, we created a BglII site in place of the SstI site that separates overdrive from the TL right border repeat; this modification increased the distance between these sequences to 36 bp. We inserted specific restriction fragments from phage lambda into this

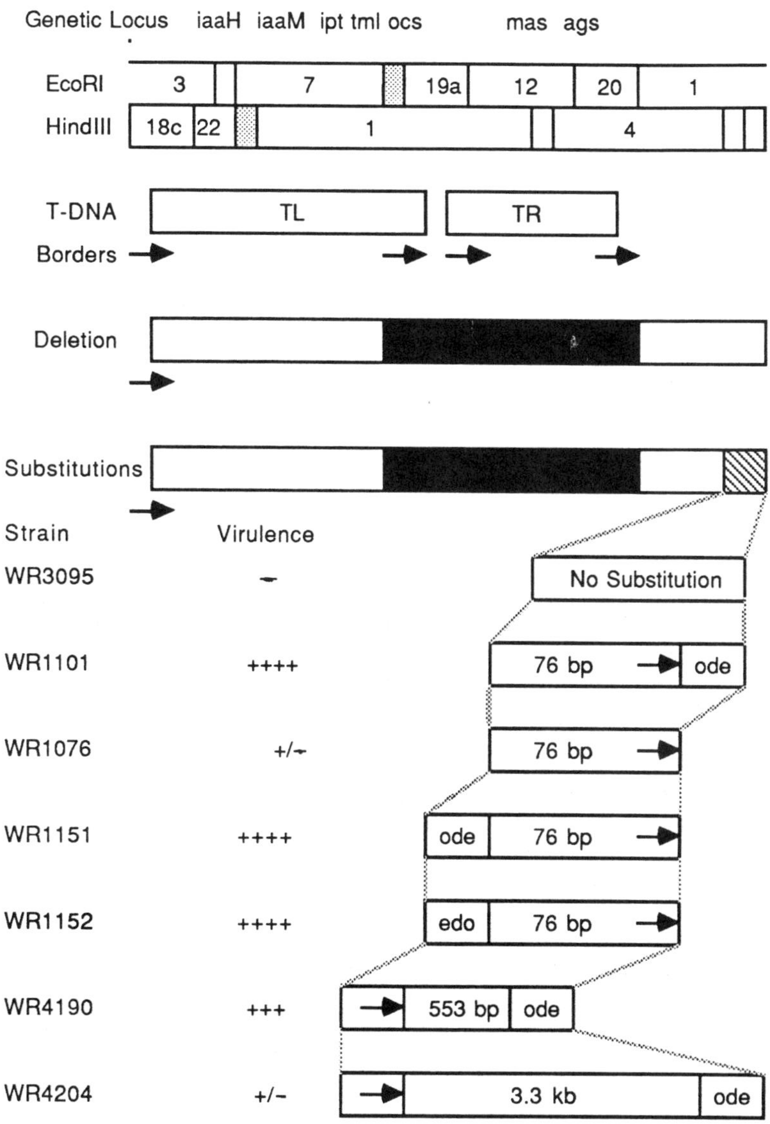

Figure 1. Border Assay System. The symbols indicate: → = border repeat; ode = <u>overdrive</u>; edo = inverted <u>overdrive</u>; ++++ = fully virulent; +++ = almost fully virulent; +/- = very weakly virulent; - = avirulent; ■ = deletion; ▨ (Continued)

= substitution; ▒ = region contains two restriction fragments. We measured virulence on carrot discs and *Kalanchoe daigremontiana* leaves. The gene symbols represent: indoleacetamide hydrolase (*iaaH*), tryptophan monooxygenase (*iaaM*), isopentenyl transferase (*ipt*), tumor morphology large (*tml*), octopine synthase (*ocs*), mannopine synthase (*mas*), and agropine synthase (*ags*).

---

*Bgl*II site, for example: (1) a 517 bp *Bcl*I fragment (lambda coordinates 8,845 to 9,362; (26), and (2) a 3,339 bp *Bam*HI-*Bcl*I fragment (lambda coordinates 5,506 to 8,845). In one resulting strain (WR4190; Fig. 1), 553 bp separated the right border repeat from *overdrive*, yet this strain exhibited essentially wild-type virulence. The other strain (WR4204), with 3,375 bp between *overdrive* and the right border repeat, exhibited weak virulence equivalent to that of an *overdrive* mutant (WR1076). We tested additional fragments from lambda with similar lengths but entirely different sequences and observed the same results; therefore, any effect of the lambda DNA on *overdrive* activity likely resulted from the length of the fragment rather than specific features within the lambda sequences. Although these fragments lacked sequences with obvious similarity to *overdrive* or the border repeat, we removed just the *overdrive* from each strain to prove the lambda DNA itself did not stimulate virulence. These control strains (WR4191 and WR4205; not shown) exhibited weak virulence. Thus, distances up to 0.5 kb did not diminish the ability of *overdrive* to stimulate T-DNA transmission, but distances of 3 kb rendered *overdrive* unable to enhance virulence.

Overdrive Increases T-Strand Accumulation.

T-DNA transmission, a process involving multiple steps, apparently initiates at the right border repeat, the site where *overdrive* acts. Therefore, it seemed likely that *overdrive* would stimulate early events that occur at the right border repeat: nicking within the repeat and subsequent T-strand production. To investigate this possibility, we compared the levels of T-strands generated, upon cocultivation with tobacco protoplasts, in strains with (WR1032) and without (WR1105) *overdrive*. The *overdrive* mutant accumulated dramatically fewer T-strands than the wild-type strain (Fig. 2). Apparently, *overdrive* promotes virulence by enhancing T-strand generation.

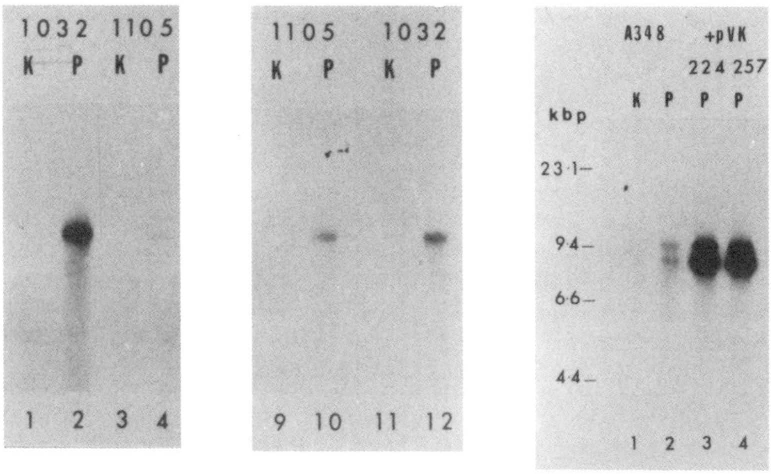

Figure 2. Influence of *overdrive* and *vir* copy number on T-strand production. We subjected uncut bacterial DNA to non-denaturing blot analysis essentially as described (16,25); we used nick-translated *EcoRI* fragment 7 as the probe. K indicates incubation of the bacteria with K3 medium (25), and P indicates induction of bacteria with tobacco protoplasts in K3 medium. Left panel: strains WR1032 and WR1105 containing only one copy of each *vir* gene; WR1032 contains *overdrive* and WR1105 lacks *overdrive*. Lanes 1 & 3 are not induced; lanes 2 & 4 are induced. WR1032 produced a very strong T-strand band (lane 2) whereas WR1105 produced a very faint T-strand band of the same mobility (lane 4). Center panel: strains WR1105 and WR1032 containing extra copies of the *vir* genes (on pVK225 or pVK224, repectively). Both WR1105(pVK225) (lane 10) and WR1032(pVK224) (lane 12) produced abundant T-strands upon induction. Right panel: The wild-type strain (A348) produced a moderate amount of T-strands upon induction (lane 2), but introduction of a *vir* cosmid (lanes 3 & 4) greatly increased T-strand accumulation. Note: we expected to see two prominent T-strand bands in this strain with the *EcoRI* fragment 7 probe because A348 carries four border repeats.

Additional Copies of Vir Genes Increase T-Strand Accumulation.

Proteins encoded by the _virD_ operon play an essential role in T-strand production (15,25,27). This process also requires: the acetosyringone receptor encoded by _virA_ and the _virG_ positive regulatory protein that activates transcription of the other _vir_ operons, including _virD_ (28). We introduced a multicopy cosmid (either pVK224 or pVK225; (29)) carrying _virG_, _virC_, _virD_, and _virE_ into strains with [WR1156 = WR1032(pVK224)] and without [WR1155 = WR1105(pVK225)] _overdrive_. Both strains exhibited wild-type virulence; upon cocultivation with tobacco protoplasts, the _overdrive_ mutant contained almost the same level of T-strands as the wild-type strain (Fig. 2). Thus, overexpression of specific _vir_ genes suppressed the need for the _overdrive_ enhancer sequence. Similarly, a wild-type strain harboring pVK224 [WR1150 = A348(pVK224)] produced significantly more T-strands upon cocultivation with tobacco protoplasts than a strain containing a single copy of each _vir_ gene (Fig. 2), but virulence appeared unchanged on carrot discs and _Kalanchoe daigremontiana_ leaves. Thus, the level of specific _vir_-encoded proteins limited T-strand production even in a wild-type strain, but the level of T-strands typically found upon induction of a wild-type strain apparently allowed maximum virulence on the hosts we examined. Presumably, the level of T-strand production restricted the virulence of _overdrive_ mutants, but other factors probably determined the maximum virulence of wild-type strains.

Genetic Interaction Between VirC and Overdrive.

Genetic analysis allows us to identify proteins that interact with the _overdrive_ enhancer sequence. One or more _vir_ proteins probably bind the enhancer and then interact with other _vir_ proteins to stimulate T-DNA transmission. Insertion mutations in _vir_ genes encoding _overdrive_-binding proteins will exhibit the same mutant phenotype (weak virulence) as an _overdrive_ deletion mutant, and a double mutant will mimic the single mutants. Insertion mutations in _virC_ or _virE_ reduce virulence (30). To determine whether strains with insertion mutations in either of these operons exhibit virulence comparable to _overdrive_ mutants, we compared the virulence of each mutant in quantitative assays. We uniformly inoculated serial slices of carrot roots with each strain as described (7), incubated the infected slices on water agar for three weeks, and excised and weighed the tumor tissue from each carrot slice. For each inoculation series (on a particular carrot) we compared the tumor mass produced by each mutant with that produced by a wild-type strain. *overdrive* and *virC* single mutants each produced tumors weighing approximately ten fold less, on average, than wild-type tumors on an adjacent carrot slice. In contrast, *virE* mutants exhibited extremely weak virulence. Therefore, *virC* mutants exhibited the phenotype expected of strains deficient in an *overdrive*-binding protein. To determine whether the *virC* locus encodes proteins that function at *overdrive*, we constructed several *virC overdrive* double mutants and compared their virulence to the single mutant parents and to a wild-type strain. The double and single mutants exhibited equivalent virulence in quantitative assays on carrot slices and in visually-scored assays on *Kalanchoe daigremontiana* leaves and stems. Thus, at least one of the two proteins encoded by the *virC* locus interacts with *overdrive*, presumably through specific DNA-protein binding.

DISCUSSION

The T-DNA border repeat-*overdrive* system resembles other site-specific recombination systems; border repeats and *overdrive* constitute separate elements that interact to promote efficient T-DNA transmission. Our results show the *overdrive* enhancer functions in either orientation, from either side of the border repeat, and without strict regard for its distance from the border repeat. Several genetic recombination pathways, for example phage lambda integration (31) and Tn*3* resolution (32), require specific flanking sequences in addition to repeat sequences directly involved in a crossover site. Site-specific inversions that mediate tail fiber switching in bacteriophages (e.g. Mu, P1, P7) and variation of *Salmonella typhimurium* flagellar antigens require inverted repeat sequences and specific flanking sequences in *cis* for efficient inversion (20-24). These flanking sequences, called recombinational enhancers, stimulate site-specific inversion independent of their position and orientation relative to the inverted repeats. Thus, precise DNA transactions, including initiation of T-DNA transfer, require multiple proteins acting at several specific sequences (33,34).

Wild-type levels of tumorigenesis require the right border repeat and a flanking sequence called *overdrive* (7,10,11). Although it plays a nonessential role, the *overdrive* sequence enhances T-DNA transmission. We investigated the influence of *overdrive* on the formation of T-strands and found that *overdrive* stimulated T-strand production, which presumably represents an early step in T-DNA transmission. Deletion of the *overdrive* sequence greatly reduced the level of T-strands that accumulated upon induction of the *vir* genes. However, introduction of additional copies of specific *vir* genes on a multicopy cosmid restored accumulation of T-strands and virulence to wild-type levels in strains without *overdrive*. This *vir*-containing cosmid also greatly increased T-strand accumulation (but not virulence) in a wild-type strain. Therefore, the *overdrive* sequence plays a quantitative role in both the generation of T-strands and virulence. When the levels of *vir* gene products limited the amount of T-strand production in wild-type strains, *overdrive* served as an enhancer. However, when overexpression of specific *vir* genes generated abnormally high levels of *vir*-encoded proteins (35), efficient T-strand production occurred even without *overdrive*. The enhancer may attract specific *vir*-encoded proteins (for example the *virD* endonuclease) to the vicinity of the right border repeat. Alternatively, *overdrive* may bind ancillary *vir*-encoded proteins which then stimulate the activity of the *virD* endonuclease (or other proteins), or specific *vir* proteins may change their conformation and activity upon binding *overdrive*. Genetic evidence indicates that *overdrive* interacts with at least one of the two proteins encoded by the *virC* operon: *overdrive virC* double mutants mimic either single mutant. Interaction between *virC*-encoded proteins and *overdrive* does not preclude binding of the *virD* endonuclease or other proteins to this sequence. Studies of sequence-specific protein binding will elucidate the exact nature of the DNA-protein interactions that occur at *overdrive* and the border repeat.

REFERENCES

1. Nester EW, Gordon MP, Amasino RM, Yanofsky MF (1984). Crown gall: a molecular and physiological analysis. Ann Rev Plant Physiol 35:387.

2. Chilton MD, Drummond MH, Merlo DJ, Sciaky D, Montoya AL, Gordon MP, Nester EW (1977). Stable incorporation of plasmid DNA into higher plant cells: the molecular basis of crown gall tumorigenesis. Cell 11:263.
3. Bevan MW, Chilton MD (1982). T-DNA of the Agrobacterium Ti and Ri plasmids. Ann Rev Genet 16:357.
4. Barker R, Idler K, Thompson D, Kemp J (1983). Nucleotide sequence of the T-DNA region of the Agrobacterium tumefaciens octopine Ti plasmid pTi15955. Plant Mol Biol 2:335.
5. Slightom JL, Tardif MD, Jouanin L, Tepfer D (1986). Nucleotide sequence analysis of TL-DNA of Agrobacterium rhizogenes agropine type plasmid. J Biol Chem 261:108.
6. Yadav NS, Vanderleyden J, Bennett DR, Barnes WM, Chilton MD (1982). Short direct repeats flank the T-DNA on a nopaline Ti plasmid. Proc Natl Acad Sci USA 79:6322.
7. Peralta EG, Hellmiss R, Ream W (1986). Overdrive, a T-DNA transmission enhancer on the A. tumefaciens tumour-inducing plasmid. EMBO J 5:1137.
8. Peralta EG, Ream LW (1985). T-DNA border sequences required for crown gall tumorigenesis. Proc Natl Acad Sci USA 82:5112.
9. Wang K, Herrera-Estrella L, Van Montagu M, Zambryski P (1984). Right 25 bp terminus sequence of the nopaline T-DNA is essential for and determines direction of DNA transfer from Agrobacterium to the plant genome. Cell 38:455.
10. van Haaren MJJ, Sedee NJA, Schilperoort RA, Hooykaas PJJ (1987). overdrive is a T-region transfer enhancer which stimulates T-strand production in Agrobacterium tumefaciens. Nucleic Acids Res 15:8983.
11. van Haaren MJJ, Pronk JT, Schilperoort RA, Hooykaas PJJ (1987). Functional analysis of the Agrobacterium tumefaciens octopine Ti plasmid left and right T-region border fragments. Plant Mol Biol 8:95.
12. Stachel SE, Nester EW (1986). The genetic and transcriptional organization of the vir region of the A6 Ti plasmid of Agrobacterium tumefaciens. EMBO J 5:1445.
13. Stachel SE, Messens E, Van Montagu M, Zambryski P (1985). Identification of the signal molecules produced by wounded plant cells that activate T-DNA transfer in Agrobacterium tumefaciens. Nature 318:624.
14. Albright LM, Yanofsky MF, Leroux B, Ma D, Nester EW

(1987). Processing of the T-DNA of Agrobacterium tumefaciens generates border nicks and linear, single-stranded T-DNA. J Bacteriol 169:1046.
15. Jayaswal RK, Veluthambi K, Gelvin SB, Slightom JL (1987). Double-stranded T-DNA cleavage and the generation of single-stranded T-DNA molecules in E. coli by a virD encoded border specific endonuclease from Agrobacterium tumefaciens. J Bacteriol 169:5035.
16. Stachel SE, Timmerman B, Zambryski P (1986). Generation of single-stranded T-DNA molecules during the initial stages of T-DNA transfer from Agrobacterium tumefaciens to plant cells. Nature 322:706.
17. Veluthambi K, Jayaswal RK, Gelvin SB (1987). Virulence genes A, G, and D mediate the double-stranded border cleavage of T-DNA from the Agrobacterium Ti plasmid. Proc Natl Acad Sci USA 84:1881.
18. Wang K, Stachel SE, Timmerman B, Van Montagu M, Zambryski P (1987). Site-specific nick in the T-DNA border sequence as a result of Agrobacterium vir gene expression. Science 235:587.
19. Yanofsky MF, Porter SG, Young C, Albright LM, Gordon MP, Nester EW (1986). The virD operon of Agrobacterium tumefaciens encodes a site-specific endonuclease. Cell 47:471.
20. Huber HE, Iida S, Arber W, Bickle T (1985). Site-specific DNA inversion is enhanced by a DNA sequence element in cis. Proc Natl Acad Sci USA 82:3776.
21. Johnson RC, Simon MI (1985). Hin-mediated site-specific recombination requires two 26 bp recombination sites and a 60 bp recombinational enhancer. Cell 41:781.
22. Kahmann R, Rudt F, Koch C, Mertens G (1985). G inversion in bacteriophage Mu DNA is stimulated by a site within the Invertase gene and a host factor. Cell 41:771.
23. Plasterk R, van de Putte P (1985). The invertibel P-DNA segment in the chromosome of Escherichia coli. EMBO J 4:237.
24. Johnson RC, Simon MI (1987). Enhancers of site-specific recombination in bacteria. Trends Genet 3:262.
25. Veluthambi K, Ream W, Gelvin SB (1988). Virulence genes, borders, and overdrive generate single-stranded T-DNA molecules form the A6 Ti plasmid of Agrobacterium tumefaciens. J Bacteriol 170:1523.
26. Sanger F, Coulson AR, Hong GF, Hill DF, Petersen GB (1982). The nucleotide sequence of bacteriophage lambda. J Mol Biol 162:729.

27. Stachel SE, Timmerman B, Zambryski P (1987). Activation of Agrobacterium tumefaciens vir gene expression generates multiple single-stranded T-strand molecules form the pTiA6 T-region: requirement of 5′ virD gene products. EMBO J 6:857.
28. Stachel SE, Zambryski P (1986). virA and virG control the plant-induced activation of the T-DNA transfer process of A. tumefaciens. Cell 46:325.
29. Knauf VC, Nester EW (1982). Wide host range cloning vectors: A cosmid clone bank of an Agrobacterium Ti plasmid. Plasmid 8:45.
30. Garfinkel DJ, Nester EW (1980). Agrobacterium tumefaciens mutants affected in crown gall tumorigenesis and octopine catabolism. J Bacteriol 144:732.
31. Nash HA (1981). Integration and excision of bacteriophage lambda: the mechanism of conservative site-specific recombination. Ann Rev Genet 15:143.
32. Kitts P, Symington L, Dyson P, Sherratt D (1983). Transposon-encoded site-specific recombination: nature of the Tn3 DNA sequences which constitute the recombination site res. EMBO J 2:1055.
33. Craig NL (1985). Site-specific inversion: enhancers, recombination proteins, and mechanism. Cell 41:649.
34. Echols H (1986). Mutiple DNA-protein interactions governing high-precision DNA transactions. Science 233:1050.
35. Rogowsky PM, Close TJ, Chimera JA, Shaw JJ, Kado CI (1987). Regulation of the vir genes of Agrobacterium tumefaciens plasmid pTiC58. J Bacteriol 169:5101.

II. MOLECULAR GENETICS OF BACTERIAL PATHOGENS

Molecular Biology of Plant–Pathogen Interactions, pages 35–48

MUTATIONAL ANALYSIS OF THE ROLE OF PECTIC ENZYMES IN THE VIRULENCE OF ERWINIA CHRYSANTHEMI[1]

Alan Collmer, Jeffrey L. Ried, Greg L. Cleveland, Sheng Yang He, and Alan D. Brooks

Department of Botany and Center for Agricultural Biotechnology, University of Maryland, College Park, Maryland 20742

The extracellular pectic enzyme complex of the phytopathogen *Erwinia chrysanthemi* EC16 comprises exo-poly-α-D-galacturonosidase (exoPG), pectin lyase (PNL), and four isozymes of pectate lyase (PL). PL is considered to be the most important of these enzymes in causing plant tissue maceration because it is the endo-cleaving pectic enzyme produced in highest levels. To evaluate the role of PL and the other pectic enzymes in soft-rot virulence, the PL-encoding *pel* genes were deleted from the *E. chrysanthemi* chromosome by marker exchange-eviction mutagenesis. *E. chrysanthemi* mutant UM1005 contained deletions affecting all four of the *pel* genes and produced less than 0.1% of the extracellular PL activity of the wild type. The mutant was able to macerate potato tuber tissue, although its virulence was substantially reduced. The mutant was also able to colonize the stem tissues of chrysanthemum, the original host of *E. chrysanthemi* EC16, and caused a delayed maceration at high inoculum levels. To identify the residual macerating factor produced by UM1005, a genomic library was constructed in pUC19, and genes encoding exoPG and PNL were cloned. The results suggest that the pectolytic capacity of *E. chrysanthemi* far exceeds the requirement for maceration and that maceration is not necessary for colonization of plant tissues by the bacterium.

---

[1]This work was supported by grants 84-CRCR-1-1366 and 87-CRCR-1-2352 from the Competitive Research Grants Office of the U.S. Department of Agriculture.

INTRODUCTION

Erwinia chrysanthemi is representative of a group of Erwinia spp. that are characterized by their high pectolytic capacity and their ability to cause maceration and necrosis (soft rots) of parenchymatous tissues in many plant hosts. Although soft-rot erwinias act as opportunistic pathogens when they cause rots in physiologically compromised storage organs, they can also be true pathogens causing systemic infections, vascular disorders, and parenchymal necroses in growing plants (1). E. chrysanthemi can cause a variety of diseases, including, for example, bacterial foot rot of rice (2), slow wilt of carnation (3), potato tuber rot (4), and stem blight of chrysanthemum (5).

The soft-rot erwinias are the most closely related of plant pathogens to the intensely studied Escherichia coli (6). Chatterjee and Starr (7) have suggested that the genetic information required for phytopathogenicity in soft-rot erwinias is superimposed through evolution in association with plants on a core of genetic information shared by other enterobacteria. The genetic similarity between these bacteria provides many experimental advantages and offers the promise that the basis of erwinia phytopathogenicity can be completely elucidated at the molecular level.

Several physiological observations have suggested that pectic enzyme production is a key factor in the virulence of E. chrysanthemi and that PL is a particularly important component: (i) pectic polymers (chains of 1,4-linked α-D-galacturonic acid and methoxylated derivatives) are structural constituents of the middle lamellae and primary cell walls of higher plants and are readily cleaved by PL (8); (ii) PL is the pectic enzyme produced in most abundance by E. chrysanthemi (9); and (iii) the PL isolated from E. chrysanthemi can substantially solubilize primary cell walls, macerate parenchymatous tissues, and kill plant cells (10,11).

Isoelectric focusing analyses employing activity-stained ultrathin polyacrylamide gels have revealed that most strains of E. chrysanthemi produce five isozymes of PL with isoelectric points that are acidic (PLa), near neutral (PLb and PLc), or alkaline (PLd and PLe) (12-15). The corresponding pel genes have been cloned into E. coli where they confer the pectolytic phenotype in various agar plate assays (16-20). The availability of cloned pel genes has facilitated several molecular approaches to the analysis of the contribution of the PL isozymes to the virulence of E. chrysanthemi. This article summarizes progress on the construction, characterization, and experimental use of E. chrysanthemi EC16 pel mutants.

RESULTS

Construction and Characterization of E. chrysanthemi Mutants with Combinations of pel Deletions.

E. chrysanthemi EC16 was chosen for this work because the strain produces only four PL isozymes (12), the encoding pel genes have been cloned and sequenced (17,21; N.T. Keen, personal communication), and the strain has been previously used in critical genetic studies (e.g., 22-24). The origins of the bacterial strains used in this work (25), procedures for bacterial matings (26), pectic enzyme assays (27), activity-stained ultrathin-layer isoelectric focusing techniques (27), and potato tuber maceration assays (25) are described elsewhere. Recombinant DNA manipulations were performed according to the protocols of Maniatis et al. (28).

We have deleted individual pel genes from the genome of E. chrysanthemi EC16 by marker-exchange mutagenesis (29) as adapted for E. chrysanthemi (26) in the following steps. (i) The target pel gene is excised from a cloned fragment of E. chrysanthemi DNA by restriction enzyme cleavage and replaced with a DNA cartridge marked with kanamycin resistance. (ii) The mutated DNA fragment, carried on vector pBR322, is transferred into E. chrysanthemi by transformation or by heterospecific mating with an E. coli donor carrying the helper plasmids R64drd11 and pLVC9. (iii) The pel deletion is then introduced into the chromosome by selection for an exchange recombination event that occurs during maintenance of the transconjugants in medium containing kanamycin but deficient in phosphate (which renders pBR322 unstable in E. chrysanthemi).

The procedure for marker-exchange mutagenesis described above enables the construction of strains with single deletions marked with kanamycin resistance and was used, for example, to construct E. chrysanthemi EC16 ΔpelE mutant UM1001 (30). To facilitate the construction of strains with a series of directed mutations without the introduction of a corresponding series of antibiotic resistance markers, we developed a technique for marker exchange-eviction mutagenesis (31). The technique employs an nptI-sacB-sacR cartridge that confers kanamycin resistance and sucrose sensitivity to E. chrysanthemi and was used to construct a family of mutants with various combinations of pel deletions (25), as described below and depicted in Fig. 1. The pelB and pelC genes used were carried on a cloned E. chrysanthemi EC16 DNA fragment in pPEL3; the pelA and pelE genes were carried on another fragment in pPEL74 (17). The nptI-sacB-sacR cartridge was first inserted in place of the pelB and pelC genes in a pPEL3 derivative. The marked deletion was then introduced into the chromosome of E. chrysanthemi AC4150, a spontaneous Nal^r derivative of EC16, by exchange recombination (selecting for kanamycin resistance) and then evicted by a second recombinational exchange with a plasmid derivative containing an unmarked deletion (selecting for sucrose tolerance). The resulting mutant, UM1003, contained a 28-bp insertion (a remnant of the cartridge) in place of the pelB and pelC genes. Strain UM1003 provided a target

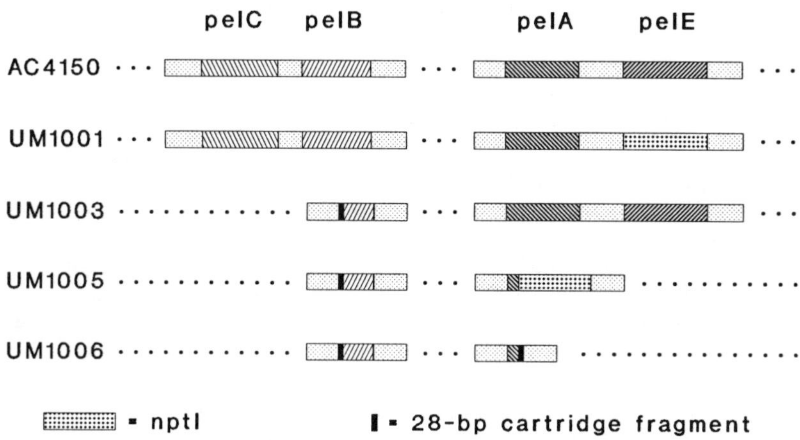

FIGURE 1. Diagram of chromosomal regions affected by pel deletions in E. chrysanthemi AC4150 (EC16 Nal^r). Mutants were constructed by in vitro replacement of respective pel genes with nptI or nptI-sacB-sacR cartridges, followed by introduction of the marked deletions into the chromosome by exchange recombination. Subsequent eviction of the cartridges in some mutants left a 28-bp cartridge fragment in the chromosome. The relative orientation of the pelC-pelB and pelA-pelE clusters in EC16 is not known.

for a series of additional directed mutations involving deletions in pPEL74 marked with nptI. The PL isozyme profiles of the mutants were determined by activity-stained isoelectric focusing gel analysis. Mutant UM1005 contained deletions in all four of the pel genes and was confirmed to produce none of the PL isozymes (25).

UM1005 was resistant to kanamycin and therefore unsuitable for further mutagenesis with nptI cartridges. The Pel^- Kan^s mutant UM1006 was constructed by (i) deleting adjacent 1.75 kb EcoRI fragments containing pelE and most of pelA from pPEL74 to produce pJR44, (ii) subcloning the E. chrysanthemi DNA insert from pJR44 as a mung bean nuclease-treated PstI fragment into a mung bean nuclease-treated BamHI site in pBR322 to produce pJR44B, (iii) conjugating pJR44B into E. chrysanthemi mutant BC501, a UM1003 derivative containing the nptI-sacB-sacR cartridge in pelE, and (iv) selection for sucrose-tolerant transconjugants. Mutant UM1006 was confirmed to be Nal^r, Kan^s, Pel^-, and able to produce exoPG and cause maceration in susceptible tissues at high inoculum levels.

Virulence of E. chrysanthemi Δpel Mutants.

The EC16 derivatives with various pel deletions were first analyzed for their ability to macerate potato tuber tissue. The maceration ability of UM1001 (ΔpelE) was 47% that of the wild type (30). The mutant could still pit pectate semisolid agar as was expected because it still produced PLa, PLb, and PLc. Surprisingly, the Pel^- mutant UM1005 was able to macerate tissue slices from potato tubers, pepper fruits, and carrots (25). It could also cause pitting in pectate semisolid agar (Fig. 2). It is important to note that the maceration ability of UM1005 was strongly affected by the inoculation procedure. For example, the amount of macerated potato tissue produced by the mutant relative to the wild type was less than 2% in whole tubers, but 21% in tuber slices (25).

The virulence of E. chrysanthemi mutant UM1005 was further explored in chrysanthemum, the original host of strain EC16. Surface-sterilized cuttings of cv. Tempter were inoculated by dipping them for 5 min in water containing test bacteria at a concentration of 5 x 10^6/ml. The cuttings were then transferred to test tubes containing sterile water and incubated at 30^oC in a humid environment.

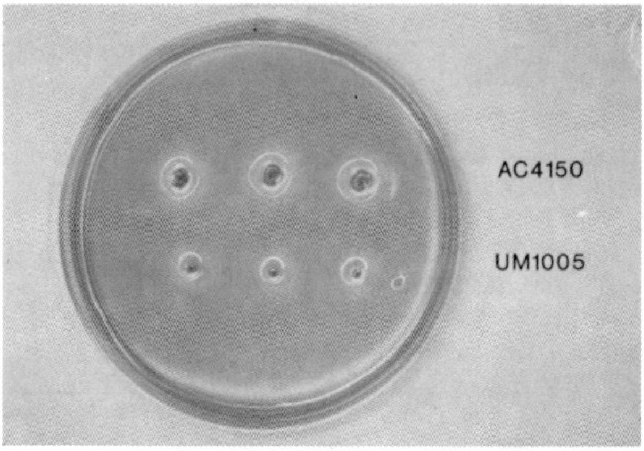

Figure 2. Pitting of pectate semisolid agar by wild-type and Pel⁻ E. chrysanthemi strains AC4150 and UM1005.

After incubation for 36 hr, stems were sliced longitudinally and examined for symptoms. Alternatively, stems were cut into 1 cm segments, and bacteria were released by crushing the tissue (32) and then counted by dilution plating. Representative bacterial colonies on dilution plates were picked to media containing appropriate antibiotics to confirm recovery of the inoculated strain.

The lower 3 cm of pith tissue in cuttings inoculated with E. chrysanthemi AC4150 was typically black and completely macerated. The pith of cuttings inoculated with UM1005 or UM1006 appeared watersoaked but was turgid and intact. With incubations longer than 48 hr and an inoculum concentration of at least 5 x 10^6, maceration was also evident in cuttings inoculated with UM1005. E. coli HB101 caused no plant reaction. As shown in Fig. 3, equally high levels of AC4150 or UM1005 could be isolated from all segments of the stem that were sampled. Substantially lower levels of E. coli were recovered from the stem.

Molecular Cloning and Mutagenesis of the E. chrysanthemi peh Gene.

ExoPG is the only extracellular pectic hydrolase produced by E. chrysanthemi (14,33). The enzyme releases digalacturonates from the nonreducing end of pectic polymers and may play an important role in bacterial utilization of pectate and in regulation of PL synthesis (33). The exoPG-

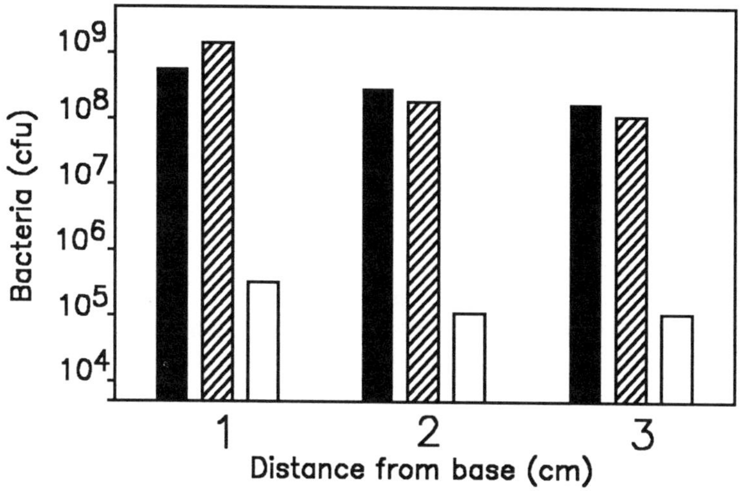

Figure 3. Bacterial populations recovered after 36-hr incubation from chrysanthemum cuttings inoculated at the base. Results represent the mean from six cuttings. Solid bars, *E. chrysanthemi* AC4150; hatched bars, *E. chrysanthemi* UM1005; open bars, *E. coli* HB101.

---

encoding *peh* gene was cloned from UM1005. *E. chrysanthemi* chromosomal DNA was partially digested with *Sau*3A, and fragments between 7 and 9 kb were isolated from a 0.7% agarose gel and ligated into *Bam*HI-digested and alkaline phosphatase-treated vector pUC19. *E. coli* HB101 transformants producing exoPG were identified by immunoblotting 2,800 transformant colonies with antibodies raised against *E. chrysanthemi* 1237 extracellular proteins and visualized with alkaline phosphatase-conjugated goat anti-rabbit antibodies. The anti-exoPG antibodies were prepared by injecting New Zealand white rabbits with proteins isolated from supernatants of strain 1237 cultures grown on pectate minimal medium. Antibody production was boosted by injections with exoPG purified by SDS gel electrophoresis.

The plasmid in one *E. coli* transformant that reacted positively in the immunoscreen was further characterized. Plasmid pPEH1 carried an 8.5 kb DNA insert and was confirmed to carry the *peh* gene by several criteria. Extracts of the clone, obtained by sonication or osmotic shock (34), caused an increase in reducing sugars from pectate without an increase in A_{235} absorbance and contained a pectic enzyme with properties identical to that of the UM1005 exoPG in activity-stained isoelectric focusing gels and in immunoblotted SDS gels (S. Y. He, unpublished results). The E. coli peh clone could also cause weak pitting in pectate semisolid agar, particularly when pH of the medium was reduced below 7.0. However, neither the E. coli clone nor pectolytic extracts caused any maceration in potato tuber tissue.

A 7.4 kb EcoRI fragment was subcloned from pPEH1 into pBR322 to produce pPEH4. The subclone was then mutagenized with TnphoA, a Tn5 derivative which can generate gene fusions producing target protein-alkaline phosphatase hybrids (35). The mutagenesis was performed in E. coli CC118 with λ::TnphoA. Mutants were screened on LB agar containing 5-bromo-4-chloro-3-indolyl-phosphate for blue colonies indicative of the fusion of alkaline phosphatase with an exported protein and on pectate semisolid agar for loss of the pitting phenotype indicative of a peh mutation. All of the four blue colonies observed in an initial mutagenesis experiment retained the ability to pit pectate semisolid agar. One white colony that no longer pitted pectate was further studied. Mutant plasmid pPEH9 was conjugated into E. chrysanthemi UM1006. The peh mutation was then introduced into the chromosome by marker exchange to produce mutant UM1009 which was Pel^- and Peh^-. Preliminary studies suggest that the mutant still retains the ability to macerate chrysanthemum stem tissue if high levels of inoculum are used.

Molecular Cloning of pnl Genes from E. chrysanthemi.

A library of E. chrysanthemi UM1005 chromosomal DNA was constructed as described above, except that size-fractionated chromosomal DNA fragments were obtained by sucrose-gradient centrifugation. The ability of UM1005 to cause pitting in pectate semisolid agar (Fig. 2) suggested that this phenotype could be used to identify clones carrying genes encoding additional pectic enzymes. Consequently, the E. coli HB101 transformants were screened for their ability to pit pectate semisolid agar. Seven of 2,000 transformants were pectolytic. Culture extracts of each of the clones produced an increase in absorbance at A_{235} with pectin, but not pectate, as a substrate (even though the clones themselves could degrade pectate in an agar medium).

Restriction mapping of the plasmids in these clones revealed two, pPNL5 and pPNL928, that had no apparent overlap in their insert DNA. The pnl gene in pPNL5 was localized by constructing restriction fragment deletion derivatives employing KpnI, EcoRI, PstI, and HindIII. Of particular interest was the observation that the pPNL5 insert contained single PstI and HindIII sites which were in a region essential for PNL activity, whereas the pPNL928 insert contained no PstI or HindIII sites at all. This indicates that although E. chrysanthemi EC16 produces very little PNL in culture (36), it carries two pnl genes.

The pPNL5 E. chrysanthemi DNA insert was subcloned into pBR322 and then inactivated by inserting the nptI-sacB-sacR cartridge into the HindIII site (via blunt-end ligation following treatment with mung bean nuclease). The mutant plasmid was then conjugated into E. chrysanthemi UM1006, and the pnl mutation was introduced into the chromosome by marker-exchange. Preliminary analysis of mutant UM1007 indicates that it is still able to pit pectate semisolid agar and can macerate chrysanthemum stem tissue if high levels of inoculum are used.

DISCUSSION

E. chrysanthemi strains isolated from various hosts in diverse geographical regions have been found to produce a characteristic set of pectic enzymes, including four or five PL isozymes (12-15). The availability of cloned pel genes enables exploration of the functional basis of the multiple PL isozymes and other pectic enzymes by: (i) biochemical characterization of single PL isozymes produced by E. coli clones; (ii) characterization of the interactions with plant tissues of pectolytic E. coli clones; (iii) directed mutagenesis of pel genes in E. chrysanthemi; and (iv) cloning from Pel$^-$ mutants and subsequent mutagenesis of additional pectic enzyme genes whose phenotype is normally masked by PL activity.

E. chrysanthemi EC16 produces only four PL isozymes because of a spontaneous deletion in pelD, as determined by sequencing of the pelA-pelE cluster (N.T. Keen, personal communication). Sequence analysis has indicated that the pelB and pelC genes are highly homologous (21). The pelE gene shares substantial homology with the pelD remnant and shows some homology with *pelA*, but it has little homology with *pelB* or *pelC* (37; N.T. Keen, personal communication).

Barras et al. (12) constructed *E. coli* clones producing single PL isozymes by cloning the two *pel* clusters and then inactivating appropriate genes by Tn*5* mutagenesis or deletion subcloning. The ability of each of the PL isozymes to induce maceration, electrolyte loss, and cell death in potato tuber disks was then determined. PLe was substantially more damaging to the plant tissue than PLb or PLc. PLa had no apparent effect on plant tissues.

Further evidence for the relative importance of PLe in plant tissue maceration is found in the phenotype of *E. coli* clones producing high levels of individual PL isozymes. Keen and Tamaki (21) subcloned the EC16 *pelB* and *pelE* genes downstream from the triple *lac* UV5 promoters. In quantitative potato tuber maceration assays, the macerating activity of the *pelE* clone was found to be 6-fold higher than that of the *pelB* clone and 1.7-fold higher than the wild-type *E. chrysanthemi* AC4150 (30). These observations indicate that production of PL, particularly PLe, at high levels is sufficient to enable an enterobacterium to macerate plant tissues.

Directed mutagenesis of the *E. chrysanthemi* EC16 *pel* genes provides further evidence for the relative importance of PLe in maceration. Loss of this one isozyme reduces the maceration ability of the bacterium to 47% of the wild type (30). In contrast, mutations in *pelB* or *pelC* have no apparent effect on the maceration ability of strain 1237 (26,38) and seem to have little effect in EC16 (Ried and Collmer, unpublished). Similar results have been found with *E. chrysanthemi* 3937, a strain pathogenic on *Saintpaulia ionantha* (39). Mutants deficient in PLd or PLe are unable to spread through the plant, and instead cause only localized maceration in the inoculated leaf. Mutants deficient in PLb and PLc are still pathogenic on the whole plant, although symptoms are delayed. Surprisingly, PLa-deficient mutants are strongly reduced in virulence in *S. ionantha* virulence tests (39).

Tests with Pel$^-$ mutant UM1005 further demonstrate that the pectolytic capacity of *E. chrysanthemi* far exceeds the requirement for the bacterium to macerate susceptible plant tissues and that individual pectic enzymes make a quantitative rather than necessary contribution to soft-rot virulence. The relationship of pectic enzyme production to virulence in these bacteria is further complicated by two additional observations. First, although extracellular pectic enzymes enable E. chrysanthemi to utilize pectate in culture, pectate utilization is apparently not required during pathogenesis: Ogl⁻ mutants blocked in oligogalacturonate catabolism are still virulent (23,40). Second, the ability of E. chrysanthemi to colonize plant tissues may be independent of tissue maceration. Thus, the populations of AC4150 and UM1005 found in the first 3-cm of chrysanthemum cuttings inoculated at the base were found to be equivalent (Fig. 3), even though only the cuttings inoculated with AC4150 were macerated at the time of assay.

Attempts to use UM1005 to protect chrysanthemum cuttings against challenge inoculation with AC4150 have so far been unsuccessful. This is not unexpected, since the mutant retains some virulence. The construction of E. chrysanthemi EC16 derivatives with additional directed mutations should ultimately yield mutants that have lost all maceration ability. Such mutants will provide the final test for the role of pectic enzymes in the maceration and colonization of plant tissues by E. chrysanthemi.

ACKNOWLEDGMENTS

We are grateful to Noel T. Keen for providing us with E. chrysanthemi EC16 pel clones and Parmjit S. Randhawa and Yoder Brothers, Incorporated, for supplying us with chrysanthemum cuttings and advice on virulence tests.

REFERENCES

1. Perombelon, MCM (1982). The impaired host and soft rot bacteria. In Mount, MS, Lacy GH (eds): "Phytopathogenic Prokaryotes," New York: Academic Press, p 55.
2. Goto, M (1979). Bacterial foot rot of rice caused by a strain of Erwinia chrysanthemi. Phytopathology 69:213.
3. Lelliott, RA (1956). Slow wilt of carnations caused by a species of Erwinia. Plant Pathol 5:19.
4. Hidalgo, OA, Echandi, E (1983). Influence of temperature and length of storage on resistance of potato to tuber rot induced by Erwinia chrysanthemi. Am Pot J 60:1.
5. Burkholder, WH, McFadden, LA, Dimock, AW (1953). A bacterial blight of chrysanthemums. Phytopathology 43:522.
6. Starr, MP (1981). The genus Erwinia. In Starr, MP, Stolp, H, Truper, HG, Balows, A, Schlegel, HG (eds): "The Prokaryotes: A Handbook on Habitats, Isolation and

Identification of Bacteria," New York: Springer-Verlag, p 1260.

7. Chatterjee, AK, Starr, MP (1980). Genetics of Erwinia species. Annu Rev Microbiol 34:645.
8. McNeil, M, Darvill, AG, Fry, SC, Albersheim, P (1984). Structure and function of the primary cell walls of plants. Annu Rev Biochem 53:625.
9. Collmer, A, Keen, NT (1986). The role of pectic enzymes in plant pathogenesis. Annu Rev Phytopathol 24:383.
10. Basham, HG, Bateman, DF (1975). Killing of plant cells by pectic enzymes: the lack of direct injurious interaction between pectic enzymes or their soluble reaction products and plant cells. Phytopathology 65:141.
11. Basham, HG, Bateman, DF (1975). Relationship of cell death in plant tissue treated with a homogeneous endopectate lyase to cell wall degradation. Physiol Plant Pathol 5:249.
12. Barras, F, Thurn, KK, Chatterjee, AK (1987). Resolution of four pectate lyase structural genes of Erwinia chrysanthemi (EC16) and characterization of the enzymes produced in Escherichia coli. Mol Gen Genet 209:319.
13. Bertheau, Y, Madgidi-Hervan, E, Kotoujansky, A, Nguyen-The, C, Andro, T, Coleno, A (1984). Detection of depolymerase isoenzymes after electrophoresis or electrofocusing, or in titration curves. Anal Biochem 139:383.
14. Ried, JL, Collmer, A (1986). Comparison of pectic enzymes produced by Erwinia chrysanthemi, Erwinia carotovora subsp. carotovora, and Erwinia carotovora subsp. atroseptica. Appl Environ Microbiol 52:305.
15. Van Gijsegem, F (1986). Analysis of the pectin-degrading enzymes secreted by three strains of Erwinia chrysanthemi. J Gen Microbiol 132:617.
16. Collmer, A, Schoedel, C, Roeder, DL, Ried, JL, Rissler, JF (1985). Molecular cloning in Escherichia coli of Erwinia chrysanthemi genes encoding multiple forms of pectate lyase. J Bacteriol 161:913.
17. Keen, NT, Dahlbeck, D, Staskawicz, B, Belser, W (1984). Molecular cloning of pectate lyase genes from Erwinia chrysanthemi and their expression in Escherichia coli. J Bacteriol 159:825.
18. Kotoujansky, A, Diolez, A, Boccara, M, Bertheau, Y, Andro, T, Coleno, A (1985). Molecular cloning of Erwinia chrysanthemi pectinase and cellulase structural genes. EMBO J 4:781.

19. Reverchon, S, Hugouvieux-Cotte-Pattat, N, and Robert-Baudouy, J (1985). Cloning of genes encoding pectolytic enzymes from a genomic library of the phytopathogenic bacterium, Erwinia chrysanthemi. Gene 35:121.
20. Van Gijsegem, F, Toussaint, A, Schoonejans, E (1985). In vivo cloning of the pectate lyase and cellulase genes of Erwinia chrysanthemi. EMBO J 4:787.
21. Keen, NT Tamaki, S (1986). Structure of two pectate lyase genes from Erwinia chrysanthemi EC16 and their high level expression in Escherichia coli. J Bacteriol 168:595.
22. Chatterjee, AK, Thurn, KK, Feese, DA (1983). Tn5 induced mutations in the enterobacterial phytopathogen Erwinia chrysanthemi. Appl Environ Microbiol 45:644.
23. Chatterjee, AK, Thurn, KK, Tyrell, DJ (1985). Isolation and characterization of Tn5 insertion mutants of Erwinia chrysanthemi that are deficient in polygalacturonate catabolic enzymes oligogalacturonate lyase and 3-deoxy-D-glycero-2,5-hexodiulosonate dehydrogenase. J Bacteriol 162:708.
24. Thurn, KK, Chatterjee, AK (1985). Single site chromosomal Tn5 insertions affect the export of pectolytic and cellulolytic enzymes in Erwinia chrysanthemi. Appl Environ Microbiol 50:894.
25. Ried, JL, Collmer, A (1988). Construction and characterization of an Erwinia chrysanthemi mutant with directed deletions in all of the pectate lyase structural genes. Mol. Plant-Microb Interact 1:32-38.
26. Roeder, DL, Collmer, A (1985). Marker-exchange mutagenesis of a pectate lyase isozyme gene in Erwinia chrysanthemi. J Bacteriol 164:51.
27. Ried, JL, Collmer, A (1985). An activity stain for the rapid characterization of pectic enzymes in isoelectric focusing and sodium dodecyl sulfate polyacrylamide gels. Appl Environ Microbiol 50:615.
28. Maniatis, T, Fritsch, EF, Sambrook, J (1982). "Molecular Cloning: A Laboratory Manual." Cold Spring Harbor, New York: Cold Spring Harbor Laboratory.
29. Ruvkun, GB, Ausubel, FM (1981). A general method for site-directed mutagenesis in prokaryotes. Nature 289:85.
30. Payne, JH, Schoedel, C, Keen, NT, Collmer, A (1987). Multiplication and virulence in plant tissues of Escherichia coli clones producing pectate lyase isozymes PLb and PLe at high levels and of an Erwinia chrysanthemi mutant deficient in PLe. Appl Environ Microbiol 53:2315.

31. Ried, JL, Collmer, A (1987). An npt-sacB-sacR cartridge for constructing directed, unmarked mutations in Gram-negative bacteria by marker exchange-eviction mutagenesis. Gene 57:239.
32. Bertoni, G, Mills, D (1987). A simple method to monitor growth of bacterial populations in leaf tissue. Phytopathology 77:832.
33. Collmer, A, Whalen, CH, Beer, SV, Bateman, DF (1982). An exo-poly-α-D-galacturonosidase implicated in the regulation of extracellular pectate lyase production in Erwinia chrysanthemi. J Bacteriol 149:626.
34. Neu, HC, Heppel, LA (1965). The release of enzymes from Escherichia coli by osmotic shock and during the formation of spheroplasts. J Biol Chem 240:3685.
35. Manoil, C, Beckwith, J (1985). TnphoA: a transposon probe for protein export signals. Proc Natl Acad Sci USA 82:8129.
36. Tsuyumu, S, Chatterjee, AK (1984). Pectin lyase production in Erwinia chrysanthemi and other soft-rot Erwinia species. Physiol Plant Pathol 24:291.
37. Barras, F, Chatterjee, AK (1987). Genetic analysis of the pelA-pelE cluster encoding the acidic and basic pectate lyases in Erwinia chrysanthemi EC16. Mol Gen Genet. 209:615.
38. Roeder, DL, Collmer, A (1987). Marker-exchange mutagenesis of the pelB gene in Erwinia chrysanthemi CUCPB 1237. In Civerolo, EL, Collmer, A, Gillaspie, AG, Davis, RE (eds): "Plant Pathogenic Bacteria: Proceedings of the Sixth International Conference on Plant Pathogenic Bacteria, Maryland, June 2-7, 1985," Dordrecht: Martinus Nijhoff, p 218.
39. Kotoujansky, A (1987). Molecular genetics of pathogenesis by soft-rot erwinias. Ann Rev Phytopathol 25:405.
40. Collmer, A, Berman, P, Mount, MS (1982). Pectate lyase regulation and bacterial soft-rot pathogenesis. In Mount, MS, Lacy, GH (eds): "Phytopathogenic Prokaryotes," New York: Academic Press, p 395.

Molecular Biology of Plant-Pathogen Interactions, pages 49-55

THE COMMON PATHOGENICITY GENES OF PSEUDOMONAS SYRINGAE PATHOVARS [1]

C. Grimm,[2] L. Rahme, R. Frederick, M. Mindrinos, P. B. Lindgren,[3] and N. J. Panopoulos

Department of Plant Pathology,
University of California,
Berkeley, CA USA 94720

ABSTRACT We have previously described a cluster of genes, designated hrp, that control the interaction between the bean halo blight pathogen, Pseudomonas syringae pv. phaseolicola, with its host (pathogenicity) and non-host plants (elicitation of the hypersensitive reaction). Structural and functional homologues of these genes occur in several members of the Pseudomonas syringae pathovar group (10). Several hrp genes, located in the left half of this ca. 20 kb cluster, are inducible either during the bacterium-plant interaction or upon transfer from nutritionally complex to nutritionally simple media. Another hrp locus, hrpS, appears to be regulatory since its predicted protein product shares

---

[1]Work summarized here was supported in part by grants DBM-8706129 and DBM-8409723 from the National Science Foundation, by Postdoctoral Fellowships to C. Grimm from the European Economic Community's Biomolecular Engineering Program and the Deutsche Forschungsgemeinschaft and by the Secretary of Research and Technology of Greece.

[2]Formerly at Institute of Molecular Biology and Biotechnology, Research Center of Crete, Heraklio, Greece.

[3]Present address: Plant Biology Laboratory, The Salk Institute, La Jolla, CA USA 92037.

significant homology to a highly conserved domain found in several prokaryotic regulatory proteins, such as NtrC, NifA, TyrR and DctD. This similarity suggests that the same basic sequence module that was utilized for the development of diverse prokaryotic regulatory systems may also have served as the progenitor sequence from which a regulatory pathogenicity gene evolved. Alternatively, the hrpS locus may have evolved from a household regulatory gene during a late stage of the evolution of P. s. phaseolicola, possibly from a saprophytic ancestor into a present-day pathogen.

INTRODUCTION

The Pseudomonas syringae taxon includes some 40 members (pathovars) that are pathogenic on many agronomically important crops, either regionally or worldwide (1). The ability of these pathogens to cause primary disease symptoms on their respective host plants ("compatible interactions") or trigger resistance responses, such as the hypersensitive reaction (HR, ref. 2) is jointly determined by at least two distinct sets of genes. One set is exemplified by the avr genes, initially cloned from P. syringae pv. glycinea (3,4). These genes determine the race/cultivar specific expression of disease symptoms in conjunction with the functionally complementary resistance gene in the host in conformity with the predictions of the gene-for-gene hypothesis (5-7). Thus, the presence of an avr gene leads to the elicitation of HR and precludes the development of disease symptoms when the host carries the corresponding resistance gene. These avr genes appear not to be required for the development of symptoms on susceptible cultivars of soybean.

Another set of genes, initially identified in P. syringae pv. phaseolicola (P. s. phaseolicola), is required for both types of reactions (7,8). These genes have been designated hrp (for hypersensitive reaction and pathogenicity). Some of the salient functional properties of these genes have been described elsewhere (8-11) and are briefly mentioned below. It is important to mention here that these genes are essential for the growth and development of the pathogen *in planta* but not *in vitro*.

Structural and functional homologues of *hrp* genes exist in several pathovars of *P. syringae*. Thus, *hrp* DNA probes from *P. s. phaseolicola* cross-hybridize with DNA sequences of several other pathovars and *hrp* mutations in this bacterium can be complemented by the correspondent genes from closely related pathovars, such as *P. s. savastanoi* and *P. s. glycinea* (10, Grimm and Panopoulos, Staskawicz and Dahlbeck, unpublished); *P. s. phaseolicola hrp*::Tn*5* mutations can be marker exchanged into the genome of certain pathovars, such as *P. s. tabaci* and *P. s. glycinea*, giving rise to Hrp$^-$ mutants and these can be complemented by the wild-type *P. s. phaseolicola* alleles (10).

Another interesting observation concerning *hrp* gene function is that the elicitation of HR in race/cultivar specific necrosis by *P. s. glycinea* on incompatible (resistant) soybean cultivars requires a fully functional *hrp* region in addition to *avr* gene function (10). This suggests that the expression of hypersensitive resistance requires *hrp* and *avr* gene products or that interactions between *hrp* genes occur at the gene or gene product level.

METHODS

A newly constructed reporter transposon, Tn*3*-Spice, carrying a promoterless ice nucleation gene was used to monitor the level of *hrp* gene expression as described elsewhere (Lindgren et al., submitted). Complementation analysis was carried out by introducing appropriate plasmids into *hrp*::Tn*5* and *hrp*::Tn*3*-Spice mutants obtained by suicide plasmid mutagenesis (9) and through marker exchange of Tn*3*-Spice insertion mutations in a plasmid clone carrying the *hrp* insert (Lindgren et al., submitted; our unpublished data). DNA sequence analysis of *hrpS* was carried out in both directions by the dideoxy method as described elsewhere (Grimm and Panopoulos, submitted). Plant inoculations and other techniques were as described in ref. 9.

RESULTS AND DISCUSSION

Genetic and Functional Analysis of hrp Genes of P. s. phaseolicola.

Previous studies (8-10) showed that the hrp genes of P. s. phaseolicola NPS3121 are organized into two linkage groups, one containing the majority of hrp genes known in this bacterium (the "hrp" cluster) and the other located at an unlinked locus. The hrp cluster spans approximately 20-22 kb, is apparently chromosomal in this strain and has been analyzed in further detail by insertional mutagenesis with a newly constructed "reporter" transposon (Lindgren et al., submitted), marker exchange and complementation analysis (our unpublished data). The region comprises at least five complementation groups/transcriptional units. Genes located in the "left" half of the cluster are expressed poorly during growth in complex media such as King's B medium and are activated upon transfer of the cultures from complex medium to minimal salts medium (data not shown) or at very early stages of infection (Lindgren et al., submitted). Thus, the hrp cluster encodes inducible functions over nearly half of its length, and transcriptional activation can apparently proceed independently of plant signal molecules. Induction is obtained in marker exchange haploids, suggesting that the inducible genes are not required for their own induction.

A regulatory hrp locus.

DNA sequence analysis has been carried out in a ca. 6 kb segment located in the right half of the hrp cluster. Computer assisted analysis of the sequence data has revealed extensive homology between the predicted amino acid sequence of the product of an hrp locus (hrpS) with several prokaryotic regulatory proteins (Grimm and Panopoulos, submitted). These include a) the NifA and NtrC proteins of nitrogen fixing Rhizobium spp. and Klebsiella pneumoniae, which regulate the expression of nitrogen fixation and nitrogen regulated operons; b) the DctD protein of Rhizobium meliloti, involved in the regulation of the dicarboxylate transport system; and c) the product of the Escherichia coli tyrR gene. The putative HrpS protein shares some 42-48% identical residues with the highly conserved domain found among these proteins. These findings strongly suggest a regulatory role for the HrpS protein.

HrpS appears to be the shortest naturally occurring member of the above family of proteins since it lacks the extended N-terminal domains found in the other members. We speculate that the progenitor gene from which the highly conserved domain of NifA, NtrC, DctD and TyrR was derived also served as the basic sequence module for the evolution of a regulatory system that controls the expression of genes which are essential to the interaction between P. syringae pathovars with plants. Alternatively, hrpS may have evolved from one of these household regulatory genes in a non-pathogenic ancestor of P. s. phaseolicola during its adaptation from a saprophytic to a pathogenic state. Nucleotide and amino acid sequence comparisons between the genes and proteins of this homology family in P. s. phaseolicola provide clues as to whether this organism existed as a saprophyte before it became a plant pathogen.

ACKNOWLEDGMENTS

We thank S. E. Lindow for allowing routine use of facilities for ice nucleation assays; T. Huynh, B. J. Staskawicz and D. Dahlbeck for sharing gene induction data with us prior to publication; G. Franz and C. Savakis for assisting us with computer analysis of sequence data; F. M. Ausubel, S. Kustu and J. Keener for discussions regarding the prokaryotic regulatory proteins.

REFERENCES

1. Dye DW, Bradbury JF, Goto M, Hayward AC, Schroth MN. (1980). International standards for naming pathovars of phytopathogenic bacteria and a list of pathovar names and phytopathogenic strains. Rev. Plant Pathol. 59:153.

2. Klement Z. (1982). Hypersensitivity. In Mount MS, Lacy GH (eds) "Phytopathogenic Prokaryotes", Vol. 2, New York: Academic Press, p 149.

3. Staskawicz BJ, Dahlbeck D, Keen NT. (1984). Cloned avirulence genes of _Pseudomonas syringae_ pv. _glycinea_ determine race-specific avirulence on _Glycine max_ (L.). Merr. Proc. Natl. Sci. USA 81:6024.

4. Staskawicz, B. J., D. Dahlbeck, N. T. Keen and C. Napoli. (1987). Molecular characterization of cloned avirulence genes from race 0 and race 1 of _Pseudomonas syringae_ pv. _glycinea_. J. Bacteriol. 169:5789.

5. Ellingboe AH. (1976). Genetics of host-parasite interactions. In Heitefuss R, Williams, PH (eds): "Encyclopedia of Plant Physiology", Vol. V, Physiological Plant Pathology, Berlin-Heidelberg: Springer-Verlag, p. 761.

6. Ellingboe AH. (1984). Genetics of host-parasite relations: an essay. In Ingram DH, Williams PH (eds): "Advances in Plant Pathology", Vol. 2, New York: Academic Press, p 131.

7. Flor, HH. (1955). Host-parasite interactions in flax rust, its genetics and other implications. Phytopathology 45:680.

8. Lindgren PB, Panopoulos NJ. (1986). Genetic

control of hypersensitivity and pathogenicity in Pseudomonas syringae pv. phaseolicola. In Bailey J (ed): "Biology and Molecular Biology of Plant-Pathogen Interactions" Berlin-Heidelberg: Springer-Verlag p 298.

9. Lindgren PB, Peet RC, Panopoulos NJ. (1986). A gene cluster of Pseudomonas syringae pv. phaseolicola controls pathogenicity on bean and hypersensitivity on non-host plants. J Bacteriol 168:512.

10. Lindgren PB, Panopoulos NJ, Staskawicz BJ, Dahlbeck D. (1987). Genes required for pathogenicity and hypersensitivity are conserved and interchangeable among pathovars of Pseudomonas syringae. Molec. Gen. Genet. 211:499.

11. Panopoulos NJ, Lindgren PB, Willis DK, Peet RC. (1985). Clustering and conservation of genes controlling the interactions of Pseudomonas syringae pathovars with plants. In Malmberg R, Crouch M, Sussex I, Ellingboe AH (eds): "Plant Cell/Cell Interactions", Current Communications in Molecular Biology, Cold Spring Harbor Laboratory, CSH, NY p 69.

III. MOLECULAR GENETICS OF FUNGAL PATHOGENS

Molecular Biology of Plant-Pathogen Interactions, pages 59–70

ELUCIDATING THE STRUCTURE AND FUNCTION OF DOUBLE-STRANDED RNA GENETIC ELEMENTS ASSOCIATED WITH BIOLOGICAL CONTROL OF CHESTNUT BLIGHT

Bradley Hillman, Brendan Rae, James Tartaglia[1], and Donald Nuss

Department of Cell and Developmental Biology
Roche Institute of Molecular Biology
Roche Research Center
Nutley, New Jersey 07110

ABSTRACT We have compared the structural properties of the dsRNA genetic elements consistently associated with a French-derived (EP713) and an American (GH2) hypovirulent strain of *Endothia (Cryphonectria) parasitica*, the chestnut blight fungus. The dsRNAs isolated from each strain consist of a large linear molecule of approximately 9 kbp and a number of smaller dsRNAs which vary in size and number. One strand of each dsRNA species contains a 3'-terminal polyadenosine moiety which is base-paired to a 5'-terminal polyuridine moiety of the complimentary strand. Molecular hybridization analysis and nuclease digestion studies suggest that most of the less-than-9 kbp dsRNAs are derived from the largest dsRNA by internal deletion events. Sequence analysis and *in vitro* expression of cDNA clones representing the 5'-end of the polyadenosine-containing strand of the EP713 dsRNAs revealed a 957 nt open reading frame (ORF1) which encodes a 29 Kd translation product. A second ORF was identified which began 68 nt upstream of the ORF1 termination codon and extended at least

---

[1]Present address: Department of Immunology, New York State Department of Health, Albany, New York 12201

1,412 nt. A similar analysis of cDNA clones corresponding to the 3'-terminus of the polyadenosine-containing strand revealed no ORFs larger than 120 codons within 1200 nucleotides of the polyadenosine moiety. Transformation experiments have been initiated using derivatives of the fungal transformation vector pDH25 bearing ORFs encoded by EP713 dsRNAs.

INTRODUCTION

The first half of this century witnessed the destruction of several billion chestnut trees in North America and Europe following the introduction of the filamentous fungus *Endothia (Cryphonectria) parasitica* (reviewed in references 1 and 2). It is understandable, therefore, that reports of the isolation of hypovirulent strains of the fungus from naturally recovering, blighted trees were received with interest. The demonstration that the hypovirulent phenotype is transmissible to virulent strains by hyphal anastomosis and that natural or artificial introduction of hypovirulent strains could result in effective biological control of the disease heightened that interest. It was subsequently demonstrated that "transmissible hypovirulence" is associated with discrete double-stranded (ds) RNA species (3,4) that differ widely among hypovirulent strains isolated in France, Italy, or the United States (5).

A clear understanding of the molecular basis of transmissible hypovirulence requires a detailed knowledge of the structural and functional properties of the hypovirulence-associated dsRNAs. To this end, we have adopted a strategy which relies on i) identification of gross structural properties by direct analysis of the molecules, ii) utilization of that information to orient and characterize cDNA clones derived from the dsRNAs, and iii) introduction of cDNA constructs representing various portions of the dsRNAs into virulent, dsRNA-free, fungal strains by DNA-mediated transformation.

RESULTS

Structural Landmarks

Structural analysis has now been performed on the dsRNAs associated with two hypovirulent strains of *E.*

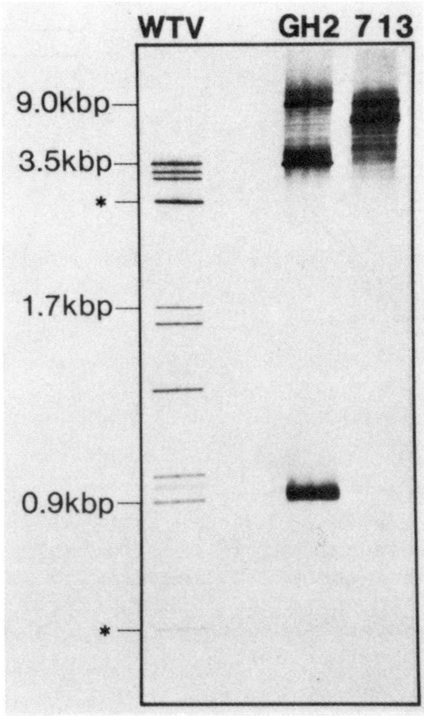

FIGURE 1. DsRNAs associated with strains GH2 (from Michigan; ref. 6) and EP713 (French-derived dsRNA in American virulent isolate; ref. 7). DsRNAs were extracted from liquid-grown fungal tissue, isolated from other cellular nucleic acids by cellulose chromatography, separated in a 7.5% polyacrylamide gel, and visualized by silver staining. Wound tumor virus (WTV) dsRNA standards are included in the left lane. Reprinted by permission of the publisher from Tartaglia and Nuss, 1988 (8), copyright 1988 by Marcel Dekker, Inc.

parasitica: the North American strain Grand Haven 2 (GH2) and the French-derived strain EP713 (Fig. 1). GH2 dsRNA consists of three major species designated L (~9 Kbp), M (~3.5 Kbp) and S (~1 Kbp). The individual dsRNAs were subjected to molecular hybridization analysis and digestion with a battery of base-specific nucleases (9) yielding the information summarized in Fig. 2. For each dsRNA only one strand, designated (+), is found in the cytoplasm in a single-stranded form. The other strand,

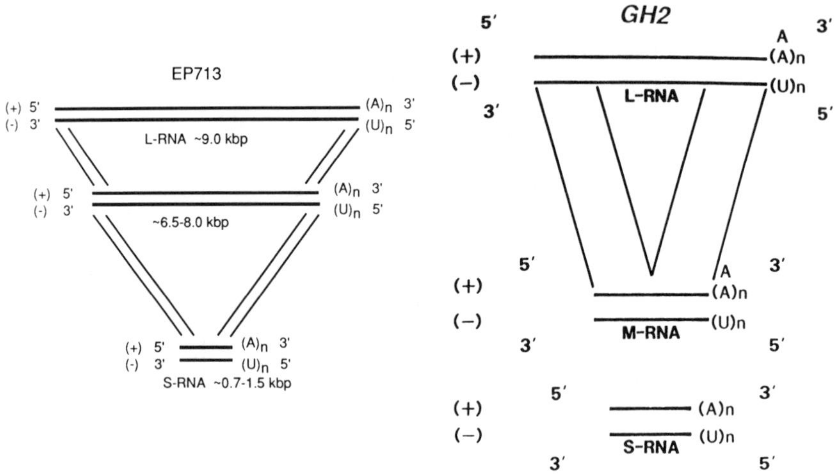

FIGURE 2. Structural characteristics of dsRNAs isolated from strains GH2 and EP713 of *E. parasitica*. The line drawing of GH2 is from Tartaglia *et al.* (9). Information for the EP713 line drawing is from Hiremath *et al.* (10) and our data. GH2 and EP713 dsRNAs share no detectable sequence homology (Tartaglia and Nuss, unpublished observation).

designated (-), is found only in a double-stranded form. In each case, the 5'-end of the (+) strand terminates in either a guanosine or an adenosine residue, while the 3'-end of the (-) strand terminates exclusively with a cytidine residue. Unexpectedly, the 3'-end of the (+) strand contains 30 to 60 adenosine residues; although a fraction of the L and M (+) strands contain only a single 3'-adenosine residue. The 5'-end of the (-) strand of each RNA contains 30 to 60 uridine residues base paired to the 3'-polyadenosine moiety. However, in 40% of these molecules, the 5'-polyuridine moiety is longer than the 3'-polyadenosine moiety resulting in a stretch of non-base paired uridine residues of undetermined length. L and M RNAs share extensive sequence homology and available evidence indicates that M RNA was derived from L RNA by one or multiple internal deletion events. S RNA did not hybridize with L or M RNAs.

The dsRNAs associated with hypovirulent strain EP713 consist of a species approximately the same size as the GH2 L RNA and additional large species in the size range of 6.5

to 8 Kbp (10). Three small dsRNAs in the range of 700-1500 bp have also been observed associated with EP713 dsRNAs (10) but they vary in concentration and are not detectable in Fig. 1. Analysis of the major large dsRNAs revealed that all species share extensive sequence homology and have identical terminal sequences (10). Recent experiments have shown that oligonucleotide probes specific for both ends of the large EP713 dsRNAs also hybridize with the 3 smaller dsRNAs indicating that the terminal regions of all EP713 dsRNAs are conserved (Hillman & Nuss, unpublished information). A 28 nt sequence corresponding to the 3'-end of the (-) strand of each large RNA species was determined by direct sequence analysis of the end-labeled dsRNAs (10). As was found for GH2 dsRNAs, the 3'-terminus of the (+) strand of each large EP713 dsRNA species consists of a polyadenosine moiety base-paired to a polyuridine moiety at the 5'-terminus of the complimentary strand. The combined results suggest that, as in the case of GH2 L and M RNAs, the 6.5-8 Kbp dsRNA species, and perhaps the smaller dsRNA species, were derived from the largest dsRNA. In this context, inspection of the silver stained gel presented in Fig. 1 reveals a large number of less intense bands. It is likely that these dsRNA species are also derived from the largest dsRNA by internal deletion events. We anticipate that much of the complexity observed for hypovirulence-associated dsRNAs will be shown to result from the generation and continued replication of defective RNAs.

Genetic Organization

The dsRNAs associated with strain EP713 provide several advantages for further characterization at the cDNA level. Firstly, dsRNAs accumulate to a 10-fold higher concentration in EP713 than in GH2. Furthermore, pigmentation and conidiation are suppressed in EP713 relative to that in the isogenic virulent strain EP155 thus providing clearly observable phenotypic differences associated with the EP713 dsRNAs (11).

Total EP713 dsRNA was used as template to construct the first generation cDNA library. The information available from direct structural analysis, including the 28 nt, 3'-terminal (-) strand sequence, was used to orient the resulting cDNA clones. Several large (in excess of 3 Kbp) cDNA clones corresponding to the 5'-terminus of the (+) strand were selected and subsequently sequenced to reveal the organization illustrated in Fig. 3 (actual sequence information and supporting data have been submitted for publication elsewhere). Because of the complications introduced by the presence of defective RNAs in the popula-

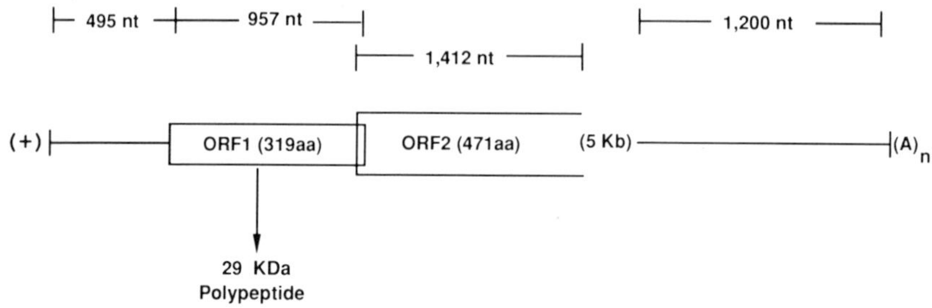

FIGURE 3. Organization of the 5'-terminal portion of the (+) strand of the largest dsRNA associated with EP713. The line drawing was compiled from information discussed in the text. No termination codon has yet been encountered in the portion of ORF2 sequenced to date. No substantial ORF has been found in the 3'-terminal 1200 nt of the EP713 (+) strand.

tion of dsRNAs used to generate the cDNA library, we have proceeded cautiously with the sequence analysis. For example, to obtain the information summarized in Fig. 3, several independent cDNA clones which extended 3 Kbp from the 5'-end of the (+) strand were sequenced completely in both orientations. In addition, much of the sequence information was confirmed by primer-directed sequencing on total melted dsRNA template. Finally, primer extension studies were performed in which sequencing primers were extended toward the 5'-terminus on templates composed of total melted dsRNA. In each case, the extension product consisted of one major cDNA of the predicted size, indicating that each of the large EP713 dsRNAs contains the 3 Kbp region represented in Fig. 3.

The 5'-proximal portion of the (+) strand of the EP713 dsRNAs contains two large open reading frames (ORF) (Fig. 3). The first consists of 319 codons and is preceded by 495 nts in which are located 6 potential initiator AUGs, all followed by one or several termination signals. The largest of these mini-cistrons extends 37 codons. The second large ORF begins 68 nt upstream of the ORF1 termination codon and extends to the end of the available sequence information, 1,412 nt.

Transcription vectors have been used to express the ORF 1 product *in vitro* and to confirm the position of the termination codon. A fragment corresponding to the 3 Kbp 5'-terminal portion of the (+) strand which contained the

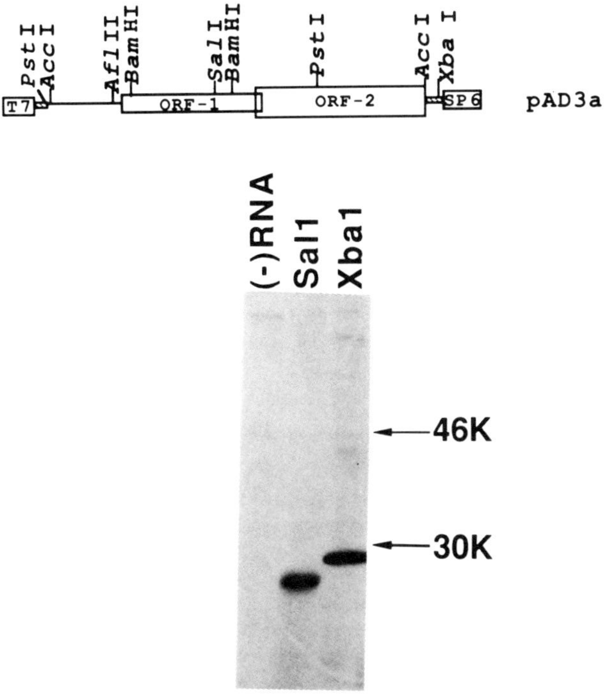

FIGURE 4. *In vitro* translation of synthetic transcripts derived from cDNA clones representing the 5' end of the large EP713 dsRNAs. Synthetic transcripts were initiated from the T7 promotor site of the cDNA clone pAD3a and terminated at SalI or XbaI. Transcripts were translated in rabbit reticulocyte lysates in the presence of ^{3}H-leucine. Products were separated on a 12.5% acrylamide gel and visualized by fluorography.

entire 5'-upstream region, ORF1, and most of the sequenced portion of ORF2 was cloned into a pGEM transcription vector. 5'-coterminal transcripts of various lengths were generated by run-off transcription and subjected to *in vitro* translation. The full-length 3 Kb transcript yielded one prominant polypeptide which migrated in PAGE with an apparent molecular weight of 29 Kd (Fig. 4). Translation of transcripts generated from the pGEM plasmid after digestion at restriction sites upstream of the predicted termination codon yielded polypeptides with altered migration rates, confirming the computer-predicted position of the termination codon.

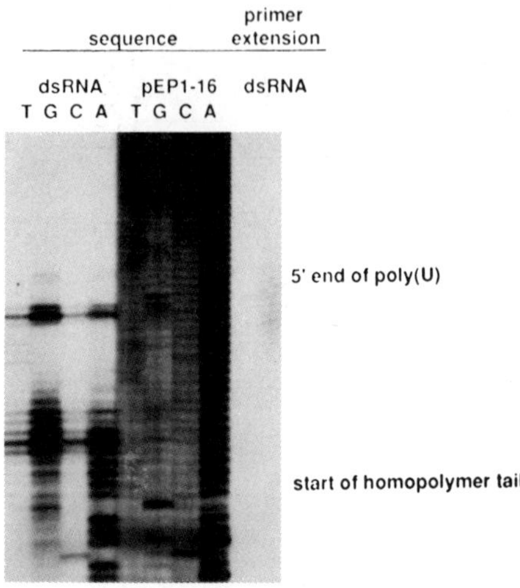

FIGURE 5. Characteristics of the homopolymer end of EP713 dsRNA. An oligonucleotide primer mapping to a region 45-62 nt from the poly (A):(U) sequence of the cDNA clone pEP9 of Hiremath *et al.* (10), and complementary to the poly (U)-bearing (-) strand was used to prime sequencing reactions on the cDNA clone pEP1-16 and on unfractionated dsRNA templates. Parallel reactions were performed without dideoxynucleoside triphosphates, permitting visualization of the 5'-terminus of the (-) strand by run-off extension. Reaction products were separated on an 8% sequencing gel. The average of 20 (U) residues on the dsRNA determined directly by Hiremath *et al.* (10) corresponds to the number observed in our extension reactions.

The 3'-end of the (+) strand of EP713 dsRNAs contains features typical of a eukaryotic mRNA. In addition to the 3' terminal polyadenosine moiety, the sequence AAUAAA, believed to function as a eukaryotic polyadenylation signal (12) is located 82-87 nt upstream of the first residue in the polyadenosine tract. Large cDNA clones corresponding to this region were identified by hybridization to the cDNA clone pEP9 described by Hiremath *et al.* (10) as potentially representing the 3'-terminal 194 nt sequences of the large EP713 dsRNAs. The origin of this clone was confirmed by performing parallel primer-extension reactions on melted EP713 dsRNAs and the pEP9 cDNA templates as shown in Fig. 5. While the sequence information derived from primer-directed sequence analysis of the dsRNA template differed slightly from the published pEP9 sequence, the information regarding

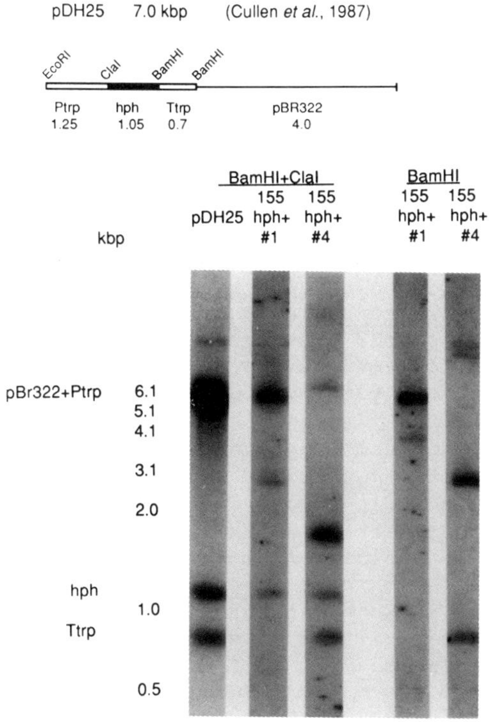

FIGURE 6. Transformation of *E. parasitica* strain 155 (virulent) with plasmid pDH25 (13). This vector contains the hygromycin phosphotransferase (hph) gene of *E. coli* fused to the trpC promotor (Ptrp) and terminator (Ttrp) elements of *Aspergillus nidulans* in a pBR322 background. Total DNA isolated from transformants grown on potato dextrose agar (PDA) was digested to completion with restriction enzymes BamHI or BamHI+ClaI and separated on a 1% agarose gel. Separated DNA was transferred to nylon membrane and probed with plasmid pDH25 that had been ^{32}P-labeled by random hexamer priming. The gene encoding hph is entirely contained within a ClaI-BamHI fragment of 1.2 kbp, and is intact in both transformants.

the average length of the polyuridine moiety found at the 5'-terminus of the (-) strand (an average of 20 residues) agreed with that derived from mobility-shift analysis of the end labeled dsRNAs (10). Computer analysis of over 1200 nts extending upstream from the polyadenosine moiety revealed no ORFs with a coding capacity in excess of 120 amino acids. The biological significance of these mini-ORFs, if any, remains to be determined. The combined 5' and 3' terminal sequence information is currently being utilized to construct a second generation cDNA library of the internal ~5 Kbp of the largest EP713 dsRNA.

Transformation of *E. parasitica*

An efficient transformation system for *E. parasitica* is required for defining the precise genetic information responsible for conferring the hypovirulence phenotype and will be useful for exploring other aspects of the molecular biology of this pathogen, e.g., the basis of vegetative compatibility. We, and others (Olin Yoder and Neal van Alfen, unpublished results), have successfully transformed *E. parasitica* with the vector pDH25 (13) which contains the *E. coli* hygromycin B phosphotransferase gene fused to the promoter and terminator regions of the *Aspergillus nidulans* TrpC gene in a pBR322 background (Fig. 6). Both stable and unstable transformants have been obtained. Unstable transformants exhibited only poor growth on medium containing 40 µg/ml hygromycin and lost the resistant phenotype after a single passage on nonselective medium. Stable transformants (~20% of the total) exhibited good growth on selective medium and retained the resistant phenotype after multiple passages on nonselective medium. Furthermore, southern analysis of DNA isolated from several stable transformants revealed integration of the vector DNA into the fungal genome (Fig. 6). Examination of a limited number of transformants has already provided evidence that rearrangement of the integrating DNA is not an uncommon event. Although considerable additional work is required to optimize transformation of *E. parasitica*, we are now in a position to introduce cDNA clones representing portions of the hypovirulence associated dsRNAs into virulent strains. Derivatives of vector pDH25 containing EP713 dsRNA ORF1 have been constructed and are presently being used to transform the isogenic *E. parasitica* strain EP155.

DISCUSSION

The RNA genetic elements associated with transmissible hypovirulence in *Endothia (Cryphonectria) parasitica* resemble the genomes of fungal viruses in terms of size, double-stranded character and absence of an extracellular infectious cycle (14). However, unlike mycovirus genomes, these dsRNAs are not associated with discrete virus particles. Consequently, they are not amenable to study by standard methodologies used in virological investigations. The capacity to construct cDNA clones that are representative of defined portions of the dsRNA genetic elements coupled with the ability to reintroduce these constructs into the fungal host by DNA-mediated transformation affords alternative avenues for elucidating the biological function of these genetic elements.

Although good progress has been made in determining the gross structural properties of the hypovirulence-associated dsRNAs , elucidation of the genetic organization of the molecules and an understanding of how the genetic information is expressed is in the early stages of development. A continual problem encountered in characterizing cDNA libraries derived from the dsRNAs stems from the presence of apparent defective RNAs in the population. In this context, overlapping cDNA clones initially thought to represent the entire 9 Kbp of the largest EP713 dsRNA were shown by comparative sequence on dsRNA and cDNA templates to contain a number of cloning artifacts (Hillman and Nuss, unpublished information). This has necessitated constant surveillance of sequence information derived from cDNA clones by confirmative sequence analysis on the dsRNA template. However, now that accurate terminal sequence information is available, it is possible, starting with small quantities of the purified 9 Kbp EP713 large dsRNA, to generate a second generation cDNA library that will be free of the cloning artifacts encountered in the first library. That work is in progress.

As sequence analysis of the hypovirulence-associated dsRNAs uncovers potential coding regions, the function of these domains can be studied by introduction of cDNA copies into virulent strains of the fungus by DNA-mediated transformation. Identification of the precise genetic information responsible for the hypovirulence phenotype could lead to the engineering of hypovirulence in other plant pathogenic fungi.

REFERENCES

1. Roane MK, Griffin GJ, Elkins JR (1986). Chestnut blight, other Endothia diseases, and the genus *Endothia*. APS Monograph, St. Paul, MN:APS Press, pp 53.

2. Anagnostakis SL (1982). Biological control of chestnut blight. Science 215:466.

3. Moffitt EM, Lister RM (1975). Application of a serological screening test for detecting double-stranded RNA mycoviruses. Phytopathology 65:851.

4. Day PR, Dodds JA, Elliston JE, Jaynes RA, Anagnostakis SL (1977). Double-stranded RNA in *Endothia parasitica*. Phytopathology 67:1393.

5. Dodds JA (1980). Revised estimates of the molecular weights of dsRNA segments in hypovirulent strains of *Endothia parasitica*. Phytopathology 70:1217.

6. Fulbright DW (1984). Effect of eliminating dsRNA in hypovirulent *Endothia parasitica*. Phytopathology 74:722.

7. Anagnostakis SL, Day PR (1979). Hypovirulence conversion in *Endothia parasitica*. Phytopathology 69:1226.

8. Tartaglia J, Nuss DL (1988). Structural properties of double-stranded RNA genetic elements of plants and plant pathogenic fungi. In Koltin Y, Leibowitz MJ (eds): "Viruses of Fungi and Simple Eukaryotes," New York:Marcel Dekker, pp 283.

9. Tartaglia J, Paul CP, Fulbright DW, Nuss DL (1986). Structural properties of double-stranded RNAs associated with biological control of chestnut blight fungus. Proc Natl Acad 83:9109.

10. Hiremath S, L'Hostis B, Gabrial SA, Rhoads RE (1986). Terminal structure of hypovirulence-associated dsRNAs in the chestnut blight fungus *Endothia parasitica*. Nucl Acids Res 14:9877.

11. Grente J (1965). Les formes hypovirulentes d'*Endothia parasitica* et les espoirs de lutte contre le chancre du chataignier. C R Seances Acad Agric Fr 51:1033.

12. Wickens M., Stephenson P (1984). Role of the conserved AAUAAA sequence: Four AAUAAA point mutants prevent messenger RNA 3' end formation. Science 226:1045.

13. Cullen D, Leong SA, Wilson LJ, Henner DJ (1987). Transformation of *Aspergillus nidulans* with the hygromycin-resistance gene, *hph*. Gene 57:21.

14. Lemke PA, Nash CH (1974). Fungal viruses. Bacteriol Rev 38:29.

Molecular Biology of Plant–Pathogen Interactions, pages 71–85

STRATEGIES FOR CLONING AVIRULENCE GENES FROM *BREMIA LACTUCAE*

Howard S. Judelson and Richard W. Michelmore

Department of Vegetable Crops, University of California, Davis 95616

ABSTRACT One of our long term goals is to clone avirulence genes from the Oomycete fungus *Bremia lactucae* that determine pathotype specificity in the disease lettuce downy mildew. Classical genetic analyses of defined lines of host and pathogen indicate that specificity in the disease is governed by a gene-for-gene interaction. Thirteen dominant avirulence genes in the fungus match 13 dominant resistance genes in the host. Restriction fragment length polymorphism loci that are linked to avirulence genes are being identified which will allow chromosome walking towards avirulence alleles. A DNA-mediated transformation system for the fungus is being developed. This technology will be used to identify avirulence alleles by transferring clones which cosegregate with avirulence genes into otherwise virulent isolates.

INTRODUCTION

The outcome of interactions between potential pathogens and their hosts is determined by factors in both the pathogen and the host. These factors may act at several levels to determine the specificity of the association. The ability to cause disease is thought to be determined by basic pathogenicity genes which encode products required for the successful infection and colonization of the host, such as cell wall degrading enzymes. The host species may also produce, or fail to synthesize, compounds which influence the challenging species. When a species is capable of causing disease, intraspecific variation often exists in the virulence of different isolates of the pathogen. Individuals in the host species also exhibit variation in their susceptibility. Populations of the pathogen frequently can be classified into pathotypes of defined specificity against a range of host cultivars. In some diseases, this level of specificity has been shown to be determined by a "gene-for-gene" interaction involving dominant alleles of major effect for resistance in the host and corresponding dominant alleles for avirulence in the pathogen (1,2). Incompatibility occurs in pairings between hosts and pathogens that contain these matching avirulence and resistance alleles. The resulting resistance involves a hypersensitive response and there is no further colonization of plant tissue. Within the same pathotype, or where a gene-for-gene interaction can not describe the disease, differences in the relative amounts of disease are mediated by genes for aggressiveness in the pathogen. Loci modifying resistance also exist in the host.

In the association between *Lactuca sativa* and the Oomycete fungus *Bremia lactucae* (lettuce downy mildew) the major determinants of specificity are involved in a gene-for gene interaction (3,4). It is the genetically best understood disease caused by an Oomycete. One of our goals is to identify and clone avirulence genes in *B. lactucae*. As prerequisites to cloning these genes, we have characterized the genetics of specificity in detail, and we are developing a DNA-mediated transformation system and a detailed genetic map for *B. lactucae*. The fungus is an obligate biotroph, and our strategies for its molecular manipulation may be relevent to other economically important fungi for which axenic culture is not possible.

STRATEGIES FOR CLONING AVIRULENCE GENES

Little is known of the products of genes conferring intraspecific specificity or of the molecular mechanisms by which specificity is determined. Strategies for the cloning of genes required for specificity, such as avirulence genes, should therefore make the minimum number of assumptions concerning the nature of the genes or their products. Methods for cloning could in theory exploit differences between avirulent and virulent isolates to perform differential cDNA or immunological screenings. However, these approaches require major assumptions concerning the temporal and spatial expression of the genes as well as whether avirulence or virulence results from an active molecular interaction. Strategies that involve mutagenesis have been used to identify disease-related genes in bacterial pathogens, but these approaches have generally identified loci involved in basic pathogenicity rather than specificity (5,6).

A strategy utilizing gene transfer technology to clone avirulence alleles was used by Staskawicz *et al.* (7) to clone genes from *Pseudomonas syringae* pv. *glycinea*. In this system no data was previously available to indicate whether avirulence or virulence resulted from an active process. DNA was therefore transferred, using cosmid libraries, from an avirulent to a virulent isolate *and* in the opposite direction. Genes from the avirulent isolate were identified that changed the race specificity of a virulent isolate; no genes from the virulent isolate could be identified that would change the specificity of an avirulent strain.

The application of this type of shotgun transformation approach to fungi will be considerably more difficult than in bacteria. The frequency of gene transfer in fungi, especially in phytopathogens, is lower than in bacteria (8-10) and many more transformants must be generated due to the larger size of eukaryotic genomes. Assuming a genome size of 5×10^7 bp, and that a library of cosmids containing on average 35 kb inserts will be used, then a minimum of 4,300 transformants will be required to ensure a 95% probability of transferring the gene of interest. A larger number of transformants will likely have to be generated since some insertions will not be active due to position effects and rearrangements. If a bidirectional transfer of DNA is performed, as with *P. syringae* (7), then twice the number of transformants will be required. As the number of transformants increases, so will the time required to screen these transformants for changes in their specificity phenotype. A shotgun cloning approach for the cloning of avirulence genes from fungi will therefore be more problematic than for bacteria.

If the genetics of the interaction are not understood, a gene transfer approach in fungi may be further complicated. This approach is most easily applied to systems exhibiting a classic gene-for-gene relationship as elucidated by Flor and others. Since avirulence is inherited as single dominant allele, it is predicted that the transfer of a single gene will provide a clear change in the phenotype of the transformant. Not all host-pathogen systems are sufficiently characterized, however, to make this assumption with confidence. Genetic analyses of specificity have generally concentrated on the host and thus more is known of resistance genes than avirulence genes. The presence of undetected genes in the pathogen may hinder the cloning of avirulence alleles. Avirulence alleles may be incompletely dominant or recessive and thus difficult to identify. Avirulence genes must be distinguished from basic pathogenicity genes or aggressiveness loci which may be important to disease development but may not determine intraspecific specificity. Also, inhibitor genes epistatic to avirulence loci may prevent the phenotypic expression of the transformed gene. Furthermore, unstable loci, as have been observed in *Phytophthora* (11), may not be suited to this type of analysis. To plan the appropriate strategy for cloning avirulence loci, therefore, it is advantageous to have a detailed undertanding of the genetics of specificity.

The classical genetics of specificity have been extensively characterized in the lettuce downy mildew interaction (3,4). These studies demonstrated that a single avirulence gene can be transferred into an otherwise virulent background and change the specificity of the recipient to avirulence. Our strategy for isolating avirulence alleles from *B. lactucae* will therefore use molecular genetic techniques to achieve changes in phenotype that classical genetics has already demonstrated to be possible. Clones of *B. lactucae* DNA containing putative avirulence alleles will be transformed into virulent isolates. Those clones which contain alleles for avirulence will change the phenotype of the recipient isolate to avirulence. Restriction fragment length polymorphism (RFLP) markers that are linked to avirulence genes are being identified. These DNA probes will be used as the starting points of short chromosome walks to avirulence genes using a cosmid library. Thus only a limited number of clones will need to be introduced into *B. lactucae*, rather than the large numbers required of shotgun approach.

GENETICS OF SPECIFICITY IN LETTUCE DOWNY MILDEW

B. lactucae and lettuce are both amenable to the genetic analysis of specificity (3). Lettuce is an inbreeding species with a generation time of approximately 90-120 days. The fungus is an outbreeding diploid with a sexual cycle of 2 months and an asexual cycle of 1 week. The interaction between host and pathogen is easily assayed in the laboratory by applying spore suspensions to week-old lettuce cotyledons. Compatible and incompatible interactions can be unambiguously scored. Associations that are incompatible result in no sporulation, while in compatatible pairings profuse sporulation occurs after 1 week.

The genetics of specificity of both host and pathogen have been analysed simultaneously (3,4,12,13, TW Ilott, SH Hulbert, and RW Michelmore, submitted). Flor's concept of a gene-for-gene relationship accurately describes the interaction. Avirulence is dominant to virulence; resistance is dominant to susceptibility. Both avirulence and resistance are determined by genes of major effect. Thirteen single dominant genes for avirulence (*Avr*) have now been characterized in *B. lactucae*. These loci are matched in lettuce by 13 dominant loci for resistance to downy mildew (*Dm*) in lettuce. Additional resistance has been identified in wild species but has not been genetically characterized. No complementation for avirulence was observed between virulence alleles in crosses between isolates of *B. lactucae*. Phenomena once thought to indicate deviation from a gene-for-gene association were shown to result from heterogeneous seed stocks, tight linkage between resistance genes, or a dominant inhibitor of avirulence epistatic to *Avr5*. Further undetected inhibitor loci which modulate the expression of dominant avirulence genes may exist in *B. lactucae*, but such loci are not common. Genes of minor effect may modify the interaction; however, these do not alter the specificity determined by the major avirulence and resistance genes.

TABLE 1

GENOTYPES OF AVIRULENCE LOCI IN ISOLATES OF *B. LACTUCAE*

Isolate	Genotype at avirulence locus[1]											
	1	2	3	4	5/8	6	7	10	13	14	15	16
NL6	*aa*	*aa*	*AA*	*aa*	*aa*	*Aa*	*AA*	*aa*	*aa*	*aa*	*AA*	*AA*
S1	*aa*	*AA*	*aa*	*aa*	*aa*	*aa*	*aa*	*aa*	*aa*	*aa*	*aa*	*AA*
CG1	*aa*	*AA*	*aa*	*aa*	*Aa*	*AA*	*aa*	*aa*	*aa*	*AA*	*aa*	*AA*
SF3	*aa*	*aa*	*aa*	*AA*	*aa*	*Aa*	*aa*	*Aa*	*aa*	*aa*	*aa*	*A–*[2]
SF5	*AA*	*aa*	*AA*	*aa*	*Aa*	*Aa*	*Aa*	*aa*	*aa*	*aa*	*aa*	*AA*
CS9	*aa*	*aa*	*aa*	*aa*	*aa*	*aa*	*aa*	*aa*	*aa*	*aa*	*aa*	*A–*[2]

[1]A = avirulent; a = virulent allele
[2]Full genotype undetermined

These studies have identified the detailed genotypes of many isolates of fungi in our collections (examples in TABLE 1). These data can be used to determine which isolates are suitable donors and recipients of transforming DNA. Chromosome walks towards avirulence alleles, performed using flanking RFLP markers as described below, will be facilitated by using a cosmid library constructed from an isolate that is homozygous for avirulence at the targeted locus. The clones will be inserted into CS9 (which has an *Avr* allele at only one locus). Our studies have also determined the resistance genotypes of the lettuce cultivars in our collection. Thus the proper lines can be chosen to screen for changes in the specificity of the recipient.

RFLP LINKAGE MAP OF *B. LACTUCAE*

DNA restriction fragment length polymorphisms have wide applications in classical and molecular genetic analyses. RFLP markers will be used as starting points for chromosome walks towards closely linked *Avr* alleles. It will therefore be necessary to transform only a limited number of clones, rather than an entire library, into virulent isolates of *B. lactucae* to identify genes encoding avirulence.

The details of RFLP mapping in *B. lactucae* will be published elsewhere (SH Hulbert, T Ilott, E Legg, SE Lincoln, ES Lander, and RW Michelmore, submitted). Polymorphisms were detected by probing genomic DNA from three parental isolates of the pathogen, digested with one of four restriction enzymes, with low copy genomic DNA or cDNA probes. The segregation of RFLPs was studied in the progeny of crosses between the parental isolates. To date the segregation of over 50 RFLP markers, plus eight *Avr* genes, has been studied using the MAPMAKER program (14). RFLPs have been assigned to 13 partial linkage groups that encompass 230 cM. Approximately half of the loci are still unlinked, but with the addition of 50 additional markers a more detailed map will be obtained. One linkage of 6.5 cM between a RFLP probe and avirulence gene *Avr6* has already been identified (Fig. 1); as the map is expanded additional and tighter linkages should be detected. Statistical analysis of the distribution of linkages, assuming a constant relationship between physical and genetic distance, indicates that in *B. lactucae* 6.5 cM equals on average approximately 160 kb. Each walking step through this region will provide new polymorphic probes which can be used to estimate the proximity to the *Avr* locus and the direction of the walk. To further facilitate chromosome walking, procedures for the electrophoretic separation of *B. lactucae* chromosomes using pulsed-field gels are being developed.

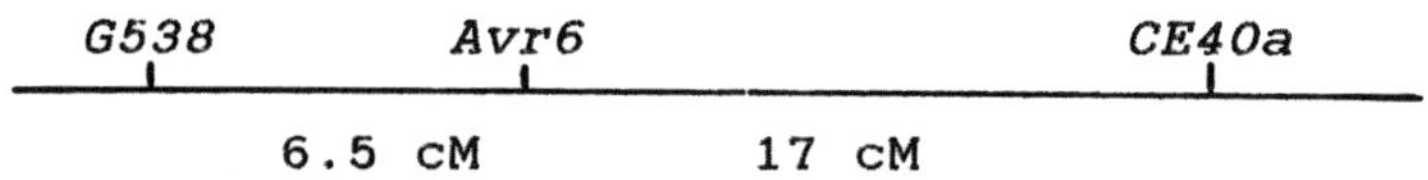

FIGURE 1. Linkage relationship between *Avr6* and flanking RFLP markers (*G538* and *CE40a*).

TRANSFORMATION OF *B. LACTUCAE*

Methods for the genetic transformation of fungi have been developed in a number of systems, including several plant pathogens (8-10). The development of a transformation system for *B. lactucae*, however, presents a number of interesting challenges. Vectors for transforming DNA have not been previously developed for the Oomycete fungi. Also, while the transformation of protoplasts is the most common method used with filamentous fungi, this will not be applicable to *B. lactucae* since this fungus is an obligate biotroph; the axenic growth conditions required to regenerate protoplasts are unknown. Spores can be harvested from infected cotyledons, germinated *in vitro* and temporarily maintained in water or buffer, but must be returned to the plant for further growth. Methods which are standard in other species for the selection of drug resistant or prototrophic transformants from the non-transformed background are similarly not feasible. To achieve the transformation of *B. lactucae*, vectors need to be constructed that will express markers for selection. The DNA must be introduced into intact spores or germlings. Finally, the selection must work *in planta*.

VECTORS FOR TRANSFORMATION

Bacterial genes which confer resistance to the drugs G418 and hygromycin B (aminoglycoside phosphotransferase II or hygromycin phosphotransferase) were chosen for incorporation into vectors for transforming DNA since spores of *B. lactucae* fail to germinate in the presence of 50 ug/ml of either compound. Prior to this study other workers had made vectors that utilized ascomycete promoters to drive the expression of these bacterial genes for the transformation of ascomycetes and basidiomycetes. Instead of using those constructs, fusions were made between promoter and polyadenylation signals from *B. lactucae* and the drug resistance genes. Foreign promoters may operate at low efficiency in this fungus; even within the ascomycetes variation has been observed in promoter structure, and the Oomycetes are taxonomically distinct from ascomycetes and other true fungi (15).

A gene encoding a 70 kDa heat shock protein (hsp70) was selected as the source of expression sequences since this gene is usually transcribed at moderate or higher levels during normal growth and heat shock conditions, and since its evolutionary conservation would facilitate cloning through the use of heterologous probes. An efficient transformation system for *Ustilago maydis* has been developed that uses a *hsp70* promoter to express a hygromycin phosphotransferase gene (8). Sequences which hybridized to a *hsp70* clone from *U. maydis* were isolated from a Lambda EMBL4 library of *B. lactucae* DNA. One clone from *B. lactucae* was analysed in detail: it was determined to be a member of a small multigene family and encoded a hsp70-related protein. Quantitative S1 protection and Northern analysis indicated that a transcript from this gene was present in RNA isolated from non-heat shocked spores, germlings, and infected lettuce cotyledons. The promoter is therefore active during all phases of the life cycle and is suitable for inclusion in the vectors for transformation. Upon heat shock, the abundance of the *hsp70* mRNA increased more than 10-fold.

Sequences of potential importance in the transcription of the *hsp70* gene were excised from the clone and incorporated into pUC19 to form a series of expression vectors. Different 5' sequences were included in various versions of the upstream portions of the vectors. The upstream boundary of the promoter constructs was a BamHI site located 590 nucleotides upstream of the intiation codon (-530 relative to the 5' mRNA terminus as determined by primer extension). The fragments extended to termini created by ExoIII deletion of the coding sequence. In one case, the endpoint of the deletion was inside the first codon of the *hsp70* open reading frame (after the A of the ATG). This will create transcriptional fusions with genes inserted into the vector. Other deletions maintained four to six codons of the *hsp70* gene and will form translational fusions. Within these promoter constructs are a canonical heat shock regulatory sequence (HSE) at -330, several CCAAT boxes, and an AT-rich "TATA" box at -35. A 550 nucleotide SalI-EcoRI restriction fragment was selected to serve as the downstream polyadenylation region. This fragment contains 114 bases of sequences present in the mature mRNA, as determined by S1 nuclease protection analysis, plus 440 bases of additional 3' sequence. A canonical polyadenylation element (AATAAA) is located 70 nucleotides from the 5' end of the fragment.

The upstream and downstream regions were connected using SmaI linkers into which genes to be expressed will be introduced. In the case of the vectors destined for translational fusions linkers of three different sizes were inserted to facilitate the expression of genes in all reading frames. The constructs also contain multiple unique cloning sites to allow the future insertion of *cos* sites or fungal DNA.

INTRODUCTION OF TRANSFORMING DNA

The traditional method of gene transfer in fungi, protoplast transformation, can not be applied to *B. lactucae* since the fungus is an obligate biotroph. Our experiments will be restricted to spores or young germlings obtained by incubating spores in water for 5-9 hours.

Preliminary experiments have indicated that electroporation might be useful in achieving transformation. DNA has been introduced into plant, bacterial, and yeast cells without the prior removal of their cell walls using this technique (16,17). The transfer of DNA in these studies was generally most efficient at voltages that resulted in the death of 20-50% of the cells. Satisfactory kill curves were generated for intact spores or germinated spores using a commercial electroporator (Biorad) capable of producing high electric fields. These kill rates were obtained at 5250 V/cm (time constant of 50 milliseconds) for spores and 1750 V/cm (time constant of 15 ms) for germlings. It may be possible to introduce DNA into electroporated spores or germlings since more than 50% of these cells internalized large amounts of the fluorescent dye calcein (MW 360) when this compound was included in the electroporation buffer. FITC-dextran (MW 1,500,000) was also taken up at lower efficiency.

DNA can be transferred into cells through intact cell walls using several additional methods. Alkali cation treatment works with adequate efficiency in *yeast* (18) and *Neurospora crassa* (9) but seemed to be ineffective in *B. lactucae*. Other methods which have not yet been tried in *B. lactucae* include microinjection (19), and high velocity bombardment of cells with DNA-coated microprojectiles (20).

SELECTION OF TRANSFORMANTS

Drug resistant transformants will be isolated using a scheme developed for selection *in planta*. This protocol allows both high efficiencies of infection and selection. Drops containing 20,000 spores or germlings each (10^6/ml) were spotted on the surface of detached, 1 week old cotyledons. Cotyledons have a high capacity for infection; mixing experiments using isolates of distinguishable genotypes in different ratios indicated that 2,000 to 6,000 independent infections will result from this inoculum density. This infection frequency is the same as that observed for single spores. One million infection events can be monitored on only 250 cotyledons. After waiting 2 days to allow for fungal penetration and phenotypic expression, the cotyledons were floated on a balanced salt solution containing 75 ug/ml of G418 or hygromycin B. The drug was imbibed into the leaf and killed the fungus. Lettuce is normally sensitive to G418, but the cotyledon appeared healthy under these conditions for several weeks (sporulation should occur in 4 days) and should be able to support the growth of drug-resistant transformants. Some evidence of slight toxicity to hygromycin B was observed. Although it is probably not required for G418, we have transformed lettuce to resistance to both drugs to obtain drug-resistant substrates for fungal growth.

To identify avirulence alleles, clones linked to *Avr* loci will be transferred into otherwise virulent isolates and drug resistant transformants will be obtained by inoculating the spores on a compatible host. The transformants will then be tested on the appropriate cultivars to determine if a change in the phenotype had been achieved.

OUTLOOK

Careful and detailed studies of the genetics of specificity in the lettuce downy mildew interaction indicate that a gene transfer approach may be used to successfully clone avirulence alleles from *B. lactucae*. The development of transformation techniques for this obligate biotroph will be more challenging than for other fungi. Our strategy of identifying clones linked to avirulence alleles by chromosome walking from RFLP markers, however, will considerably facilitate the identification of clones containing an avirulence locus once transformation is achieved.

The traditional focus of studies in the specificity of plant-pathogen interactions has been on the host. An understanding of both avirulence and resistance is necessary to fully understand specificity. It will be important to isolate both avirulence genes and the resistance genes with which they interact. The isolation of avirulence genes and the identification of their products may ultimately be used to describe the matching resistance factors. The cloning of avirulence genes is thus complementary to the study of resistance genes in plants.

ACKNOWLEDGMENTS

We thank Scot Hulbert and Terrence Ilott for sharing unpublished results, and David Francis and Rick Kesseli for their critical reading of the manuscript. This work was supported by USDA grants USDA-87-CRCR-12458-I and USDA-85-CRCR-1-1561, and by a grant to HSJ from the McKnight Awards for Interdisciplinary Research in Plant Biology.

REFERENCES

1. Flor HH (1956). Complementary genetic systems in flax and flax rust. Adv Genet 8:29.
2. Crute I (1985). The genetic bases of relationships between microbial parasites and their hosts. In Fraser RSS (ed): "Mechanisms of Resistance to Plant Diseases," Boston: Martinus Nijhoff/Dr. W. Junk, p. 80.
3. Michelmore RW, Ilott TW, Hulbert SH, Farrara BF (1988). The Downy Mildews, In Sidhu GS, Williams PH, Ingram DS (eds): "Advances in Plant Pathology, Volume 6, Genetics of Pathogenic Fungi," New York: Academic Press (in press).
4. Crute IR, Johnson AG (1976). The genetic relationship between races of *Bremia lactucae* and cultivars of *Lactuca sativa.* Ann Appl Biol 83:125.
5. Lindgren PB, Peet RC, Panapoulos NJ (1986). A gene cluster of *Pseudomonas syringae* pv. *phaseolicola* controls pathogenicity on bean and hypersensitivity on non-host plants. J

Bacteriol 168:512.
6. Niepold F, Anderson D, Mills D (1985). Cloning determinants of pathogenesis from *Pseudomonas syringae* pathovar *syringae*. Proc Natl Acad Sci USA 82:406.
7. Staskawicz BJ, Dahlbeck D, Keen NT (1984). Cloned avirulence gene of *Pseudomonas syringae* pv. *glycinea* determines race-specific incompatibility on *Glycine max*. Proc Natl Acad Sci USA 81:6024.
8. Wang J, Holden DW, Leong SA (1988). Gene transfer system for the phytopathogenic fungus *Ustilago maydis*. Proc Natl Acad Sci USA 85:865.
9. Dhawale SS, Paietta JV, Marzluf GA (1984). A new, rapid and efficient transformation procedure for *Neurospora*. Curr Genetics 8:77.
10. Parsons KA, Chumley FG, Valent B (1987). Genetic transformation of the fungal pathogen responsible for rice blast disease. Proc Natl Acad Sci USA 84:4161.
11. Black W (1954). Late blight resistance work in Scotland. Am Pot J 31:93.
12. Farrara BF, Ilott TW, Michelmore RW (1987). Genetic analysis of factors for resistance to downy mildew(*Bremia lactucae*) in species of lettuce (*Lactuca sativa* and *L. serriola*). Plant Path 36:499.
13. Norwood JM, Crute IR (1984). The genetic control of avirulence in *Bremia lactucae*. Plant Pathol 33:385.
14. Lander ES, Green P (1987). Construction of multilocus genetic linkage maps in humans. Proc Natl Acad Sci USA 84:2363.
15. Gunderson JH, Elwood H, Ingold A, Kindle K, Sogin ML (1987). Phylogenetic relationships between chlorophytes, chrysophytes, and oomycetes. Proc Natl Acad Sci USA 84:5823.
16. Hofmann GA and Evans GA (1986). Electronic genetic-physical and biological aspects of cellular electromanipulation. IEEE Eng Med Biol (December):6.
17. Hashimoto H, Morikawa H, Yamada Y, Kimura A (1985). A novel method for transformation of intact yeast cells by electroinjection of

plasmid DNA. Appl Micro Biotechnol 21:336.
18. Ito H, Murata K, Kimura A (1984). Transformation of intact yeast cells treated with alkali cations or thiol compounds. Agric Biol Chem 48:341.
19. Crossway A, Hauptli H, Houck CM, Irvine JM, Oakes JV, Perani LA (1986) Micromanipulation techniques in plant biotechnology. Biotechniques 4:320.
20. Klein TM, Wolf, ED, Wu R, Sanford JC (1987). High-velocity microprojectiles for delivering nucleic acids into living cells. Nature 327:70.

Molecular Biology of Plant–Pathogen Interactions, pages 87–102

GENE EXPRESSION RESULTING FROM THE EARLY SIGNALS IN PLANT-FUNGUS INTERACTION[1]

P.E. Kolattukudy, G.K. Podila, E. Roberts and M.D. Dickman

Ohio State Biotechnology Center, The Ohio State University, 206 Rightmire Hall, Columbus, Ohio

ABSTRACT Fungal spores of virulent pathogens that land on the plant surface generate a small amount of cutin monomers using the small amount of cutinase present on the spore. The unique cutin monomers trigger cutinase gene expression allowing the germinating spore to penetrate the cuticular barrier. Cutinase cDNA and gene from several fungal pathogens were cloned and sequenced. Transcription of cutinase gene by isolated nuclei of *Fusarium solani pisi* was activated by unique cutin monomers and a soluble protein factor. The 5' - portion of the cutinase gene showed promoter activity when used to regulate a hygromycin resistance gene in the transformants of *Fusarium* and *Colletotrichum*. Upon penetration of the cuticle the fungal pathogen must penetrate pectinaceous barriers. Hydrolases and lyases involved in this process were purified. Specific inhibition of pectate lyase protected pea stem against *F. solani pisi*. The lyase cDNA and gene were cloned. To limit the ingress of the pathogen, the plant reinforces its cell walls by suberization. A highly anionic peroxidase involved in this process was purified and its cDNA and gene were cloned and sequenced. The timely expression of this peroxidase gene may be a key factor in the plant's defense against pathogens.

[1]Supported by a grant DMB-8306835 from the National Science Foundation.

INTRODUCTION

Fungal spores land on the plant surface which is protected by the cuticle. The major structural component of the cuticle is an insoluble polyester called cutin which is composed of hydroxy-and hydroxyepoxy fatty acids (1). To seek an answer to the long standing controversy (2,3) concerning whether penetration of pathogenic fungi into plants is an enzyme-assisted process, we searched for cutinase, the enzyme postulated to be involved in this process. Cutinase has been purified from a variety of fungal pathogens (3,4). These enzymes were characterized, active sites were mapped, and antibodies were prepared. Cutinase was shown to be essential for pathogenesis in several host-pathogen pairs by conducting bioassays in which inhibition of cutinase by specific antibodies and/or specific active-site directed chemicals were found to protect the host (3). These pairs included apple seedlings against *Venturia inaequalis*, corn against *Colletotrichum graminicola* and pepper against *C. capsici*. Cutinase inhibition was demonstrated to be an effective method to protect plants against fungal attack in the field by showing that papaya fruits in the plantation were protected by biweekly sprays of an organic phosphate inhibitor of cutinase (5).

CLONING CUTINASE cDNA AND GENE

Cutinase cDNA was first cloned from *Fusarium solani pisi* (*Nectria hematococca*) and sequenced (6). About 40% of the protein, including peptides containing the labeled members of the catalytic triad, was sequenced and all of these sequences matched with sequence derived from the cDNA sequence. Cutinase could be induced in glucose-grown *C. capsici* with cutin hydrolysate and the mRNA of induced culture was used to prepare cDNA in λgt11. Cutinase cDNA was isolated, subcloned and sequenced (7). Direct amino acid sequencing of peptides derived from ^{14}C-carboxymethylated protein gave two stretches of amino acids that matched with the amino acid sequence derived from the nucleotide sequence. The sequence of cutinase from *C. gloeosporioides* was also determined. These se-

```
C. gloeosporioides      met lys phe leu ser val leu ser
C. capsici              met lys phe leu ser ile ile ser
F. solani f. sp. pisi   met lys phe phe ala leu thr thr

leu ala ile thr leu ala ala ala ala pro val glu val ... ... glu thr gly val ala
leu ala val ser leu val ala ala ala pro val glu val gly leu asp thr gly val ala
leu leu ala ala thr ala ser ala leu pro thr ser asn pro ala gln ... ... ... ...

... leu glu thr arg gln ser ... ... ser thr arg asn glu leu glu thr gly ser ser
asn leu glu ala arg gln ser ... ... ser thr arg asn glu leu glu ser gly ser ser
glu leu glu ala arg gln leu gly arg thr thr arg asp asp leu ile asn gly asn ser

ser ala cys pro lys val ile tyr ile phe ala arg ala ser thr glu pro gly asn met
ser asn cys pro lys val ile tyr ile phe ala arg ala ser thr glu pro gly asn met
ala ser cys arg asp val ile phe ile tyr ala arg gly ser thr glu thr gly asn leu

gly ile ser ala gly pro ile val ala asp ala leu glu arg ile tyr gly ala asn asn
gly ile ser ala gly pro ile val ala asp ala leu glu ser arg tyr gly ala ser gln
gly ... thr leu gly pro ser ile ala ser asn leu glu ser ala phe gly lys asp gly

val trp val gln gly val gly gly pro tyr leu ala asp leu ala ser asn phe leu ...
val trp val gln gly val gly gly pro tyr ser ala asp leu ala ser asn phe ile ile
val trp ile gln gly val gly gly ala tyr arg ala thr leu gly asp asn ala leu ...

pro asp gly thr ser ser ala ala ile asn glu ala arg arg leu phe thr leu ala asn
pro glu gly thr ser arg val ala ile asn glu ala lys arg leu phe thr leu ala asn
pro arg gly thr ser ser ala ala ile arg glu met leu gly leu phe gln gln ala asn

thr lys cys pro asn ala ala ile val ser gly gly tyr ser gln gly thr ala val met
thr lys cys pro asn ser ala val val ala gly gly tyr ser gln gly thr ala val met
thr lys cys pro asp ala thr leu ile ala gly gly tyr ser gln gly ala ala leu ala

ala gly ser ile ser gly leu ser thr thr ile lys asn gln ile lys gly val val leu
ala ser ser ile ser glu leu ser ser thr ile gln asn gln ile lys gly val val leu
ala ala ser ile glu asp leu asp ser ala ile arg asp lys ile ala gly thr val leu

phe gly tyr thr lys asn leu gln asn leu gly arg ile pro asn phe glu thr ser lys
ser ala ile thr lys asn leu gln asn leu gly arg ile pro asn phe ser thr ser lys
phe gly tyr thr lys asn leu gln asn arg gly arg ile pro asn tyr pro ala asp arg

thr glu val tyr cys asp ile ala asp ala val cys tyr gly thr leu phe ile leu pro
thr glu val tyr cys ala leu ala asp ala val cys tyr gly thr leu phe ile leu pro
thr lys val phe cys asn thr gly asp leu val cys thr gly ser leu ile val ala ala

ala his phe leu tyr gln thr asp ala ala val ala ala pro arg phe leu gln ala arg
ala his phe leu tyr gln ala asp ala ala thr ser ala pro arg phe leu ala ala arg
pro his leu ala tyr gly pro asp ala arg gly pro ala pro glu phe leu ile glu lys

ile gly
ile gly
val arg ala val arg gly ser ala
```

Figure 1. Primary structure of cutinases deduced from cloned cDNA sequences. Homology between them is shown by solid lines between the homologous residues. The vertical bar indicates the position of the single intron in cutinase gene. The catalytic triad residues and the 4 Cys residues of the disulphide bridges are boxed.

quences revealed homology in regions apparently critical for activity (Fig. 1). The most notable feature was the conservation of the locations of the members of the catalytic triad and the strictly conserved locations of the 4 Cys involved in the two disulphide bridges that we showed were essential for activity. However, only 43% of the total amino acid residues were conserved between the species.

With the cDNA as the probe, cutinase genomic clones were obtained from genomic libraries prepared from *F. solani pisi*, *C. gloeosporioides* and *C. capsici*. They were sequenced. Cutinase genes have one intron of 51-57 bp towards the 5'-end of the coding region (7,8). The transcription initiation and termination sites were determined by S1 mapping. Cutinase genes showed transcriptional start sites with a core of CAGAC that is repeated within 11 to 21 nucleotides.

INDUCTION OF CUTINASE BY UNIQUE CUTIN MONOMERS

Contact with cutin was found to induce cutinase production in the spores of *F. solani pisi* (9). Chemically prepared cutin hydrolysate also induced cutinase in *Fusarium* spores. The unique cutin monomers, dihydroxy-C_{16} acid and the trihydroxy-C_{18} acid, showed the greatest cutinase-inducing activity. Experiments with several compounds structurally related to these fatty acids suggested that both the ω-hydroxyl and a mid-chain hydroxyl are required for cutinase-inducing activity. Immunological measurement of cutinase and determination of cutinase-specific RNA levels by dot-blot hybridization with ^{32}P-labeled cutinase cDNA showed that the cutinase gene transcripts could be detected within 15 min after addition of the inducers (9). These results strongly suggest that the fungal spore senses that it is in contact with the plant by the production of small amounts of cutin monomers catalyzed by the low level of cutinase carried by the spore, and that these monomers induce the synthesis of cutinase needed for penetration of the fungus into the plant. This conclusion is consistent with a finding that spores of only the highly virulent isolates of *F. solani pisi* carry cutinase, albeit at low levels. The inducibility of the cutinase in the spore correlates extremely well with virulence. For example, *F. solani pisi* isolates 8,29 and 23, that

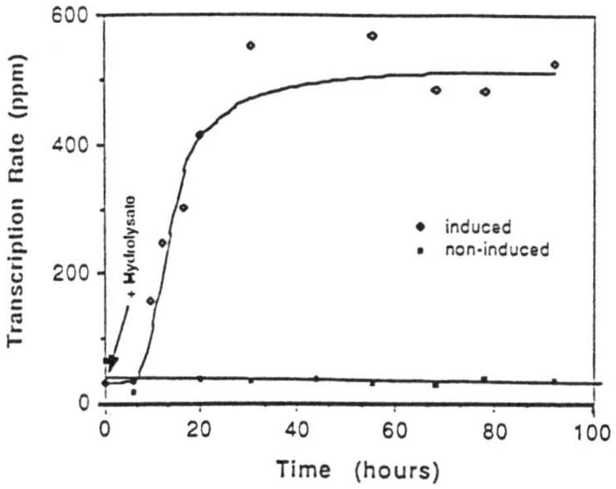

Figure 2. Nuclear runoff showing cutinase gene transcript formation in *F. solani pisi* after different periods of induction with cutin hydrolysate.

showed inducibility as shown by enzyme and transcript levels, were highly virulent on intact pea stem whereas isolates 1,30,34 and 95 that did not show inducibility were avirulent (C.P. Woloshuk and P.E. Kolattukudy, unpublished, cited in Ref. 7).

How the unique cutin monomers induce cutinase is a major unanswered question. Nuclear run-off experiments showed that the regulation is at the level of transcription (Fig. 2). A breakthrough in studying the underlying mechanism was our recent finding that cutin monomers selectively stimulate transcription of cutinase gene in isolated nuclei (G.K. Podila, M.B. Dickman and P.E. Kolattukudy, manuscript submitted). When nuclei isolated from uninduced culture were incubated with ^{32}P-UTP, little label was incorporated into cutinase transcripts recovered by hybridization with cutinase cDNA. When both a cutin monomer and an aliquot of soluble fungal extract were added together, a major increase in the incorporation of label into cutinase transcript was observed; neither the soluble extract nor the cutin monomer alone could activate transcription of cutinase gene. The transcription-stimulating activity of soluble extract was macromolecular, heat sensitive and protease sensitive.

To test whether the stimulation of cutinase gene transcription in isolated nuclei by the cutin monomer and the protein factor is the result of some generalized effect or a specific activation of cutinase gene, the effect of cutin monomer and the protein factor on the transcription of actin gene was examined. While actin gene is transcribed in the fungal nuclei, labeling of actin gene transcripts was unchanged by the addition of cutin monomer and the protein factor under conditions that caused large stimulation of cutinase gene transcription (G.K. Podila, M.D. Dickman and P.E. Kolattukudy, manuscript submitted). These results strongly suggested that the observed stimulation of cutinase gene transcription was a selective stimulation. The cutinase transcript produced by the isolated nuclei had the same size as the mRNA indicating normal initiation and termination of transcription.

If the activation of cutinase gene expression observed in the isolated nuclei is relevant to the mechanism by which the fungal spore senses its contact with the plant surface, the isolated nuclear preparation should show a requirement for the

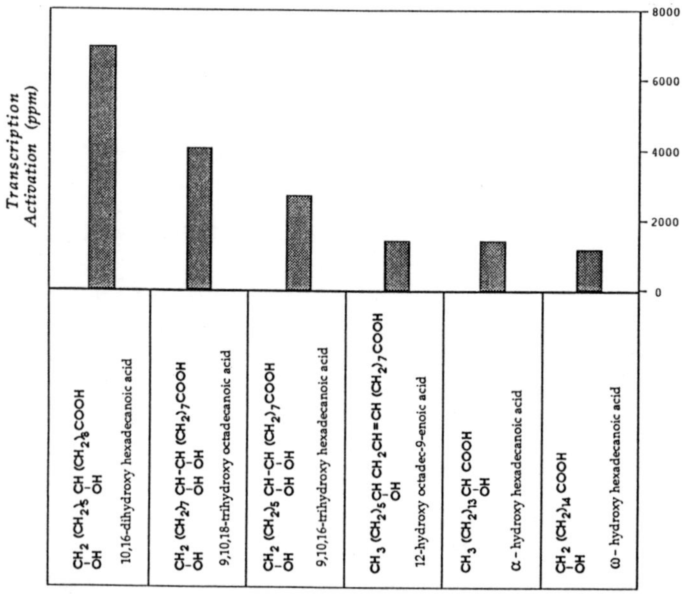

Figure 3. Cutinase transcription activating efficiency of cutin monomers and some analogues. Each hydroxy fatty acid was tested with a protein factor in isolated nuclei from *F. solani pisi* and the transcript that hybridized was measured (G.K. Podila, M.D. Dickman and P.E. Kolattukudy, manuscript submitted).

structural elements of the unique monomers of cutin. To test this possibility, several analogues of cutin monomer were tested (Fig. 3). When the mid-chain hydroxyl group of 10,16-dihydroxyhexadecanoic acid was removed, the transcription-stimulating effect decreased dramatically. The ω-hydroxyl group was found to be essential for the transcription-activation effect as ricinoleic acid, which does have a mid-chain hydroxyl group but lacks an ω-hydroxyl, could not substitute for the cutin monomer. 9,10,18-Trihydroxyoctadecanoic acid, another unique cutin monomer, also stimulated cutinase transcription. 9,10,16-Trihydroxyhexadecanoic acid, a molecule very similar to the trihydroxy-C_{18} cutin monomer, showed some stimulation of cutinase gene transcription. Thus, cutinase gene transcription activation requires the unique structural elements found in the cutin monomers which have not been found heretofore elsewhere in nature.

FUNCTIONAL ANALYSIS OF CUTINASE REGULATION BY TRANSFORMATION

Functional analysis of the gene activation involves identification of regulatory regions of the gene. We initiated such an effort by developing a transformation system for *F. solani pisi* and *C. capsici*. A plasmid containing promoterless hygromycin resistance gene was used to test for promoter activity of the flanking regions of cloned cutinase gene from *F. solani pisi* (Fig. 4 top left). Selection on hygromycin-containing medium gave transformants of *F. solani pisi* and *C. capsici* (Fig. 4 top right). Southern blot analyses showed integration of the plasmid into the fungal genome (Fig. 4 bottom). This approach with constructs containing different portions of the 5'- flanking region of cutinase gene, showed that the 360 bp segment immediately 5'- to the translation initiation of cutinase (Pvu 1 Bgl 1 fragment), (Fig. 4 top left) has promoter activity. With this transformation system, cutinase gene from *F. solani pisi* T-8 was introduced into *F. solani pisi* isolate T-30 that does not penetrate intact pea stem. Transformants that showed a high level of cutinase also showed a high degree of infection of intact pea stems (Table 1). Some transformants showed no

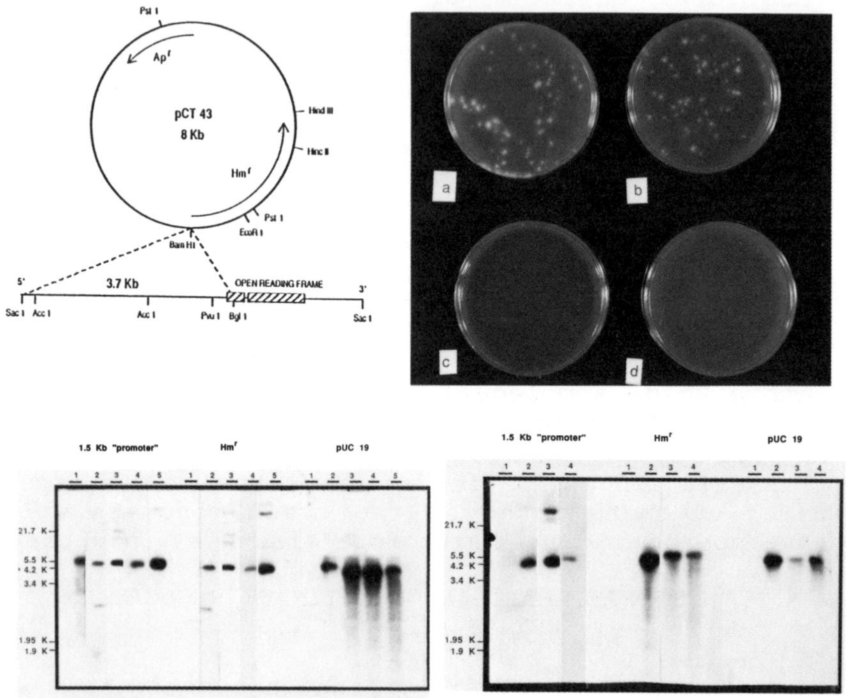

Figure 4. Top Left: The hygromycin resistance gene-containing vector that was used to test promoter activity of the 5'-flanking regions of cutinase gene. Cutinase gene is shown on the bottom. Top Right: Transformants of *F. solani pisi* and *C. capsici* growing on hygromycin containing medium. Transformants generated with the hygromycin resistance gene under the control of 1.5 kD upstream region of *Fusarium* cutinase gene are shown on top (a, *F. solani pisi*, b, *C. capsici*) and corresponding transformants containing hygromycin resistance gene without the cutinase promoter are shown in the bottom, c and d. Bottom: Southern hybridization of *Pst*-digests of genomic DNA from hygromycin resistant transformants generated by pCT 43. Left, *F. solani pisi*, right, *C. capsici*. The three labeled probes used are indicated on top.

---

cutinase, not even the low level found in the wild type, and these transformants were avirulent.

TABLE 1
Cutinase Activity and Infectivity of Transformants of *F. solani pisi* T-30

Transformant	Cutinase Activity % of Isolate T-8	Infection %
T-30 Field Isolate	25	20
T-30 Transformant 5	0	10
T-30 Transformant 9	91	80
T-30 Transformant 19	43	70
T-30 Transformant 20	30	30

Assays were done on pea stem sections with intact cuticle (1). (M.D. Dickman and P.E. Kolattukudy, manuscript in preparation.)

Mycosphaerella, a wound pathogen of papaya, was transformed with *F. solani pisi* T-8 cutinase gene. These transformants infected papaya fruits without needing wounds whereas the wild type could not (M.D. Dickman and P.E. Kolattukudy, unpublished). Thus, the role of cutinase in pathogenesis was confirmed using gene transfer.

PECTIN DEGRADING ENZYMES

Once the fungal pathogen breaches the cuticular barrier, it encounters carbohydrate barriers that must be penetrated. To study this process, we examined the nature of the pectin degrading enzymes produced by *F. solani pisi*. The spores produce three types of enzymes - a basic hydrolase, an acidic hydrolase and a lyase (M.S. Crawford and P.E. Kolattukudy, unpublished). When the organism was grown on pectin, a pectate lyase (EC 4.2.2.2) was released into the medium. This lyase was purified to apparent homogeneity (10). The enzyme cleaved polygalacturonate chains in an endo fashion. The isoelectric point of this 26 kDa enzyme was 8.3 and the optimum pH for activity was 9.4. Western blot analysis of the extracellular culture fluid showed a single band at 26 kDa. Following *in vitro* translation of poly(A)$^+$RNA, a 29-kDa precursor polypeptide was precipitated by the antibodies.

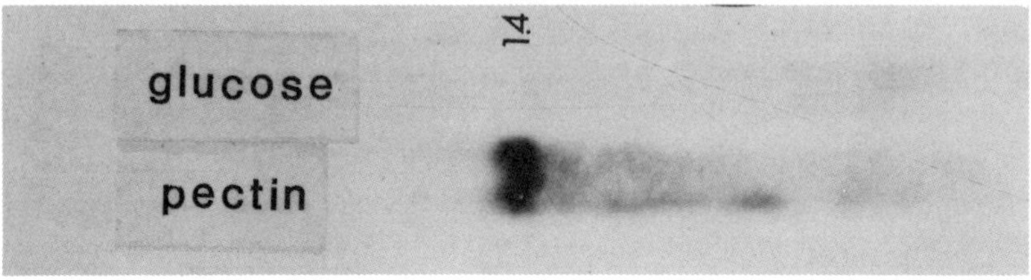

Figure 5. Northern blot showing the appearance of a pectate lyase transcript upon growth of *F. solani pisi* in the presence of pectin. A 150 kb fragment of cloned cDNA was used as the probe (M.S. Crawford and P.E. Kolattukudy, unpublished).

Antibodies inhibited both the catalytic activity of the enzyme and the ability of the fungus to infect pea stems, strongly suggesting that this lyase is involved in pathogenesis.

The two hydrolases were also purified to homogeneity (M.S. Crawford and P.E. Kolattukudy, manuscript in preparation). The molecular weights, the pI, pH optima and other properties were determined, and antibodies have been prepared against each enzyme. A λgt11 cDNA library was constructed with poly(A)$^+$RNA from induced cultures and the library was screened with anti-pectate lyase antibody. A clone containing a partial lyase cDNA was obtained that specifically hybridized with a 1.4 Kb mRNA only from the induced cells (Fig. 5). This partial cDNA clone was used to screen a genomic library of the pathogen. Two fragments of 3 Kb and 1.2 Kb derived from these clones, that specifically hybridized with the cDNA probe and oligonucleotide probes synthesized on the basis of N-terminal amino acid sequence, have been cloned (M. San Francisco and P.E. Kolattukudy unpublished). Thus, it is possible to examine the molecular basis of penetration of the carbohydrate layers.

SUBERIZATION - A PLANT RESPONSE TO FUNGAL INVASION

Plants reinforce cell walls to limit the ingress of pathogens which digest these walls with extra-cellular enzymes. Deposition of suberin in the cell wall achieves this goal. Suberization involves deposition of an aromatic matrix, somewhat similar to lignin, on the cell wall and attachment

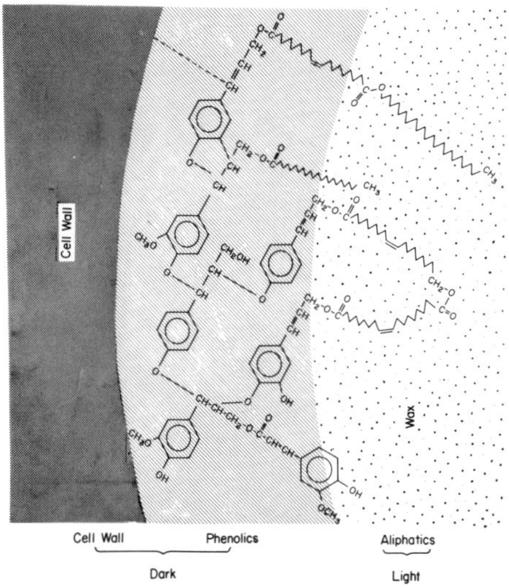

Figure 6. Proposed model for suberin structure.

of aliphatic polyester domains to the phenolic matrix (Fig. 6)(11). Evidence indicates that a highly anionic peroxidase is involved in the polymerization that generates the aromatic matrix (8) and that this peroxidase may be a key factor that regulates suberization. For example, the severe inhibition of suberization in bean roots caused by Fe deficiency was associated with a severe decrease in the anionic peroxidase activity (12). Restoration of suberization by Fe was accompanied by restoration of the peroxidase activity. The abscisic acid (ABA)-induced suberization in potato tissue culture was accompanied by induction of the anionic peroxidase but not the ω-hydroxy acid dehydrogenase involved in the synthesis of the aliphatic components of suberin (13).

The highly anionic peroxidase (EC 1.11.1.7) from wound-healing slices of *Solanum tuberosum* was purified to homogeneity (14). This 47 kDa peroxidase, with a pI of 3.15, was found to be a glycoprotein containing about 17% carbohydrate. An anionic peroxidase was also isolated from abscisic acid-treated callus tissue culture of *S. tuberosum* by the above purification procedure. The two enzymes were shown to be immunologically indistinguishable, whereas the major cationic peroxidase from wound-healing slices did not cross-react with this antibody. The anionic enzyme from both sources showed very similar specific activities when assayed with a range of substrates, whereas the specific activities found for the cationic isozyme isolated from wound-healing slices were quite different (14).

Immunocytochemically it was demonstrated that this highly anionic peroxidase is present only in the walls of the suberizing cells (not in the parenchyma cells) and only during suberization (15). The production of this suberization-associated anionic peroxidase in wound-healing tissue was also demonstrated by an immunobinding dot blot assay which showed that the largest increase in the enzyme level occurred between 4 and 6 days of wound-healing. These results support the hypothesis that this anionic peroxidase is involved in the deposition of the aromatic polymeric domain of suberin.

cDNA containing the coding region of the suberization-associated anionic peroxidase from potato has been cloned and sequenced (16). The amino acid sequence of two tryptic peptides matched exactly with two segments of the amino acid sequence deduced from the nucleotide sequence of the cloned cDNA (Fig.7). The identity of the cloned cDNA was further supported by hybrid-selected translation and immunological recovery of the product with antibodies prepared against the purified anionic peroxidase. This anionic peroxidase was barely detectable at 2 days after wounding, and reached a maximal level at 8 days after wounding. Using the cDNA for the anionic peroxidase as a probe, it was shown that the mRNA for the enzyme was induced in suberizing potato. The mRNA levels increased from an undetectable level in control tuber tissue to a maximal level in suberizing tuber tissue aged for four days. In suberizing tomato fruit the peroxidase mRNA showed induction and the level reached a maximum in three days. The data suggest that the induction of the peroxidase by wounding is preceded by transcriptional activation of the peroxidase gene or by increased stabilization of the mRNA. The time course of increase in mRNA for the anionic peroxidase was consistent with its postulated role in suberization (16). The observation that the peroxidase transcripts appeared only in potato slices placed under a suberizing environment (air), but not in one that promotes cell division (10% CO_2), strongly supported the postulated role for the peroxidase in suberization (P.E.

```
                                                                        TG      2

AGC TTT GTG GCA CTT GCA CTT GCA GGT GTT GCT ATT TAT AGA AAT ACT TAT GAA GCC ATC    62
ser-phe-val-ala-leu-ala-leu-ala-gly-val-ala-ile-tyr-arg-asn-thr-tyr-glu-ala-ile-   20

ATC ATG AAT AAC GGA TCA CTA CTC CAA AAT GCT TCT CCA CAT TTC GAT TCG TTG GAA TCA   122
ile-met-asn-asn-gly-ser-leu-leu-gln-asn-ala-ser-pro-his-phe-asp-ser-leu-glu-ser-   40

GGC GTA GCC AGT ATT TTA ACC TTA AAT AAT AAG AAG AGA AAT TCA GAC ATG TAC TTG AGA   182
gly-val-ala-ser-ile-leu-thr-leu-asn-asn-lys-lys-arg-asn-ser-asp-met-tyr-leu-arg-   60

CAG CAG CTA ACT CCG GAG GCA TGC GTT TTC TCA GCT GTA CGA GGA GTT GTG GAC AGT GCT   242
gln-gln-leu-thr-pro-glu-ala-cys-val-phe-ser-ala-val-arg-gly-val-val-asp-ser-ala-   80

ATT GAT GCA GAA ACA CGC ATG GGA GCT TCT CTT ATT CGT CTC CAC TTC CAT GAC TGC TTC   302
ile-asp-ala-glu-thr-arg-met-gly-ala-ser-leu-ile-arg-leu-his-phe-his-asp-cys-phe-  100

GTT GAT GGT TGT GAT GGA GGT ATT CTG CTA GAT GAT ATT AAT GGA ACA TTT ACA GGG GAA   362
val-asp-gly-cys-asp-gly-gly-ile-leu-leu-asp-asp-ile-asn-gly-thr-phe-thr-gly-glu-  120

CAA AAC TCA CCA CCC AAC GCC AAC TCA GCC AGA GGT TAT GAA GTA ATA GCA CAA GCT AAA   422
gln-asn-ser-pro-pro-asn-ala-asn-ser-ala-arg-gly-tyr-glu-val-ile-ala-gln-ala-lys-  140

CAA AGT GTC ATA GAT ACA TGC CCC AAC ATA TCT GTA TCT TGT GCT GAC ATA TTA GCT ATT   482
gln-ser-val-ile-asp-thr-cys-pro-asn-ile-ser-val-ser-cys-ala-asp-ile-leu-ala-ile-  160

GCT GCT CGT GAT TCG GTT GCT AAA TTA GGA GGA CAA ACT TAT AAC GTT GCA TTA GGG AGA   542
ala-ala-arg-asp-ser-val-ala-lys-leu-gly-gly-gln-thr-tyr-asn-val-ala-leu-gly-arg-  180

AGC GAT GCT AGA ACG GCC AAC TTT ACT GGT GCT TTA ACT CAA CTT CCA GCT CCA TTC GAC   602
ser-asp-ala-arg-thr-ala-asn-phe-thr-gly-ala-leu-thr-gln-leu-pro-ala-pro-phe-asp-  200

AAC CTA ACT GTC CAA ATA CAG AAA TTC AAC GAT AAA AAT TTC ACC CTC CGT GAA ATG GTT   662
asn-leu-thr-val-gln-ile-gln-lys-phe-asn-asp-lys-asn-phe-thr-leu-arg-glu-met-val-  220

GCG CTA GCT GGT GCG CAC ACG GTA GGT TTC GCC AGG TGT TCT ACC GTT TGC ACC AGC GGT   722
ala-leu-ala-gly-ala-his-thr-val-gly-phe-ala-arg-cys-ser-thr-val-cys-thr-ser-gly-  240

AAC GTT AAT CCT GCC GCA CAA CTC CAA TGC AAC TCG TCC GCC ACG CTT ACT GAT TCT GAT   782
asn-val-asn-pro-ala-ala-gln-leu-gln-cys-asn-ser-ser-ala-thr-leu-thr-asp-ser-asp-  260

TTG CAA CAA TTG GAT ACT ACT CCT ACT ATG TTC GAC AAA GTT TAC TAC GAT AAC TTA AAC   842
leu-gln-gln-leu-asp-thr-thr-pro-thr-met-phe-asp-lys-val-tyr-tyr-asp-asn-leu-asn-  280

AAC AAC CAA GGT ATA ATG TTT TCG GAT CAA GTT TTG ACC GGG GAT GCT ACA ACT GCT GGT   902
asn-asn-gln-gly-ile-met-phe-ser-asp-gln-val-leu-thr-gly-asp-ala-thr-thr-ala-gly-  300

TTT GTA ACG GAT TAT AGC AAC GAT GTT AGC GTT TTC CTT GGA GAT TTT GCT GCT GCC ATG   962
phe-val-thr-asp-tyr-ser-asn-asp-val-ser-val-phe-leu-gly-asp-phe-ala-ala-ala-met-  320

ATC AAG ATG GGA GAC TTG CCT CCA TCC GCG GGC GCT CAA TTG GAA ATT CGT GAT GTT TGT  1022
ile-lys-met-gly-asp-leu-pro-pro-ser-ala-gly-ala-gln-leu-glu-ile-arg-asp-val-cys-  340

AGC AGG GTT AAT CCC ACT TCT GTG GCT TCT ATG TGA AATTCCGAAATTTTAAGTAACTTATCTCTGA  1089
ser-arg-val-asn-pro-thr-ser-val-ala-ser-met-STOP                                  351

TGTTTTCTTCAAAATAAAAGAATCACTGGCTCCAGAATGTGGTTTTGGTATTTGTTTTGTAATCCTTTCAGTATTATGA  1168

TCAGTTGATGCCATGCATATATGTAACAAAATATATGAATATTGTTTTCCTTGTGTGCTAAAAAAAAAAAAAA        1240
```

Figure 7. The nucleotide sequence of a cloned cDNA for the anionic peroxidase from potato and the deduced amino acid sequence. The underlined portions show the match with amino acid sequence of peptides obtained from the peroxidase from wound-healing potato tuber.

Kolattukudy, R. Mohan, R. Boyd and G. Laties, unpublished results). Combined GLC/MS analysis of the coating of vascular cells observed in tomato lines resistant to *Verticillium albo-atrum* (17) showed that this apparently protective layer contains suberin (P.E. Kolattukudy and J. Robb, unpublished). To test whether this resistance reaction involves the highly anionic peroxidase, transcript levels of the anionic peroxidase were measured after inoculation of tomato petioles with *V. albo-atrum*. In the resistant line, the transcript level appeared one day earlier than in the near isogenic susceptible line. This difference in the time-course of appearance was also reflected in the appearances of the peroxidase transcripts in wound-healing fruits from the two tomato lines (P.E. Kolattukudy, R. Mohan and J. Robb, unpublished). To investigate how the expression of the gene for the anionic peroxidase is regulated, we cloned the tomato gene using a potato cDNA that encodes this enzyme as a probe. Two homologous genes for the anionic peroxidase were found and they were sequenced. (E. Roberts and P.E. Kolattukudy, manuscript submitted). The mRNAs predicted from the gene sequences are 96% and 87% identical to the potato peroxidase mRNA. Both genes consist of three exons interrupted by two introns, and the positions of the introns with respect to the coding sequences are conserved between the two genes (Fig. 8). There might be two copies of each gene in both potato and tomato. Only one gene is expressed in suberizing tomato fruits aged for 3 days, as demonstrated by primer extension analysis.

CONCLUSIONS

Fungal spores that land on plants communicate with the host to recognize it, and consequently turn on genes necessary to penetrate the defensive barriers of the host. The plant erects new bar-

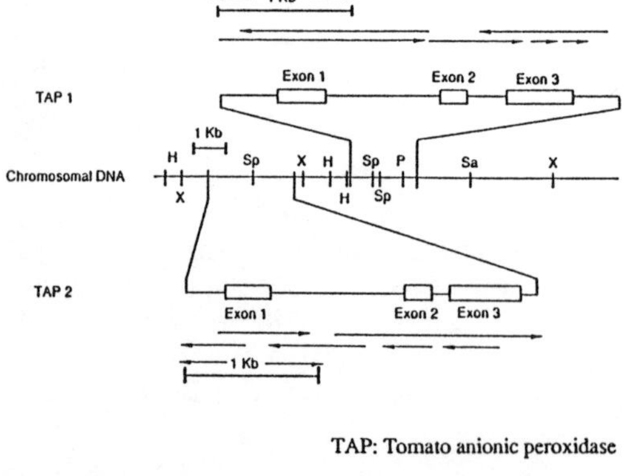

Figure 8. Organization of two homologous genes for anionic peroxidase in tomato. Tap_1 is known to be expressed during wound healing (E. Roberts and P.E. Kolattukudy, manuscript submitted).

riers as a consequence of fungal attack. With the availability of cloned cDNA and genes that are involved in the early events of fungal pathogenesis, it has become possible to investigate the molecular mechanisms involved in the early phase of plant-fungus interaction. Understanding of the molecular basis of such interactions could help to interfere with the process to protect plants against fungal attack.

ACKNOWLEDGMENTS

We thank Linda Rogers and Barbara Hartley for assistance in preparing this manuscript.

REFERENCES

1. Kolattukudy PE (1980). Biopolyester membranes of plants. Cutin and suberin. Science 208: 990.
2. Van den Ende G, Linskens HF (1974). Cutinolytic enzymes in relation to pathogenesis. Ann Rev Phytopathol 12: 247.
3. Kolattukudy PE (1985). Enzymatic penetration of the plant cuticle by fungal pathogens. Ann Rev Phytopathol 23: 223.
4. Kolattukudy PE (1984). Cutinases from fungi and pollen. In Börgstrom B, Brockman H (eds): "Lipases," Amsterdam: Elsevier/North Holland, p 471.
5. Kolattukudy PE, Ettinger WF, Sebastian J (1987). Cuticular lipids in plant-microbe interactions. In Stumpf PK, Mudd JB, Nes WD (eds): "The Metabolism, Structure, and Function of Plant Lipids," New York: Plenum Press, p 473.
6. Soliday CL, Flurkey WH, Okita TW, Kolattukudy PE (1984). Cloning and structure determination for cutinase, an enzyme involved in fungal penetration of plants. Proc Natl Acad Sci USA 81: 3939.
7. Ettinger WF, Thukral SK, Kolattukudy PE (1987). Structure of cutinase gene, cDNA, and the derived amino acid sequence from phytopathogenic fungi. Biochemistry 26: 7883. Biochemistry of Plants Vol. 9 Lipids: Structure and Function," New York: Academic Press, p 291.
8. Kolattukudy PE (1987). Lipid-derived defensive polymers and waxes and their role in plant-microbe interaction. In Stumpf PK (ed): "The

Biochemistry of Plants Vol. 9 Lipids: Structure Function," New York: Academic Press, p 291.

9. Woloshuk CP, Kolattukudy PE (1986). Mechanism by which contact with plant cuticle triggers cutinase gene expression in the spores of *Fusarium solani* f. sp. *pisi*. Proc Natl Acad Sci USA 83: 1704.
10. Crawford MS, Kolattukudy PE (1987). Pectate lyase from *Fusarium solani* f. sp. *pisi*: purification, characterization, *in vitro* translation of the mRNA, and involvement in pathogenicity. Arch Biochem Biophys 258: 196.
11. Kolattukudy PE, (1977). Lipid polymers and associated phenols, their chemistry, biosynthesis and role in pathogenesis. In Loewus FA, Runeckles VC (eds): "Recent Advances in Phytochemisry Vol. 2," New York: Plenum, p 185.
12. Sijmons PC, Kolattukudy PE, Bienfait HF (1985). Iron deficiency decreases suberization in bean roots through a decrease in suberin-specific peroxidase activity. Plant Physiol 78: 115.
13. Cottle W, Kolattukudy PE (1982). Abscisic acid stimulation of suberization: induction of enzymes and deposition of polymeric components and associated waxes in tissue cultures of potato tuber. Plant Physiol 70: 775.
14. Espelie KE, Kolattukudy PE (1985). Purification and characterization of an abscisic acid-inducible anionic peroxidase associated with suberization in potato (*Solanum tuberosum)*. Arch Biochem Biophys 240: 539.
15. Espelie KE, Franceschi VR, Kolattukudy PE (1986). Immunocytochemical localization and time course of appearance of an anionic peroxidase associated with suberization in wound-healing potato tuber tissue. Plant Physiol 81: 487.
16. Roberts E, Kutchan T, Kolattukudy PE (1988). Cloning and sequencing of cDNA for a highly anionic peroxidase from potato and the induction of its mRNA in suberizing potato tubers and tomato fruits. Plant Molec Biol, in press.
17. Street PFS, Robb J, Ellis BE (1986). Secretion of vascular coating components by xylem parenchyma cells of tomatoes infected with *Verticillium albo-atrum*. Protoplasma 132: 1.

IV. MOLECULAR GENETICS OF VIRAL PATHOGENS

Molecular Biology of Plant–Pathogen Interactions, pages 105–116

CONSTRUCTION AND TESTING OF BROME MOSAIC AND COWPEA CHLOROTIC MOTTLE VIRUS HYBRIDS[1]

Richard F. Allison and Paul Ahlquist

Institute for Molecular Virology
and Department of Plant Pathology
University of Wisconsin, Madison, WI 53706

ABSTRACT Brome mosaic virus (BMV) and cowpea chlorotic mottle virus (CCMV) are related viruses whose 8 kb genomes are divided among three separate messenger-sense RNAs. Despite close morphological and genetic similarities, BMV systemically infects grasses, including cereal grains, while CCMV infects legumes. Complete cDNA clones of both genomes have been constructed from which infectious *in vitro* transcripts can be produced, allowing direct manipulation of either virus by recombinant DNA techniques. Such molecular genetic approaches have been used to study both *cis*-and *trans*-acting elements in BMV RNA replication, demonstrating that the viral replicons are sufficiently flexible to be extensively engineered for a variety of experimental purposes. Definition of signals directing viral RNA replication and gene expression has allowed construction of BMV derivatives which replicate and express selected nonviral genes in infected cells. Viable recombinant viruses have also been made by designed exchange of selected genes and gene segments between BMV and CCMV to study the molecular basis underlying specialization of these similar viruses for divergent hosts. Current results suggest that host specificity determinants may be encoded by multiple RNAs in these tripartite genomes.

---

[1]This research was supported by NIH under grant GM35072 and by NSF under a Presidential Young Investigator Award to P.A. (Grant DMB-8451884). R.F.A. was supported by NIH Viral Oncology Training grant CA09075.

INTRODUCTION

The overwhelming majority of plant viruses and many important viral pathogens of humans and animals encapsidate messenger-sense ssRNA (1). Despite the economic and clinical significance of these (+) strand RNA viruses, relatively little is known about the actual mechanisms by which such viruses express their genes, replicate, and interact with their hosts. Our laboratory is studying these issues using plant bromoviruses as model systems. Recent sequence comparisons and functional studies show that the bromoviruses share fundamental similarities not only with many other plant viruses, but also with the animal alphaviruses (2,3). In addition to conserved features representative of many viruses, a number of specific bromovirus characteristics, including their tripartite genome organization, make them attractive models for studying RNA virus functions.

Brome mosaic virus (BMV) and cowpea chlorotic mottle virus (CCMV) are closely related members of the bromovirus group (4,5). Despite their extensive morphological and genetic similarity, the systemic host ranges of the two viruses are markedly distinct: BMV infects monocotyledonous plants, while CCMV infects dicotyledonous plants. Combined study of BMV and CCMV thus offers particular opportunities for investigating host specificity. As described below, biologically active viral cDNA clones have now been constructed for both BMV and CCMV, allowing alteration or exchange of any chosen sequence between these two viruses. This approach provides an important component in direct studies of the molecular basis for host specificity in these viruses.

Studies of virus adaptation to specific hosts by either molecular or classical genetic approaches must involve testing the interaction of different host and virus genotypes. In such tests, revealing the full spectrum of virus genes contributing to host adaptation depends on finding sufficient genetic variation among different hosts to perturb all of the relevant virus/host interactions. Not surprisingly, recent experiments suggest that multiple virus genes can influence virus/host interactions governing successful systemic infection (6,7). Consequently, the wide divergence between BMV and CCMV host ranges should provide a valuable genetic perspective for characterizing host range determinants. The normal systemic hosts of BMV and CCMV, barley and cowpea, should provide sufficient genetic variation to reveal virtually any

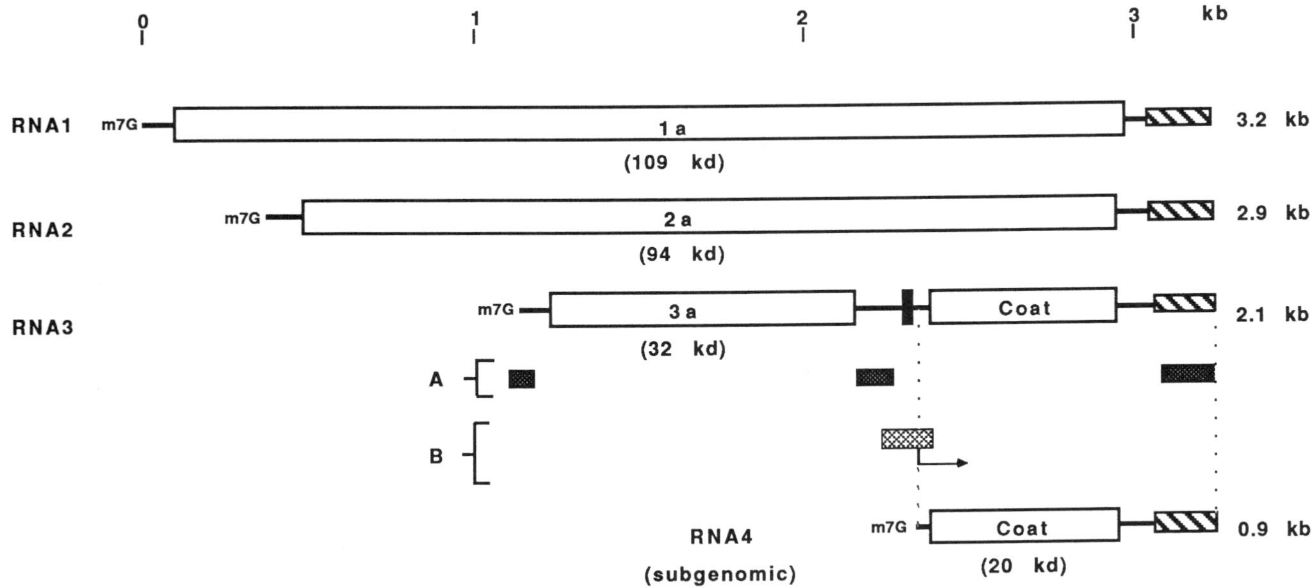

Fig. 1 - Schematic of genomic RNAs 1, 2 and 3 of brome mosaic virus. Open boxes represent expressed open reading frames, with the molecular weight of the encoded protein indicated below each frame. The conserved 3' region of each RNA is shown by a striped box. The filled box between RNA3 open reading frames maps the intercistronic oligo(A) tract of RNA3. The shaded boxes below RNA3 (bracket A) map segments required in cis for RNA3 amplification in BMV infected cells (27). The crosshatched box below RNA3 (bracket B) maps sequences directing subgenomic RNA4 production (30). The structure of subgenomic RNA4 is indicated at the bottom of the figure using the same conventions as for the genomic RNAs.

requirements for host-specific adaptation of genes or regulatory sequences in these viruses.

Bromovirus Characteristics

Bromovirus virions are nonenveloped icosahedra around 28 nm in diameter, whose capsids are composed of 180 copies of a 20 kD coat protein (8). These virions segregate into three fractions in density gradients. Each density fraction corresponds to virions encapsidating one of three different genomic RNA species, denoted RNA1, RNA2 and RNA3 (3.2, 2.9 and 2.1 kb respectively). All three of these RNAs contain distinct genetic information and all three must co-infect a cell to initiate productive infection. Particles that contain RNA3 also contain a subgenomic viral mRNA, RNA4 (0.9 kb). RNA4 is encoded by the 3' portion of RNA3 and directs translation of the viral coat protein.

Bromovirus genome organization. The complete sequence of BMV, the best characterized member of the bromoviruses, has been determined (9,10) and is diagramed in Fig. 1. The 5' end of each BMV RNA is capped with m7GpppG. However, unlike typical eukaryotic mRNAs, the 3' ends are not polyadenylated, but rather terminate with a highly conserved 200 base sequence to which several regulatory functions have been attributed. During replication, this region controls initiation of negative strand RNA synthesis (11,12). This region also folds into a tRNA-like structure (13,14) which is recognized and modified by the normal cellular tRNA nucleotidyl transferase and aminoacyl tRNA synthetase, and binds a translation elongation factor (15). Although RNAs from a number of other plant viruses are also aminoacylated, the function of this modification is still the subject of speculation (16). As well as having possible functions in translation, replication or encapsidation of virus, this modification may discourage degradation of viral RNA by cellular RNase.

Each of the three BMV genomic RNAs serves as messenger for a different noncapsid protein. The 3a protein (32 kD) encoded by the 5' end of RNA3 appears similar in several respects (17) to the tobacco mosaic virus 30 kD protein which is required for systemic spread of infection in whole plants (18,19). The 1a (109 kD) and 2a (94 kD) proteins encoded by RNAs 1 and 2 are trans-acting factors in viral RNA replication. In protoplast studies RNAs 1 and 2 are both required and together sufficient to direct RNA replication (20,21). Moreover, using the cDNA expression system described below, a variety of mutations have been engineered into these genes which cause viral RNA replication to become temperature sensitive (P. Kroner, P. Traynor and P. Ahlquist, unpublished results). The 1a and 2a proteins share extensive sequence similarities with proteins encoded by many other RNA viruses of both plants and animals (2,3).

Biologically active BMV cDNA clones. BMV was the first RNA virus for which infectious transcripts were synthesized *in vitro* from cloned cDNA (22,23). High specific infectivity of such BMV transcripts depends on eliminating extraneous nonviral nucleotides from the 5' end and on the presence of a 5' cap (22,24). Similar results have now been found for a number of other RNA viruses (25,26). Since RNA4 is produced from RNA3, a mixture of *in vitro* transcripts from cDNA clones of RNAs 1, 2 and 3 alone is highly infectious to both whole barley plants and barley protoplasts. The ability to synthesize such infectious transcripts allows the viral genome to be altered in any predesigned way by recombinant DNA techniques. As described below, this approach has facilitated many studies of virus function.

Cis-Acting Signals in BMV RNA Replication and Gene Expression

The temperature sensitive mutations noted above should be valuable in studying the trans-acting functions of the 1a and 2a genes in viral RNA replication. RNA replication also involves *cis*-acting elements which direct the action of these gene products to the appropriate viral templates. To map the *cis*-acting domains required for amplification of BMV RNA3 in infected cells, a variety of deletions and rearrangements were introduced into the cloned RNA3 sequence (27). Either of the two RNA3 open reading frames can be deleted, in whole or in part, without significantly affecting the replication of RNA3 as observed in barley protoplasts. However, efficient RNA3 amplification requires subsets of each of its three noncoding regions (Fig. 1). These regions must then contain the specific signals which initiate (+) and (-) strand RNA synthesis during RNA replication, as well as any sequences required to ensure stability of the product RNA. As noted above, the 3' terminal sequences are known from *in vitro* work to direct (-) strand initiation (11,12), and the 5' terminal sequences are thought to have a similar role in (+) strand synthesis.

The role of the required intercistronic sequences is currently less clear. Interestingly, all of these regions contain elements related to tRNAs and/or their RNA polymerase III promoters, suggesting that replication of these viruses might involve host factors normally interacting with genes transcribed by RNA polymerase III or with the RNA transcripts of such genes (27,28).

Subgenomic RNA4, the mRNA for coat protein expression, is produced by internally initiated transcription from RNA3 (-) strands (29). The promoter sequences which direct this synthesis in vivo have been characterized in our laboratory (30). Full subgenomic promoter activity was mapped to an approximately 120 base segment located immediately upstream of the coat gene. This region contains several imperfect direct repeats, and deletion studies indicate that these are required for full promoter activity. The promoter sequences can be moved as a functional "cassette" to direct production of novel subgenomic RNAs from a variety of insertion points in RNA3. Insertion of the cassette at multiple sites yields multiple subgenomic RNAs from a single RNA3 derivative.

Expression of Foreign Genes in BMV Derivatives

The above studies characterizing cis-acting sequences involved in RNA3 amplification and subgenomic mRNA synthesis demonstrated that a surprising range of genomic modifications produced successfully replicating BMV derivatives. To explore this flexibility further, several foreign genes have been inserted and expressed from different locations in the BMV genome. The first of these was the popular reporter gene for chloramphenicol acetyl transferase, or CAT. When inserted under control of the BMV subgenomic promoter in place of the normal coat gene, the CAT gene was replicated as part of the chimeric RNA3 and high levels of CAT enzyme were expressed (21,31). More recently the coat gene and assembly origin of the cowpea strain of tobacco mosaic virus (TMV) have been inserted into RNA3. In vitro, the resulting hybrid RNA3 is replicated by BMV genes but expresses and is packaged in the TMV coat protein to make rod-shaped particles rather than the usual BMV icosahedra (R. Sacher, R. French and P. Ahlquist, unpublished results).

BMV/CCMV SEQUENCE EXCHANGES

The BMV/TMV hybrid described above showed that, even for dissimilar RNA viruses, it is possible to construct replicating hybrids displaying features from both parents. This suggested that gene exchanges between BMV and more closely related viruses might provide the basis for informative experiments to map specific functions, including host specificity determinants, to particular viral genes. As noted in the Introduction, the closest known relative of BMV is cowpea chlorotic mottle virus (CCMV). CCMV shares the tripartite genome organization and virion morphology characteristics described above for BMV, and its capsid is antigenically related to that of BMV. Both viruses replicate in barley protoplasts and share the local lesion host, Chenopodium hybridum. The most obvious difference between them is that BMV systemically infects grasses, including barley, wheat and other cereal grains, while CCMV infects legumes.

Construction and sequencing of biologically active CCMV cDNA clones

Using improved approaches adapted from prior experience with BMV, complete cDNA copies of each of the three CCMV genomic RNAs have now been synthesized and cloned adjacent to a modified T7 promoter (R. Allison, M. Janda and P. Ahlquist, unpublished results). The complete mixture of in vitro transcripts from these clones shares the infectious properties of CCMV virion RNAs. Specifically, such transcripts are highly infectious to cowpea plants, undergo replication in barley protoplasts and initiate the formation of local lesions on C. hybridum.

We have now sequenced biologically active cDNA clones of CCMV RNAs 2 and 3, including the region encompassing the previously sequenced RNA4 (5). Since CCMV RNA1 has also recently been sequenced (J. Bujarski, personal communication), the complete genome of this virus has now been characterized. Amino acid sequence similarity between the encoded CCMV proteins and their BMV analogs ranges from 53 to over 70% (unpublished results). While the genomic organization of CCMV is largely homologous to BMV, some interesting apparent rearrangements occur in the noncoding regions of RNA3.

Reassortment of BMV and CCMV RNA Components

Since bromovirus genomes are divided among three separate RNAs, initial mapping of at least some functions can be achieved by reassorting specific RNA components between BMV and CCMV. Infectious in vitro transcripts from BMV and CCMV cDNA clones provide a dramatic advantage over the natural virion RNAs for such reassortments. In practice, the difficulty of separating bromovirus virion RNAs into individual component fractions is substantial, particularly for RNAs 1 and 2. Demonstrated or potential cross-contamination can thus create a significant level of uncertainty clouding many conclusions. The clonal purity of in vitro transcripts removes these uncertainties.

Transcripts from the BMV and CCMV clones replicate in barley protoplasts and cause local lesions on C. hybridum, yet maintain their host specificity on whole plants. These three systems thus offer a convenient means for testing different aspects of the biological activity of the various RNA combinations. Accordingly, we have tested all possible single component exchanges between the BMV and CCMV genomes in these systems (R. Allison, M. Janda and P. Ahlquist, unpublished results). A full account of these results will be published elsewhere. In brief, however, exchanges of RNAs 1 and 2 do not appear to be viable, while exchanges of RNA3 produce surprisingly functional genomes. Heterologous mixtures of RNAs 1 and 2 fail to induce detectable RNA replication in protoplasts. Since RNAs 1 and 2 encode two viral proteins involved in RNA replication, this suggests that the 1a and 2a proteins may require co-adaptation to effectively carry out the complete RNA replication cycle.

In contrast, for both RNA3 exchanges, the factors encoded by RNAs 1 and 2 replicate the heterologous RNA3 in protoplasts, and the RNA3-encoded coat protein is expressed and packages the heterologous RNA1 and 2. Thus signals for RNA replication, subgenomic mRNA synthesis and packaging must be conserved to a large degree between BMV and CCMV. Both RNA3-exchange hybrids also produce macroscopic local lesion infections in Chenopodium, indicating at least limited cell to cell spread of infection. These results contrast with those of Bancroft, who observed local lesion infections with BMV RNAs 1 and 2 and CCMV RNA3, but not the converse combination (32).

Neither of the replicating hybrid RNA combinations induced detectable systemic spread of infection to uninoculated leaves of either barley or cowpea plants, the natural systemic hosts of the two parent viruses. The inability of, e.g., CCMV RNA3 to support BMV systemic infection of barley clearly suggests that one or more determinants of bromovirus host specificity reside on RNA3. Conversely, the inability of the same combination to systemically infect cowpea suggests that host specificity also involves adaptations of RNAs 1 and/or 2. Thus, it appears that bromovirus host specificity is not a feature of a single viral RNA.

BMV/CCMV Gene Exchanges

To further map and characterize determinants of host specificity and other virus functions, we have begun to exchange selected genes and gene segments between BMV and CCMV. Using standard recombinant DNA approaches with the biologically active viral cDNA clones, such changes can of course range from specific point mutations to transfer of entire open reading frames. Despite the early stages of the work, a number of existing BMV/CCMV recombinant viruses, like the more classical reassortant hybrids, replicate and package their RNA in protoplasts and induce local lesion infections of Chenopodium. Further exchanges of this nature will likely be a productive approach for the study of both host specificity and more defined virus functions such as RNA replication.

ACKNOWLEDGEMENT

We thank the following colleagues for experimental contributions and valuable discussions: Roy French, Michael Janda, Robert Sacher, Philip Kroner, Radiya Pacha, Pat Traynor and Douglas Richards. We thank Craig Thompson for excellent technical assistance.

REFERENCES

1. Matthews REF (1982). Classification and nomenclature of viruses. Intervirology 17:no.1-3.
2. Ahlquist P, Strauss E, Rice C, Strauss J, Haseloff J, Zimmern D (1985). Sindbis virus proteins nsP1 and nsP2 contain homology to nonstructural proteins from several RNA plant viruses. J Virol 53:536.
3. Goldbach R (1987). Genome similarities between plant and animal RNA viruses. Microbiol Sci 4:197.
4. Rybicki EP, Von Wechmar MB (1981). The serology of the bromoviruses. 1. Serological interrelationships of the bromoviruses. Virology 109:391.
5. Dasgupta R, Kaesberg P (1982). Complete nucleotide sequences of the coat protein messenger RNAs of brome mosaic virus and cowpea chlorotic mottle virus. Nucleic Acids Res 10:703.
6. Saito T, Meshi T, Takamatsu N, Okada Y (1987). Coat protein gene sequence of tobacco mosaic virus encodes a host response determinant. Proc Natl Acad Sci USA 84:6074.
7. Knorr D, Dawson WO (1988). A point mutation in the tobacco mosaic virus capsid protein gene induces hypersensitivity in Nicotiana sylvestris. Proc Natl Acad Sci USA. 85:170.
8. Lane L (1981). Bromoviruses. In Kurstak E, (ed): "Handbook of Plant Virus Infections and Comparative Diagnosis," Amsterdam: Elsevier/North-Holland Biomedical Press, p 333.
9. Ahlquist P, Luckow V, Kaesberg P (1981). Complete nucleotide sequence of brome mosaic virus RNA3. J Mol Biol 153:23.
10. Ahlquist P, Dasgupta R, Kaesberg P (1981). Nucleotide sequence of the brome mosaic virus genome and its implications for viral replication. J Mol Biol 172:369.
11. Ahlquist P, Bujarski J, Kaesberg P, Hall T (1984). Localization of the replicase recognition site within brome mosaic virus RNA by hybrid-arrested RNA synthesis. Plant Mol Biol 3:37.
12. Miller WA, Bujarski J, Dreher T, Hall T (1986). Minus-strand initiation by brome mosaic virus replicase within the 3' tRNA-like structure of native and modified RNA templates. J Mol Biol 187:537.
13. Ahlquist P, Dasgupta R, Kaesberg P (1981). Near identity of 3' RNA secondary structure in bromoviruses and cucumber mosaic virus. Cell 23:183.

14. Rietveld K, Pleij C, Bosch L (1983). Three-dimensional models of the tRNA-like 3' termini of some plant viral RNAs. EMBO J 2:1079.
15. Bujarski J, Ahlquist P, Hall T, Dreher T, Kaesberg P (1986). Modulation of replication, aminoacylation and adenylation in vitro and infectivity in vivo of BMV RNAs containing deletions within the multifunctional 3' end. EMBO J 5:1769.
16. Haenni A, Joshi S, Chapeville F (1982). tRNA-like structures in the genomes of RNA viruses. Prog in Nucl Acid Res and Mol Biol 27:85.
17. Haseloff J, Goelet P, Zimmern D, Ahlquist P, Dasgupta R, Kaesberg P (1984). Striking similarities in amino acid sequence among nonstructural proteins encoded by RNA viruses that have dissimilar genomic organization. Proc Natl Acad Sci USA 81:4358.
18. Deom CM, Oliver JJ, Beachy RN (1987). The 30-kilodalton gene product of tobacco mosaic virus potentiates virus movement. Science 238:389.
19. Meshi T, Ishikawa M, Motoyoshi R, Semba K, Okada Y (1986). In vitro transcription of infectious RNAs from full-length cDNAs of tobacco mosaic virus. Proc Natl Acad Sci USA 83:504.
20. Kiberstis P, Loesch-Fries LS, Hall T (1981). Viral protein synthesis in barley protoplasts inoculated with native and fractionated brome mosaic virus RNA. Virology 112:804.
21. French R, Janda M, Ahlquist P (1986). Bacterial gene inserted in an engineered RNA virus: efficient expression in monocotyledenous plant cells. Science 231:1294.
22. Ahlquist P, French R, Janda M, Loesch-Fries LS (1984). Multicomponent RNA plant virus infection derived from cloned viral cDNA. Proc Natl Acad Sci USA 81:7066.
23. Ahlquist P, Janda M (1984). cDNA cloning and in vitro transcription of the complete brome mosaic virus genome. Mol Cell Biol 4:2876.
24. Janda M, French R, Ahlquist P (1987). High efficiency T7 polymerase synthesis of infectious RNA from cloned brome mosaic virus cDNA and effects of 5' extensions on transcript infectivity. Virology 158:259.
25. Dawson W, Beck D, Knorr D, Grantham G (1986). cDNA cloning of the complete genome of tobacco mosaic virus and production of infectious transcripts. Proc Natl Acad Sci USA 83:1832.

26. Rice CM, Levis R, Strauss JH, Huang HV (1987). Production of infectious RNA trnascripts from Sindbis virus cDNA clones: Mapping of lethal mutations, rescue of a temperature sensitive marker, and in vitro mutagenesis to generate defined mutants. J Virol. 61:3809.
27. French R, Ahlquist P (1987). Intercistronic as well as terminal sequences are required for efficient amplification of brome mosaic virus RNA3. J Virol 61:1457.
28. Marsh L, Hall T (1988). Cold Spring Harbor Symposia on Quantitative Biology 52 (in press).
29. Miller WA, Dreher T, Hall T (1985). Synthesis of brome mosaic virus subgenomic RNA in vitro by internal initiation on (-) sense genomic RNA. Nature 313:68.
30. French R, Ahlquist P (1988). Characterization and engineering of sequences controlling in vivo synthesis of brome mosaic virus subgenomic RNA. J. Virol 62 (in press).
31. Ahlquist P, French R, Bujarski J (1987). Molecular studies of brome mosaic virus using infectious transcripts from cloned cDNA. Adv Virus Res 32:215.
32. Bancroft JB (1972). A virus made from parts of the genomes of brome mosaic and cowpea chlorotic mottle viruses. J Gen Virol 14:223.

Molecular Biology of Plant–Pathogen Interactions, pages 117–127

THE INTERACTION OF MODIFIED VIRUSES WITH THEIR HOSTS[1]

W. O. Dawson and P. Bubrick

Department of Plant Pathology,
University of California
Riverside, California 92521

ABSTRACT A series of mutants of tobacco mosaic virus (TMV) with insertions and/or deletions in the coat protein gene was made by modification of the cDNA of the genome (pTMV204) followed by *in vitro* transcription. All mutants constructed multiplied as free-RNA viruses and moved efficiently in inoculated leaves of Xanthi tobacco. This included mutants that had the entire coat protein gene removed or deletions that extended 28 nucleotides into the 3'-non-translated region, as well as the bacterial chloramphenicol acetyltransferase gene substituted for the coat protein gene. The mutants moved systemically only to a limited extent. Most of the mutants produced coat protein-related polypeptides *in vivo*. The size and amount of protein found in inoculated leaves varied considerably among different mutants. In general, polypeptides that contained the normal coat protein carboxy terminus tended to accumulate in greater amounts.

---

[1]This work was supported in part by grants from USDA (85-CRCR-1-1795), NSF (DMB-8607638), and US-Israel BARD (I-882-85).

Three types of symptoms were observed in mutant-infected Xanthi tobacco: latency, yellowing, and necrosis. Most mutants that produced no or low amounts of coat protein induced no symptoms. The mutant that retained the carboxy terminus of the coat protein induced yellowing symptoms. Two mutants induced necrotic local lesions in Xanthi tobacco as well as almost all host plants tested. These results demonstrate the multifunctional role of the coat protein gene of TMV.

We know little about how viruses cause disease, although this may be one of the key questions in plant virology. There are several types of virus-host interactions in plants, some of which lead to reduced growth and disease, some lead to active resistance mechanisms that prevent disease, whereas others result in little or no disease either because the virus-host interaction is not detrimental or because of the reduced ability of the virus to replicate and invade plant tissue. As we develop the ability to modify the genomes of plants and viruses, we are at the threshold of an understanding of this virus-host relationship and factors that result in diseases of plants. Here we discuss the effects of alterations of the genome of tobacco mosaic virus (TMV) on its ability to induce disease symptoms or resistant responses in different plants.

Tobacco mosaic virus (TMV) has a genome consisting of one RNA molecule of 6395 nucleotides that contains three open reading frames producing four proteins. The 126 kd and 183 kd proteins presumably are involved in replication of RNA, the 30 kd protein is involved in cell-to-cell movement, and the 17.5 kd protein is structural. However, there are many more virus-associated functions and phenotypes than there are proteins produced, suggesting that some sequences of the TMV genome must be able to serve multiple functions.

We have begun a systematic examination of function-sequence relationships of TMV relative to the virus-induced response in different hosts. We began by examining the coat protein gene. Through recombinant DNA techniques we have analyzed both spontaneous and *in vitro* constructed mutants which lead to altered symptoms or novel virus-plant responses.

INDUCTION OF SYMPTOMS IN SYSTEMIC HOSTS

The first virus-host interaction examined was the effect of *in vitro* constructed coat protein mutants on the systemic host, Xanthi tobacco (1). A series of deletion or insertion mutations in the coat protein gene was made by digestion of the cDNA of TMV at the unique Acc I site in the coat protein gene, followed by insertion of a Xho I linker either before or after Bal 31 digestion (Fig. 1). *In vitro* transcripts of the resulting cDNA were used to infect plants. All of the mutants constructed were infectious, replicating as free-RNAs instead of virions. Alterations in the coat protein gene did not greatly reduce the ability of TMV to infect and replicate in inoculated leaves of intact plants. All mutants were able to undergo localized cell-to-cell movement, but compared to wild type were diminished in their ability to systemically invade plants. The entire coat protein gene (cp S3-28) or even 28 nucleotides beyond the coat protein gene into the 3' non-translated region could be removed (cp 35 and cp 5-35) without destroying the capability of replication. Similar results were obtained when the size of the genome was increased by substituting a larger foreign gene, chloramphenicol acetyltransferase (787 nucleotides)(S3-CAT-28), for the coat protein gene (478 nucleotides).

Most of the mutants produced altered coat proteins of reduced size *in vivo*. The amounts of proteins found in cells varied among the different mutants. Proteins that retained the normal C-terminus tended to accumulate in higher amounts than proteins that had this region deleted, suggesting that the C-terminal region of the coat protein may lend stability. However, there was large variation in amounts of accumulation of different mutant proteins that retain the normal C-terminus. Mutants cp 4, cp 25, and cp 27 produced much less protein than mutants cp 35-5 and cp +2. Mutants cp 5 and cp +2 differ only by 4 nucleotides and the sub-genomic mRNAs would be expected to differ by only these 4 nucleotides, yet the amount of cp +2 coat protein produced was substantially higher than that of cp 5. In vivo pulse labeling experiments suggested that the differences in amounts of proteins produced was due to differential rates of synthesis and not to different stabilities in vivo. The sequences involved in the regulation of coat protein synthesis are presently under investigation.

The most surprising result of these experiments was the extent to which the coat protein gene was involved in production of symptoms in Xanthi tobacco. Most of the symptoms produced were distinctive and individual mutants could be identified by their symptomatology. When the sequences of the altered regions of TMV RNA were compared to the symptoms induced, there were no immediately obvious correlations. However, there was some correlation between the protein structure and symptoms produced (Table I and Fig. 1). Most of the mutants that produced proteins with the normal C-terminal region deleted, either because the 3' portion of the gene was deleted (cp 28, cp 35, cp 5-35, cp S3-28, and cp S3-CAT-28) or because the reading frame was lost (cp 5 and cp 10), were symptomless. This effect could be reversed in cp 28 and cp 35 by artificially adding in frame 3' tails from other deletion mutants (e.g. cp 28-5, cp 28-27, cp 35-5); these mutants now produce the normal carboxyl tail of the coat protein and display distinct symptoms. All of the mutants that produced the normal C terminal region of the coat protein induced some degree of yellowing. We do not know whether this is a direct effect of the normal C terminal region of the protein on chloroplasts, or whether some secondary effect like protein stability or concentration affects chloroplasts. The yellowing in inoculated leaves probably results from damage to mature chloroplasts, in contrast to the abnormal development of chloroplasts that culminates in mosaic symptoms in developing leaves.

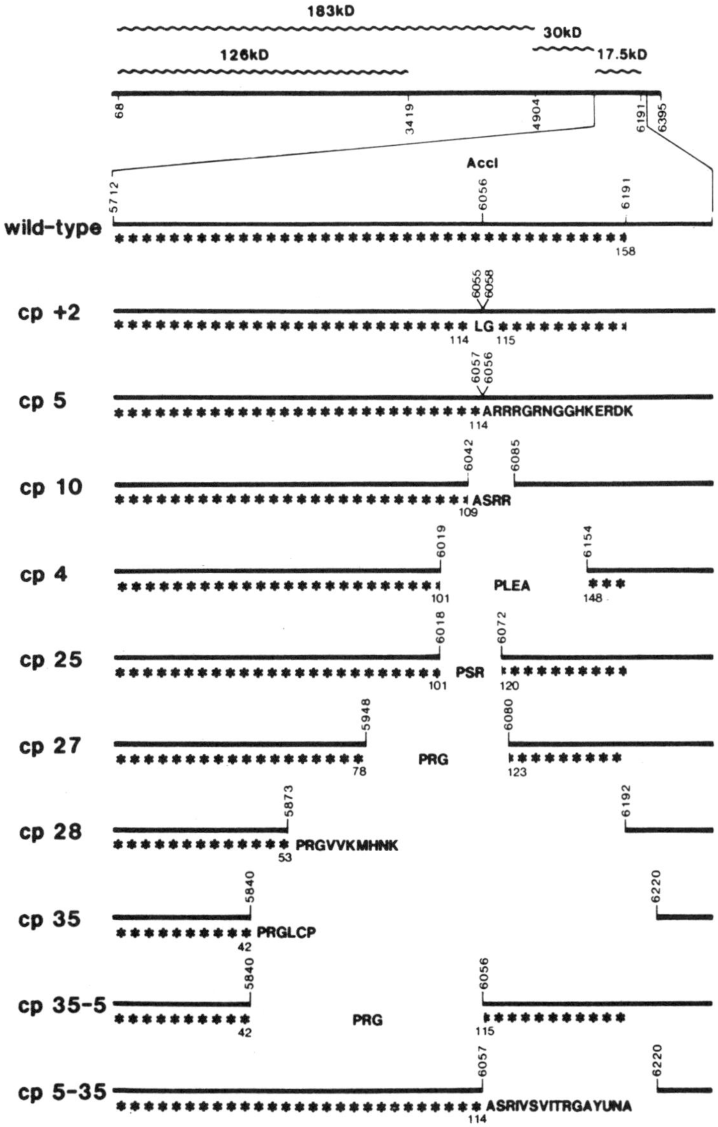

Fig. 1. Comparison of the coat protein produced and the insertion and/or deletions in the coat protein gene of TMV predicted from the sequence of the cDNA construct. The RNA is diagrammed above the protein.

TABLE 1
DESCRIPTION OF COAT PROTEIN DELETION MUTANTS

	Deletion[a] 5'	3'	Reading[b] frame	Symptoms on Xanthi tobacco
cp 5	+1	+1	-	none
cp +2	1	1	+	yellowing
cp 10	14	26	-	necrosis
cp 10-25	14	15	+	necrosis
cp 10-27	14	23	-	necrosis
cp 4	37	97	+	yellowing
cp 4-10	37	26	+	yellowing
cp 25	38	15	+	yellowing
cp 27	108	23	+	necrosis
cp 27-5	108	+1	+	necrosis
cp 27-10	108	26	-	necrosis
cp 28	164	135		yellowing
cp 28-27	164	23	+	yellowing
cp 35	216	163		none
cp 35-5	216	+1	+	yellowing
cp 5-35	+1	163	-	none
cp S3-28	345	135		none
cp S3CAT28	345	135		none
TMV 204	0	0	+	mosaic

There also was some correlation between the amount of altered coat protein that accumulated in cells and the amount of yellowing symptoms in leaves. The largest amount of protein accumulated in leaves infected with mutants cp 35-5, cp 25, cp 4, and cp +2 and, with the exception of cp +2, these mutants induced greater degrees of yellowing. The least amount of protein was found in leaves infected with mutants cp 5, cp 28, cp 35, and cp 5-35, which induced no yellowing symptoms in Xanthi. Mutants that did not produce any coat protein (S3-28) or produced a foreign protein (S3-CAT-28) also induced no symptoms similar to earlier reports (2,3). The proteins that were produced by the mutants probably accumulated as free protein in contrast to that in wild type infected leaves which is mostly associated with virions. This relatively large amount of free protein of altered structure may be the primary factor that adversely affects the infected plants.

INDUCTION OF THE HYPERSENSITIVE REACTION

One type of resistance to plant virus diseases is due to the hypersensitive reaction (HR). In response to the virus, the localized area of infection becomes necrotic and the virus does not spread from this area. We have examined the interaction of TMV with different species of *Nicotiana* which have different genes or alleles that produce local lesions in response to TMV infection. All naturally occurring strains of TMV induce HR in plants with the N gene from *N. glutinosa* (which was bred into *N. tabacum* cv. Xanthi nc). *N. tabacum* cv. Xanthi, which has the corresponding n allele, is susceptible to essentially all strains of TMV resulting in a systemic mosaic disease. Other species of *Nicotiana*, for example *N. sylvestris*, contain the closely linked or allelic gene, N', that localizes some strains of TMV but not others.

Interaction of TMV with nn plants.

Remarkably, two of the coat protein deletion mutants, cp 10 and cp 27, induced distinct necrotic lesions on inoculated leaves of Xanthi which has the nn genotype and normally does not respond hypersensitively to TMV (1). This demonstrated that the coat protein gene of TMV could be involved in production of the hypersensitive reaction in plants in which wild type TMV normally does not induce local lesions. The lesions produced on inoculated leaves of Xanthi were slightly larger and occurred later (5 days) than lesions produced on Xanthi nc (3 days). When inoculated plants were maintained at 25 C, the virus usually was restricted to the necrotic areas and did not move systemically. Occasionally the virus would move systemically, resulting in systemic yellowed and necrotic areas. These two mutants also induced HR on tobacco plants carrying the N or N' gene.

It is difficult to correlate the mutations among the different deletion mutants with their ability to induce necrosis. Both mutants cp 10 and cp 27 have deletions in the region where the coat protein binds to the RNA during assembly (amino acids 90-123). However, several of the other mutants have deletions in this area. Mutants cp 27 and cp 10 are deleted to similar extents in the region 3' of the Acc I site (23 and 26 nucleotides, respectively), but mutant cp 27 retains the correct reading frame and maintains the normal C terminus, while cp 10 does not. There are mutants with deletions smaller or larger than either mutant as well as deletions between cp 10 and cp 27 which do not induce HR. Hybrid combinations between mutants that do and do not induce necrosis demonstrate that only the 5' portion of the deletions of cp 10 and cp 27 are required to induce HR. Disruption of the reading frame of cp 27, or in frame changes of cp 10 do not alter the reaction. All of the deletion or insertion mutants also were examined in *N. sylvestris* which carries the N' gene. Only mutants cp 10 and cp 27 produced necrosis in this plant. Additionally, both mutants were examined in a series of other hosts and both induced local lesions in almost all of these plants (1). However, cp 10 failed to induce lesions in tomato and cp 27 failed to induce lesions in *N. glauca*. These data suggest that two different domains may be involved in the induction of this resistance reaction in different plants.

Interaction of TMV with N'N' plants.

Another approach toward examination of viral sequences involved in induction of plant resistance responses was to examine spontaneous mutants derived from our cloned virus. Our common strain of TMV (U1) does not induce HR in *N. sylvestris*, but mutants that do induce HR can be easily isolated. We isolated such a mutant and characterized nucleotide alterations responsible for the phenotypic change (4). The mutant, TMV

204-D1, was cloned as cDNA and segments of the mutant genome were substituted into the complete wild type genome by replacing corresponding sequences of the wild type. Infectious RNA from the hybrid constructs was tested for ability to induce HR (Fig. 2). Initially, the mutation was found to occur in the 3' half of TMV. Progressively smaller sections of the mutant cDNA were substituted into the wild type genome until the mutation was localized between nucleotides 5972 and 6206 (pDK24). Sequence analysis of this region revealed point mutations at nucleotides 6157 (C to U) and 6199 (A to G). The mutation at 6157 changed a serine to phenylalanine at position 148 of the coat protein whereas nucleotide 6199 occurred just outside of the coat protein gene in the 3' non-translated region. When each point mutation was individually substituted into the wild type background, transcripts containing only the alteration at 6157 (pDK32) produced local lesions in _N. sylvestris_, whereas transcripts containing only the alteration at 6199 (pDK31) produced systemic mosaic symptoms.

This demonstrates that a single nucleotide change in the coat protein gene can be responsible for the induction of HR in _N. sylvestris_. The single nucleotide alteration has clearly changed the virus-host interaction from a systemic mosaic disease to a resistant reaction.

Interaction of TMV with NN plants.

All mutants induced local lesions in Xanthi-nc tobacco and _N. glutinosa_ which have the N gene for resistance to TMV. This included the mutant with no coat protein gene and the mutant with the chloramphenicol acetyltransferase gene in place of the coat protein gene. This demonstrates that the coat protein gene is not required for induction of HR in plants with the N gene.

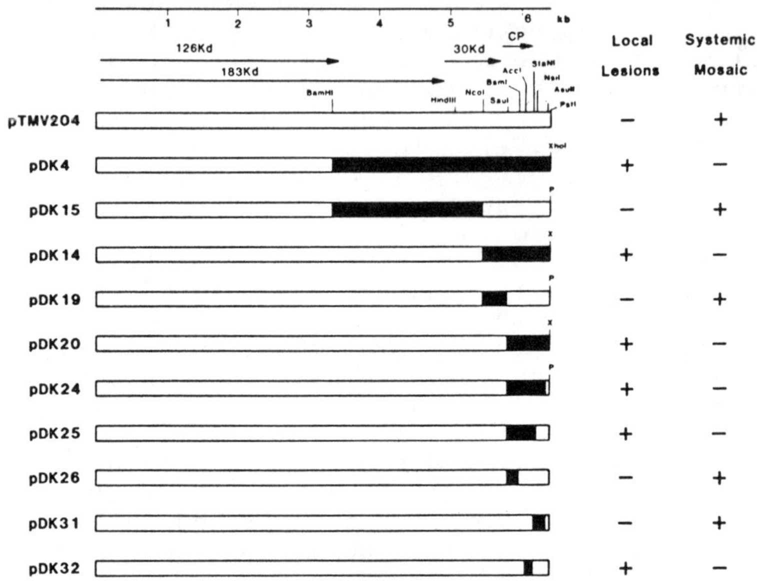

Fig. 2. Composition and symptomatology of wild type and hybrid TMV genomes. Dark portions of genomes show sequences from the mutant that induces local lesions in *N. sylvestris*. Light portions of genomes represent sequences from the wild type virus. Symptoms produced in *N. sylvestris* inoculated with transcripts from cDNA are indicated beside each genome.

These experiments demonstrate that the coat protein gene of TMV is multifunctional. Not only is this gene responsible for the structural features and long distance movement of the virus, but it also appears to be intimately involved with the physiological interactions between the virus and its host. These interactions include alterations of the normal host physiology that results in disease or induction of resistance responses that limit disease. The range of functions associated with alterations in the coat protein gene appears to depend upon how the plant interprets changes in viral RNA or protein.

REFERENCES

1. Dawson, WO, Bubrick, P, Grantham G (1988). Modification of the TMV coat protein gene affects replication, movement and symptomatology. Phytopathology (in press).
2. Sarkar, S, Smitamana P (1981). A truly coat-protein-free mutant of tobacco mosaic virus. Naturwissenschaften 68:145-147.
3. Takamatsu, N, Ishikawa, M, Meshi, T, Okada, Y (1987). Expression of bacterial chloramphenicol acetyltransferase gene in tobacco plants mediated by TMV-RNA. EMBO J. 6:307-311.
4. Knorr, DA, Dawson WO (1988). A point mutation in the tobacco mosaic virus capsid protein gene induces hypersensitivity in _Nicotiana sylvestris_. Proc. Natl. Acad. Sci. USA 85:170-174.

Molecular Biology of Plant–Pathogen Interactions, pages 129–140

MOLECULAR GENETIC AND FUNCTIONAL ANALYSIS OF A PLANT VIRUS PROTEINASE AND ITS ROLE IN POLYPROTEIN PROCESSING

William G. Dougherty, James C. Carrington, T. Dawn Parks, and Susan M.Cary

Department of Microbiology,
Oregon State University,
Corvallis, Oregon 97331

ABSTRACT Tobacco etch virus (TEV), a potyvirus, has a single-stranded RNA genome. The RNA is organized as a single open-reading frame that potentially could encode a 346,000 dalton (d) polyprotein. Processing of this polyprotein has been characterized using molecular genetic, immunological and biochemical approaches. The TEV small nuclear inclusion protein (49,000 d) is a viral-encoded proteinase. Monospecific antiserum to this viral protein specifically inhibits proteolytic activity. The 49,000 d protein is 430 amino acids in length and contains, near the carboxy terminus, the conserved Cys-15 amino acids-His motif present in all viral encoded cysteine-like proteinases. A molecular genetic analysis of the sequence encoding this protein has been completed.

During TEV genome expression, this proteinase autocatalytically releases from the polyprotein and processes the polyprotein at

---

WGD would like to thank the National Science Foundation and the Competitive Grants Office of the United States Department of Agriculture for support.

JCC is a National Institute of Health Postdoctoral Fellow.

three other sites. Cleavage occurs between the dipeptide Gln-Ser or a Gln-Gly contained within the conserved sequence
Glu - Xaa - Xaa - Tyr - Xaa - Gln - Gly/Ser.
This seven amino acid sequence is essential in defining a cleavage site, as shown by insertion and cleavage of synthetic sites and by site-directed mutagenesis of an authentic site. Understanding mechanisms of viral proteinase recognition may be useful in the design of new virus control strategies.

INTRODUCTION

Members of the potato virus Y group of pathogens, or potyviruses, comprise one of the largest known group of plant viruses(1)(2). While the host range of a particular potyvirus is quite narrow or restrictive, this group, with over a 100 different members, represents a continuum of viral pathogens with the potential to infect most, if not all, commercially grown crop species.

A typical potyvirus is a unicomponent, flexuous rod-shaped virion approximately 750nm in length and 12 nm in diameter(1). The viral genome is a single-stranded RNA molecule nearly 10,000 nucleotides in length. The nucleotide sequence of tobacco etch virus [TEV]- and tobacco vein mottling virus [TVMV]-RNA has been determined(3)(4). A single open-reading-frame is present in this sequence and it spans nearly the entire length of the genomic RNA. Additionally, subgenomic mRNAs are not detected in TEV-infected plant tissue(5). This has led to the proposal that the TEV genome is expressed as a single polyprotein which is proteolytically processed into functional gene products.

In this article, we will summarize current information about the 49,000 dalton (d) TEV-encoded proteinase and the role it plays in processing the TEV polyprotein. This is an unusual protein, as it aggregates in the nucleus of infected cells with another virus-encoded protein(6). These nuclear inclusion bodies can be readily purified and are abundant sources of proteolytic activity(7)(8). The amino acid sequence recognized by this proteinase also is distinguished in that it is conserved(9) and can be moved as a cassette into foreign sites(10). The potential of targeting this proteinase for virus control or exploiting the specificity of this proteolytic reaction is discussed.

MATERIAL AND METHODS

The cloning of TEV cDNA sequences and their expression in cell-free transcription and translation systems has been reported(3)(8). The pTL-series of expression vectors has been constructed for this purpose and used through out our studies(11). These plasmid vectors permit site-directed mutagenesis and cell-free transcriptional expression of cDNA sequences. Using this approach, transcripts of wild-type or mutated cDNA sequences are translated in a rabbit reticulocyte lysate and proteinase and synthetic polyprotein substrates can be made(8)(12). In many studies, purified nuclear inclusion bodies are the source of proteolytic activity(7)(8). Polyprotein precursors and their processed products are separated by SDS-polyacrylamide gel electrophoresis and detected by fluorography(13).

RESULTS AND DISCUSSION

The 49,000 d TEV Proteinase

The 49,000 d TEV-encoded nuclear inclusion protein is a proteinase. The region of the TEV genome that codes for this protein is schematically presently in Figure 1. The location of this gene between a putative VPg and RNA-dependent, RNA-polymerase (replicase) coding sequence maintains a genetic motif found in picornaviruses and comoviruses(14)(15).

A number of structure-function relationships have been elucidated and can be summarized as follows.

First, the TEV 49,000 d proteinase is formed by autocatalytic or *cis* processing events(12). Cleavage is between the dipeptide glutamine-glycine

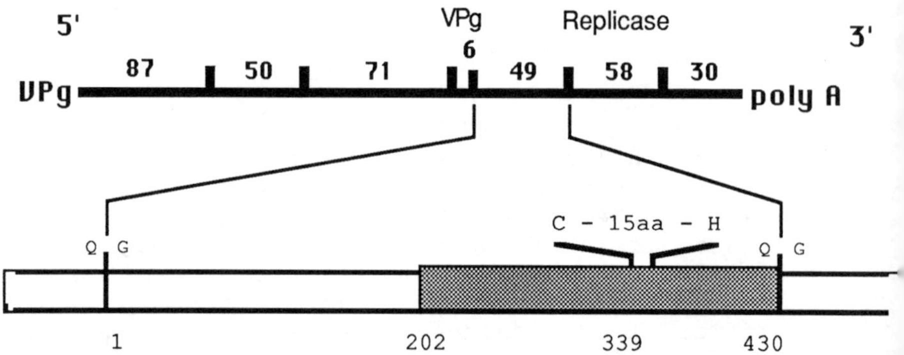

Figure 1. Schematic representation of the TEV genom and 49,000 d proteinase. The proposed TEV genetic organization is present at the top of the figure with estimated molecular weight of the TEV protei The essential features of the TEV proteinase are present below. The protein is 430 amino acids in length and is formed by autocatalytic cleavage events between glutamine(Q)-glycine(G) dipeptides The domain responsible for proteolytic cleavage i stippled. The conserved cysteine(C)-histidine(H) motif is presented.

and results in the formation of a protein which is 430 amino acids in length [Figure 1](12)(16). Proteolytic activity is associated with the 49,000 d protein made in a cell-free system or isolated from infected plant cells as a component of the nuclear inclusion body(8). Cleavage site mutations [glutamine to proline] prevent the proteinase from autocatalytically releasing from the polyprotein precursor, but do not inhibit proteolytic activity, as the proteinase is still able to process substrates in a bimolecular or *trans* reaction(16).

Second, deletion and site-directed mutational analyses reveal that proteolytic activity is associated with the carboxy-terminal half of this protein [Figure 1](8). The amino terminal 202 amino acids have been deleted and the remaining 228 amino acids comprising the carboxy-terminal half maintain the same activity and specificity as the 49,000 d protein. Deleting 30 amino acids from the carboxy terminus of the 49,000 d protein completely eliminates proteolytic activity. Within this carboxy terminal half, the amino acid motif cysteine - 15 amino acids - histidine is present(3). A similar conserved sequence, present in the 3C proteinase of picornaviruses and the 24,000 d proteinase of cowpea mosaic virus, has been suggested to be important in proteolysis(17). A single amino acid substitution in which the cysteine (amino acid 339) has been replaced with alanine totally eliminates proteolytic activity associated with this protein, and supports the hypothesis that these sequences contribute to functional activity(12). Overall, it would appear that the 49,000 d TEV protein may be a multifunctional protein comprised of two separate domains. The role of the N-terminal domain in the TEV replication cycle remains to be determined.

Finally, we have been able to inhibit the activity of this proteinase with antiserum specific for the 49,000 d protein derived from nuclear inclusion bodies. Antisera to other virus-specific proteins have no effect on proteolytic activity(8).

Cleavage Sites Recognized by the 49,000 d TEV Proteinase

Naturally occurring cleavage sites. The 49,000 d proteinase cleaves the TEV polyprotein at five unique positions(8)(13)(16). The sequence surrounding these five cleavage sites is presented in Table 1. The sequence surrounding the cleavage site is notable in that, in addition to the conservation of the dipeptide glutamine-glycine or glutamine-serine between which cleavage occurs [position -1 and +1 relative to the scissile bond], the -3 [tyrosine] and the -6 [glutamic acid] positions are strictly conserved. Additionally, an amino acid with a neutral side chain [leucine, isoleucine or valine] is always in the -4 position(8)(9).The extented sequence similarity surrounding naturally occuring TEV cleavage sites is not evident at the cleavage sites of other viral-encoded polyproteins(15)(18). Cleavage at these five sites has been demonstrated experimentally in three ways. First, polyprotein substrates have been synthesized from transcripts derived from specific TEV cDNA sequences. Addition of the 49,000 d proteinase to these substrates mediates cleavage into lower molecular weight products(8)(12)(16).

TABLE 1. Amino acids present at TEV polyprotein cleavage sites processed by the 49,000 d TEV proteinase.

Protein Junction	Amino acid Sequence	
50kD - 71kD	-R-E-I- I-Y-T-Q	S-L-D-D-Y-V-T-
71kD - 6kD	-L-E-T- I-Y-L-Q	S-D-S-E-V-A-K-
6kD - 49kD	-N-E-P-V-Y-F-Q	G-K-K-N-Q-K-H-
49kD - 58kD	-N-E-L-V-Y-S-Q	G-E-K-R-K-W-V-
58kD - 30kD	-T-E-N-L-Y-F-Q	S-G-T-V-D-A-G-
	- 6 -3 -1	+1

↑ CLEAVAGE SITE

Second, site-directed mutagenesis has permitted the replacement of glutamine at the -1 position with proline, leucine, or arginine. In all cases tested, this single amino acid replacement eliminates cleavage at the five sites(16). Finally, microsequence analysis has been conducted on some of the processed products(12)(16). By these three criteria functional cleavage sites have been mapped to five locations on the TEV polyprotein. We have been unable to demonstrate 49,000 d proteinase mediated cleavage in other regions of the TEV polyprotein (unpublished observations).

Engineered-cleavage sites and a delination of the minimal sequence necessary to define a cleavage site. We have been able to demonstrate that seven amino acids [position -6 thru +1] are required to define a functional TEV polyprotein cleavage site. This has been accomplished in two related experimental approaches(10). First, cDNA encoding 25 amino acids present at the 50,000/71,000 d TEV cleavage site has been inserted in the middle of the capsid protein gene while maintaining the capsid protein gene reading frame. This 25 amino acid sequence encodes 18 amino acids on the amino-terminal side of the scissile bond and 7 amino acids on the carboxy-terminal side of the bond. The polyprotein derived from this engineered cDNA sequence is specifically processed by the TEV 49,000 d proteinase at the naturally-occurring site and the newly inserted cleavage site. The second experimental approach has been to insert different peptide sequences into a TEV polyprotein via recombinant DNA techniques. These sequences maintain the open reading frame of the polyprotein and code for 1) an authentic seven amino acid cleavage site sequence [position -6 thru +1], 2) only the glutamine-serine [position -1 and +1] between which cleavage occurs or 3) only the serine in the +1 position. The 49,000 d proteinase is able to process the engineered polyprotein substrate in which the authentic seven amino acid cleavage site sequence was inserted. The other two oligonucleotide linkers did not generate a functional polyprotein cleavage site.

Site-directed mutagenesis of an authentic TEV cleavage site. The role of the conserved amino acids [at positions -6, -3, -1 and +1] in defining a functional cleavage site has been examined(9). The junction between the 58,000 d replicase and the 30,000 d capsid protein gene products has been selected for study and the plasmid pTL-8595 has been used. A series of different polyprotein substrates has been generated using site-directed mutagenesis and cell-free transcription and translation. These polyprotein substrates, which have a number of different amino acid replacements made at the four conserved positions, have been tested in a cell-free assay which permits quantitation of processing. The results suggest that the conserved amino acids in the -6, -3 and -1 are essential in defining an optimal cleavage site. Some amino acid replacements permit cleavage but at a greatly reduced rate. The -1 position [glutamine] tolerates changes the least and most polyprotein substrates containing an amino acid other than glutamine in this position are not processed. The +1 position, in which serine and glycine are found naturally at this junction, tolerates a number of different amino acid replacements. Polyprotein substrates in which the serine has been replaced with isoleucine or asparagine appear to be processed even more rapidly.

The cell-free analyses of this TEV polyprotein cleavage site are providing valuable insight into the role of these conserved amino acids in defining a cleavage site. However, substantial work remains in determining the effect of these amino acid replacements *in vivo* during virus replication.

Future Directions

The 49,000 d TEV proteinase may provide unique opportunities in bioengineering and in designing new control strategies for potyviruses. Both initiatives rely on the specificity of the cleavage reaction. Few viral proteinases have been described which can be purified in large quantities (gram amounts) and have a cleavage site recognition sequence which is seven amino acids in length.

In the area of bioengineering, it should be possible to accurately process a fusion protein. A gene of interest could be constructed that when expressed as a protein would consist of a bacterial or yeast amino acid sequence - seven amino acid TEV cleavage site sequence cassette - the protein of interest. This fusion protein could be treated with TEV proteinase and an authentic (or modified by a single N-terminal amino acid) protein would be released. This approach may be particularly useful when biological properties or activities are being examined or when the authentic product is toxic to the host cell.

More important is the opportunity this proteinase presents in the control of potyviral infections. Two different approaches may be taken; in one, the aim would be to disrupt the proteinase activity while, in the other, the specificity of the proteinase would be exploited to activate a resistance mechanism.

Most attempts to design effective viricides for plant viruses have been too costly and for the most part ineffectual. Most viricides tested have been nucleotide or base analogs(19). Uptake by the plant with preferential incorporation into rapidly replicating viral RNA, rather than into host nucleic acids, is the desired result. Frequently, there is a fine line between effectiveness and toxicity. The TEV proteinase has an unusual degree of specificity and it should be possible to design compounds which target this proteinase for inactivation and hence, interruption of the viral replication cycle.

The alternative approach uses the viral proteinase and the specificity it shows to activate a lethal event. An example is as follows. A plant would be engineered to constitutively express a precursor protein which would be inactive because 1) it is targeted to a cellular compartment where it would be unable to act, or 2) it would be in an inactive precursor form. An essential aspect of this precursor is that it contains a functional TEV cleavage sequence. Infection by TEV would result in early rounds of translation in which the TEV polyprotein is made and processed by the viral-encoded proteinase. In addition to cleaving the TEV polyprotein, the 49,000 d proteinase should also cleave the inactive engineered precursor, resulting in an activated protein. This protein should be lethal to the cell. In a sense, the final phenotype would be to develop a hypersensitive type response in which virus replication would be limited to a single (or a few) cell(s).

This is one example of how basic biological information is important and can be applied to control practical plant pathological problems.

ACKNOWLEDGEMENTS

WGD would like to thank Stephen Johnson and Dennis Hruby for their comments and stimulating discussion about pathogen derived resistance. This is Oregon Agriculture Experiment Station Technical Paper Number 8478.

REFERENCES

1. Hollings, M., Brunt, A. (1981). Potyviruses. In Kurstak, E. (ed):"Handbook of Plant Virus Infection," Amsterdam, Elsevier/North Holland, p 731.
2. Edwardson, J.R. (1974). Some Properties of the Potato Virus Y Group. Fla. Agri. Expt. Stat. Mono. Series 4., Gainesville, p394.
3. Allison, R.F., Johnston, R.E., Dougherty, W.G. (1986). The nucleotide sequence of the coding region of tobacco etch virus genomic RNA: evidence for the synthesis of a single polyprotein. Virology 154:9.
4. Domier, L.L., Franklin, K.M., Shahabuddin, M., Hellmann, G.M., Overmeyer, J.H., Hiremath, S., Siaw, M.F.E., Lomonossoff, G.P., Shaw, J.G., Rhoads, R.E. (1986). The nucleotide sequence of tobacco vein mottling virus RNA. Nucleic Acids Res. 14: 5417.

5. Dougherty, W.G. (1983). Analysis of viral RNA isolated from tobacco leaf tissue infected with tobacco etch virus. Virology 131: 473.
6. Knuhtsen, H., Hiebert, E., Purcifull, D.E. (1974). Partial purification and some properties of tobacco etch virus induced intranuclear inclusions. Virology 61: 200.
7. Dougherty, W.G., Hiebert, E. (1980). Translation of potyvirus RNA in a rabbit reticulocyte lysate: identification of nuclear inclusion proteins as products of tobacco etch virus RNA translation and cylindrical inclusion protein as a product of the potyvirus genome. Virology 104: 174.
8. Carrington, J.C., Dougherty, W.G. (1987). Small nuclear inclusion protein encoded by a plant potyvirus genome is a protease. J. of Virology 61: 2540.
9 Dougherty, W.G., Carrington, J.C., Cary, S.M., Parks, T.D. (1988). Biochemical and mutational analysis of a plant virus polyprotein cleavage site. EMBO J. 7: in press.
10 Carrington, J.C., Dougherty, W.G. (1988). A viral cleavage site cassette: identification of amino acid sequences required for tobacco etch virus polyprotein processing. Proc. Natl. Acad. Sci. USA. 85: in press.
11. Carrington, J.C., Parks, T.D., Cary, S.M., Dougherty, W.G. (1987). Vectors for cell-free expression and mutagenesis of protein coding sequences. Nucleic Acids Res. 15: 10066.
12. Carrington, J.C., Dougherty, W.G. (1987) Processing of the tobacco etch virus 49K protease requires autoproteolysis. Virology 160: 355.
13. Laemmli, U.K. (1970). Cleavage of structural proteins during the assembly of the head of bacteriophage T4. Nature (London) 227: 680.
14. Palmenberg, A.C. (1987). Genome Organization, translation, and processing in picornaviruses. In Rowlands, D.J., Mayo, M.A., Mahy, B.W.J. (eds) "The Molecular Biology of the Positive Strand RNA Viruses". New York, Academic Press. p1.

15. Wellink, J., van Kammen, A.(1988). Proteases involved in the processing of viral polyproteins. A Brief Review. Arch. Virol. 98: 1.
16. Carrington, J.C., Cary, S.M., Dougherty, W.G. (1988). Mutational analysis of tobacco etch virus polyprotein processing: cis and trans proteolytic activities of polyproteins containing the 49-kilodalton proteinase. J. of Virology in press.
17. Argos, P. Kamer, P., Nicklin, M.J.H., Wimmer, E. (1984). Similarity in gene organization and homology between proteins of animal picornaviruses and a plant comovirus suggest common ancestry of these virus families. Nucleic Acids Res. 12: 7251.
18. Toyoda, H., Nicklin, M.J.H., Murry, M.G., Wimmer, E. (1986). Proteolytic processing of the poliovirus polyprotein by two virus-encoded proteinases. In Inouye, M., Sarma, R. (eds) "Protein Engineering: Application in Science, Medicine and Industry". New York, Academic Press. p.156.
19. Dawson, W.O., Boyd, C. (1987). Modifications of nucleic acid precursors that inhibit plant virus multiplication. Phytopathology 77: 477.

Molecular Biology of Plant-Pathogen Interactions, pages 141-152

GENES AND SEQUENCES INVOLVED IN THE REPLICATION OF THE COWPEA MOSAIC VIRUS RNAs

Rik Eggen, Jan Verver, Pieter Vos, Joan Wellink, Ab van Kammen and Rob Goldbach

Departments of Molecular Biology and Virology, Agricultural University, Binnenhaven 11, 6709 PD Wageningen, The Netherlands

ABSTRACT A model is presented in which a number of B-RNA-encoded proteins form a membrane-bound RNA replication complex that is active during only one single round of replication. This "once-only" use of viral replication proteins is based on a number of observations and may explain the formation of cytopathological inclusions containing bulk amounts of viral proteins that seem not to be involved in viral replication. To study the genome sequence requirements for replication full-length cDNA clones of both B-RNA and M-RNA have been constructed from which infectious transcripts were obtained by transcription *in vitro*. The introduction of a first point mutation in a putative replication signal demonstrates the great potential of these clones. The clones were also applied to study the proteolytic processing of the viral polyproteins. By introducing specific deletions in the B cDNA clone it is shown that CPMV encodes only one protease (the 24K protein) while a second protein (the 32K protein) is required as co-factor for the cleavage of a Q/M cleavage site *in trans*.

INTRODUCTION

The genetic information of the bipartite RNA genome of cowpea mosaic virus (CPMV), type member of the comoviruses, is expressed via the production of long polyproteins from which mature, functional proteins are generated by proteolytic processing (see Fig. 1 and for recent reviews refs. 1 and 2).

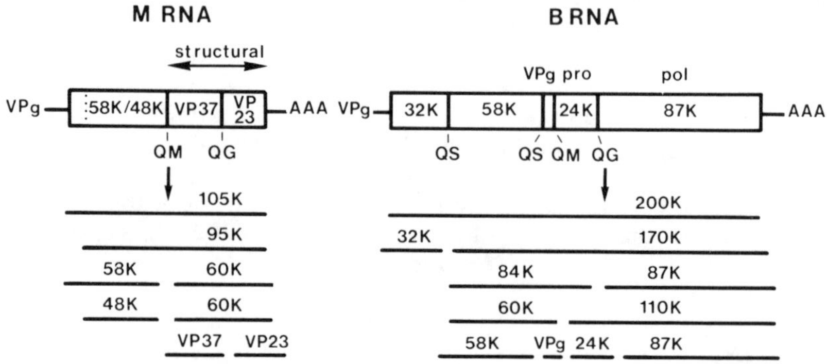

FIGURE. 1. Genetic map of CPMV RNAs. All proteins indicated in the figure have been identified in infected cells, with the exception of the M-RNA-encoded 105K, 95K and 58K proteins which only have been observed upon in vitro translation of M-RNA.

Both the shorter M-RNA (3481 nucleotides) and the longer B-RNA (5889 nucleotides) possess a small protein, denoted VPg, covalently bound to the 5'-end and a poly(A) tail at the 3'-end. Together with the potyviruses (see chapter of W. G. Dougherty et al.) and nepoviruses the comoviruses represent the so-called picorna-like plant viruses, i.e. plant viruses genetically related to the picornaviruses of animals (3-5). With regard to the genetic map it is known that M-RNA encodes the two capsid proteins VP37 and VP23. B-RNA is able to replicate independently of M-RNA in cowpea protoplasts and is therefore considered to encode all functions required for viral RNA replication (6). B-RNA, however, cannot move from cell-to-cell in the absence of M-RNA and therefore the overlapping 58K and 48K proteins encoded by M-RNA have been proposed to be involved in cell-to-cell movement of the virus (6, 7). This conclusion has been strengthened by the observation that all transport mutants (i.e. mutants inducing small local lesions on Phaseolus vulgaris cv. Pinto) map on M-RNA (C.P. de Jager, unpublished results) and by results obtained with another comovirus, red clover mottle virus, showing that the transport function of tobamoviruses may complement B-RNA, enabling it to spread through tobacco leaves (8). Furthermore B-RNA encodes the viral (24K) protease, which, in collaboration with the 32K protein (see below), achieves the complete proteolytic processing of the viral polyproteins.

RESULTS

Proteins involved in viral RNA replication

As quoted above all viral functions involved in CPMV RNA replication appear to be encoded by the B-RNA. This conclusion has been further substantiated by the discovery (3) that four of the B-RNA-coded proteins show significant sequence homology to non-structural picornaviral proteins, that have also been implied in RNA replication. These proteins are the comoviral 58K membrane-bound protein, VPg, the 24K protease and the 87K core polypeptide of the viral polymerase (see Fig. 1), corresponding to the picornaviral proteins 2C, VPg, 3C and 3D. Moreover, these conserved proteins are encoded by a similarly arranged gene set in the respective viral genomes and all four appear to be involved in a membrane-bound RNA replication complex in both comoviruses (9) and picornaviruses (10). Partial purification of active, membrane-detached replication complexes from CPMV-infected cowpea leaf tissue revealed the involvement of the B-RNA-encoded 110K protein (i.e. the covalent combination of the 24K protease and 87K polymerase domains), together with two host-encoded proteins of 68K and 57K (11). However, for CPMV there seems to be a discrepancy between the amount of 110K protein (and 87K protein) in infected cells and the actual CPMV replicase activity measured. While the amount of viral 110K polypeptide found in actively RNA-replicating complexes is hardly detectable by silver staining (11) bulk amounts of this protein are found in amorphous inclusions in infected cowpea cells (12, 13). Clearly we have to face the possibility that the CPMV polymerase molecules have a very limited activity. Indeed, the translation expression mechanism used by the virus (polyprotein processing) implies the production of a surplus of polymerase molecules. For each progeny RNA molecule the production of a VPg molecule is required. Since VPg and the viral core polymerase (110K and 87K protein) are produced from a common polyprotein they are produced in equimolar amounts. Hence, on average a polymerase molecule only needs to synthesize a single RNA molecule to keep step with the production of VPg. In view of this it is feasible that viral polymerase molecules lose their activity upon releasing their first template by not being capable to

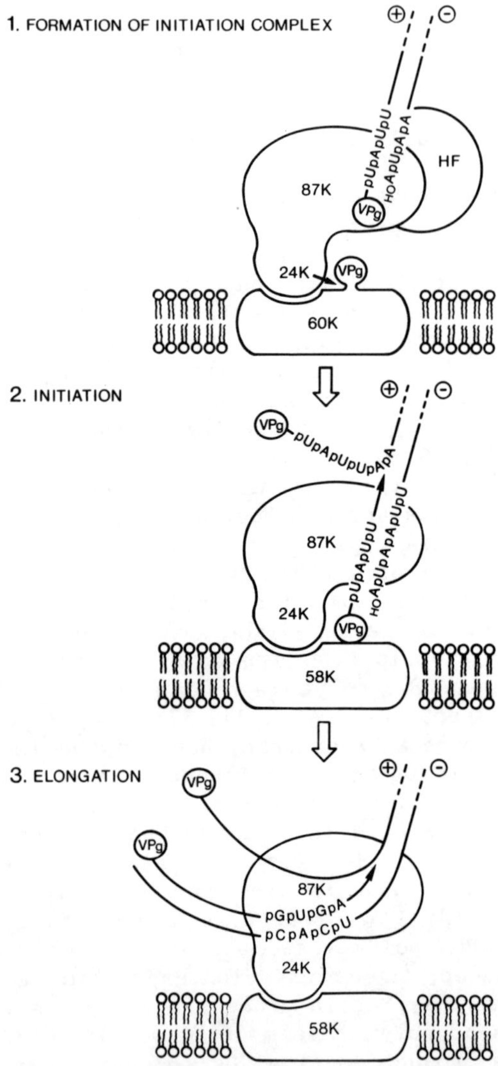

FIGURE 2. Model of a membrane-bound CPMV RNA replication model. For details see text.

initiate a second time. Such restriction of the polymerase activity would nicely match with the observation that isolated CPMV replication complexes contain polymerase molecules which are only able to complete nascent chains copied from their endogeneous template and do not seem able to accept added template molecules.

Therefore, to add a little speculation to this chapter in Fig. 2 a model for the CPMV RNA replication is presented which starts from the principle that the polymerase and all other viral proteins involved serve only once. With regard to the reactions occurring during initiation the model is partly based on the mechanism proposed by Takegami et al (10) for poliovirus RNA synthesis. The model of Fig. 2, which shows only plus-strand synthesis, accommodates most of the characteristic features of the CPMV replication complex as emerged from extensive experimental work, and proposes the following steps:

1. Formation of an initiation complex.
   A complex is formed between the B-RNA-coded 60K and 110K proteins at one hand, and between the 110K protein, possibly a host factor (HF) and template RNA at the other hand. The 60K protein is tightly associated to the membranes of the numberous vesicles formed in the cytopathic structures in the cytoplasm of infected cells (7, 14) and serves for membrane-attachment and VPg supply. The 110K protein contains the 24K protease domain which, at the onset of RNA synthesis, is able to release VPg by cleavage at a glutamine-serine site (cf. Fig. 1). VPg may become uridylated prior to initiation as has been suggested by Takegami et al (10) for poliovirus. Since the 60K and 110K proteins are derived, as neighbours, from the same 170K precursor the formation of an initiation complex may start with the binding of this precursor protein to the membranes, while cleavage to give the 60K and 110K proteins only occurs after binding. As a template the double-stranded end of an RI molecule is shown in the model.
2. Initiation.
   Following the release of (uridylated) VPg from the 60K protein by the action of the 24K protease, the 87K polymerase domain in the 110K protein starts plus strand synthesis thereby driving the pre-existing (nascent) plus-strand chain out of the RI molecule.
3. Elongation.
   While remaining attached to the 58K protein the 87K domain

of the 110K protein continues to synthesize the plus-strand. When the chain is completed the template is released and the activity of the remaining membrane-bound protein complex has ceased due to the absence of VPg sequences necessary for initiation.

The model of Fig. 2 may also account for the synthesis of minus strand which starts on the 3'-poly(A) tail of virion RNA. It implies a role for VPg as primer, a supposition which needs to be tested. Furthermore the model proposes that the 60K protein plays a role in binding the replication complex to the membranes.

The hypothesis that the bulk of B-RNA encoded replication proteins in infected cowpea cells are just dead-end molecules, clustered in cytoplasmic inclusions, has been recently confirmed by analysis of the intracellular levels of these proteins in another host of CPMV, _Chenopodium amaranticolor_ (15). While in both cowpea and _Chenopodium_ similar amounts of virus are produced and similar levels of viral RNA synthesizing activity are measured, in the latter host the non-structural proteins are hardly or even not detectable. Hence, the accumulation of non-structural proteins is not stringently interrelated to the synthesis of virus RNA or virus particles. The model of "once-only" use of replication proteins as presented in Fig. 2 may also hold for potyviruses, another group of picorna-like plant viruses, of which some members deposit large amounts of polymerase and protease molecules in the nuclei of infected cells.

Infectious transcripts from cDNA-clones

As another approach to unravel the mechanism of viral RNA replication and to identify the genes and sequences involved in this crucial process, we have aimed for the construction of full-length cDNA clones that generate infectious transcripts upon _in vitro_ transcription. Using the T7 system and a truncated T7 promoter, _in vitro_ transcripts were obtained containing only two or even one non-viral G residues at the 5'-end and, as a result of cleavage of the clones with a restriction enzyme (ClaI) for run-off transcription, 5 extra nucleotides added to the 40 residues-long poly(A) tail (Table 1). The highest level of infectivity was observed with transcripts containing only one extra G, either capped or uncapped. While the infectivity of B cDNA transcripts could be tested independently from M-RNA (Table 1), transcripts of full-length M cDNA clones could only be tested in the presence of B clone transcripts. The number of protoplasts in

Table 1

INFECTIVITY OF IN VITRO TRANSCRIPTS OF cDNA CLONES FROM B-RNA

CLONE	TERMINI OF TRANSCRIPT	% PROTOPLASTS PRODUCING B-RNA ENCODED PROTEINS [a]
pTB35	X_{35}-UAUU------A_{40}UAUCG	0.2
pTB2G	GG-UAUU------A_{40}UAUCG	5
pTB2G-cap	m^7GpppGG-UAUU------A_{40}UAUCG	10
pTB1G	G-UAUU------A_{40}UAUCG	25
pTB1G-cap	m^7GpppG-UAUU------A_{40}UAUCG	40
pTB1G-40	G-UAUU------$A_{40}X_{400}$	25
control:		
CPMV B-RNA[b]	VPg-UAUU------A_{50-140}	20

[a] For each test a portion of 2.5×10^6 cowpea protoplasts was transfected with 50 μg of RNA.

[b] As a control a portion of protoplasts was transfected with 1 μg of natural B-RNA.

which the transcripts of both M and B clones started replication and hence resulted in complete virus multiplication was therefore much lower, i.e. approximately 1%. Even so enough virus could be recovered from these transfected protoplasts to induce (wild type) systemic infections in cowpea plants upon mechanical inoculation. The availability of DNA clones of both M- and B-RNA expressing infectivity provide a very good starting point to map the sequences involved in replication (e.g. replicase binding sites). As a first step in this aim a point mutation was introduced in an eleven base sequence (UUUUAUUAAAA) which is conserved (except for a U to G exchange) in the 3'-terminal ends of both the minus and plus strands of B- and M-RNA and may, therefore, represent a replicase-binding site (2). Moreover, in the 3'-ends of the plus-strands this motif may form a stable hairpin. The point mutation involved an A to T change by which a (TTTAAA) cleavage site for the restriction enzyme AhaIII was created in the cDNA clone and an A to U change in the transcript. Transcripts of this mutant clone were viable, although the infectivity dropped to 17% (compared to 40% for wild type, see Table 1) and is a first indication for a crucial function of the modified sequence. The creation of the AhaIII-site within this sequence allows further mapping of terminal sequence requirements by chewing and by linker insertion. These studies are currently in progress.

Two viral proteins involved in proteolytic processing

The availability of a full-length cDNA-clone of the B-RNA has also created the possibility to study the involvement of viral proteins in the proteolytic processing of the viral polyproteins. For this purpose infectivity of modified clones is not required since proteolytic processing can be readily studied *in vitro* by translation of T7 transcripts in a rabbit reticulocyte lysate (16). Based on antibody inhibition studies (17) and expression of cloned viral genes *in vitro* (18) and in *E. coli* (19), it has been previously proposed that two different viral proteases are involved in cleavage of the polyproteins, the B-RNA-encoded 32K protein representing a protease recognising the Q/M cleavage sites and the 24K protein recognising the Q/G and Q/S cleavage sites. By introducing specific deletions in their coding regions within a B cDNA clone the role of these two proteins in the proteolytic processing events has now been further analysed. By introduction of a small (87 base pair) deletion in the coding region of the 24K protein (without disturbing the open reading frame) a slightly shorter primary translation product was obtained of which proteolytic processing was completely blocked. Introduction of a (360 bp) deletion in the 32K protein coding region, on the other hand, did not influence the proteolytic processing of the primary translation product. This result unequivocally demonstrates that the 24K protein bears the proteolytic activity responsible for all cleavages (at Q/M, Q/S and Q/G sites) in the B polyprotein, while the 32K protein is not involved. However, for cleavage of the Q/M site in the M-RNA-encoded polyproteins (see Fig. 1) the presence of intact 32K polypeptide is essential, although this protein itself does not have any proteolytic activity. Strikingly, the presence of functional 32K protein results in cleavage at the Q/M site in the M polyproteins solely, while in the absence of this protein the 24K protease cleaves the Q/G site but not the Q/M site in these polyproteins. It is tempting to assume that the 32K protein acts here as a modulator of the activity of the 24K protease, giving a logical and desired order in the cleavages. Indeed it makes sense if in vivo the M polyproteins are first cut at the Q/M site and then only at the Q/G site, since the release of a 60K common precursor to both capsid proteins (see Fig. 1) would greatly facilitate the virion assembly process, e.g. by the formation of procapsids built up by these 60K precursors. Immunological analyses have shown that such precursors indeed occur in infected cowpea cells (20). Likewise also in the B polyprotein a Q/M site is found, which for correct VPg release should be cleaved prior to the Q/S cleavage used to release this protein at its N-terminus (Fig. 1). Therefore it is very attractive to propose that not the 24K protease alone, but a tight complex between this protease and the 32K protein represents the proteolytic entity during polyprotein processing. In such complex the 24K protein is the sole protease, while the 32K protein modulates its activity and gives order in the cleavage reactions. In this context it is worthwhile noting that as a first event during polyprotein processing the 32K protein is released from nascent polypeptide chains and becomes tightly bound to the protease (Fig. 3 and ref. 17, 21).

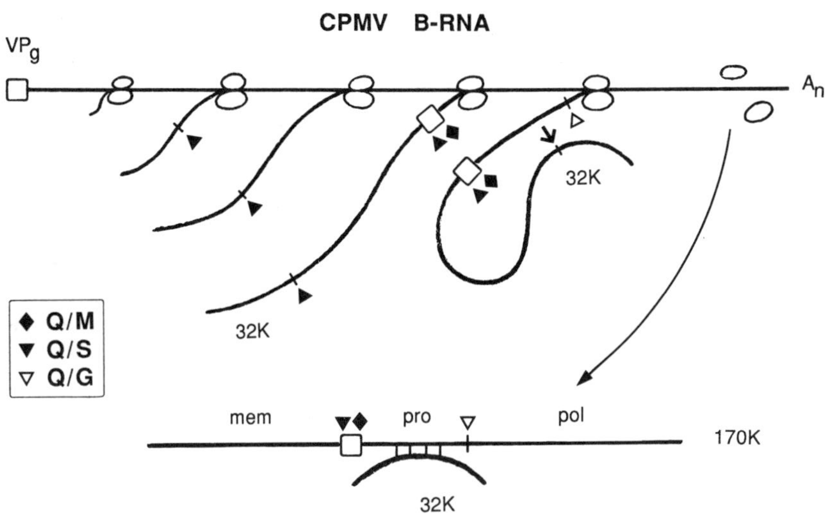

FIGURE 3. The formation of a complex between the 24K protease (pro) and the 32K product. The primary cleavage of (Legend continued on the following page.)

the B-RNA-encoded polyprotein, by which the 32K protein becomes attached to the protease, occurs already in nascent polypeptide chains (21). Mem, membrane-bound protein (58K); pol, 87K polymerase core polypeptide. It is proposed that the complex between protease and 32K protein represents the proteolytic entity during polyprotein processing (see text).

DISCUSSION

In spite of all our efforts, extending over a period of more than 15 years, the enzymology and mechanism of CPMV RNA replication still seems to be a black box. The unravelling of this crucial process has been hampered by the failure to isolate a replication complex that accepts exogenously added templates. The information available to date leads to the concept that the replication proteins of CPMV act only once and are not able to initiate RNA synthesis a second time. This idea should be further tested now and one of the approaches to be followed is to isolate viral precursor polypeptides (from infected cells or from expression vectors) since proteolytic processing (e.g. the release of VPg) and the various steps in RNA replication (e.g. initiation) may occur strictly hand-in-hand. The preliminary results obtained with infectious transcripts from viral cDNA clones are also promising and mutagenesis of these clones may provide another break-through in the analysis of the CPMV replication process. The availability of these clones has already resulted in a thorough insight in the proteolytic events that occur during maturation of the viral proteins. One of the interesting results obtained sofar is the finding that for CPMV only one viral protease (the 24K protein) is responsible for polyprotein processing, while a second viral protein (the 32K protein) acts as co-factor for cleavage at Q/M *in trans* and possibly even as a more generally involved regulatory protein charged with the ordering of all proteolytic cleavage reactions.

ACKNOWLEDGEMENTS

The authors thank Hetty Geitenbeek for excellent typing of the manuscript, Oliver Richards for critical reading of the text and Geertje Rezelman for technical assistance. This work was supported by the Netherlands Foundation for Chemical Research (SON) with financial aid from the Netherlands Organisation of Pure Research (NWO).

REFERENCES

1. Goldbach R, Van Kammen A (1985). Structure, replication and expression of the bipartite RNA genome of cowpea mosaic virus. In Davies JW (ed): "Molecular Plant Virology" vol II Boca Raton: CRC Press, p 86.
2. Goldbach R (1988). Comoviruses: Molecular biology and replication. In Harrison BD, Murant AF (eds): "The Plant Viruses: Viruses with bipartite genomes and isometric particles" New York, Plenum, in press.
3. Franssen H, Leunissen J, Goldbach R, Lomonossoff G, Zimmern D (1984). Homologous sequences in non-structural proteins from cowpea mosaic virus and picornaviruses. EMBO J 3:855.
4. Goldbach RW (1986). Molecular evolution of plant RNA viruses. Ann Rev Phytopathol 24:289.
5. Goldbach R (1987). Genome similarities between plant and animal RNA viruses. Microbiological Sciences 4:197.
6. Goldbach RW, Rezelman G, Van Kammen A (1980). Independent replication and expression of B-component RNA of cowpea mosaic virus. Nature 286:297.
7. Rezelman G, Franssen H, Goldbach RW, Ie T, Van Kammen A (1982). Limits to the independence of bottom component RNA of cowpea mosaic virus. J gen Virol 60:335.
8. Malyshenko SI, Lapchic LG, Kondakova OA, Kuznetzova LL, Taliansky ME, Atabekov JG (1988). Red clover mottle comovirus B-RNA spreads between cells in tobamovirus-infected tissues. J gen Virol 69:407.
9. Van Kammen A, Eggen HIL (1987). The replication of cowpea mosaic virus. BioEssays 5:261.
10. Takegami T, Kuhn RJ, Anderson CW, Wimmer E (1983). Membrane-dependent uridylation of the genome-linked protein VPg of poliovirus. Proc Natl Acad Sci USA 80:7447.
11. Dorssers L, Van der Krol S, Van der Meer J, Van Kammen A, Zabel P (1984). Purification of cowpea mosaic virus RNA replication complex: identification of a virus-encoded 110,000-dalton polypeptide responsible for RNA chain elongation. Proc Natl Acad Sci USA 81:1951.
12. Rezelman G, Goldbach RW, Van Kammen A (1980). Expression

of the bottom component RNA of cowpea mosaic virus in cowpea protoplasts. J Virol 36:366.

13. Wellink J, Van Lent J, Goldbach R (1988). Detection of viral proteins in cytopathic structures in cowpea protoplasts infected with cowpea mosaic virus. J gen Virol 69:751.
14. Assink AM, Swaans H, Van Kammen A (1973). The localisation of virus-specific double-stranded RNA of cowpea mosaic virus in subcellular fractions of infected Vigna leaves. Virology 53:384.
15. Eggen R, Kaan A, Goldbach R, Van Kammen A. Cowpea mosaic virus RNA replication in crude membrane fractions of cowpea and Chenopodium amaranticolor. J gen Virol, submitted.
16. Vos P, Verver J, Van Wezenbeek P, Van Kammen A, Goldbach R (1984). Study of the genetic organisation of a plant viral RNA genome by in vitro expression of a full-length DNA copy. EMBO J 3:3049.
17. Franssen H, Moerman M, Rezelman G, Goldbach R (1984). Evidence that the 32,000 dalton protein encoded by bottom-component RNA of cowpea mosaic virus is a proteolytic processing enzyme. J Virol 50:183.
18. Verver J, Goldbach R, Garcia JA, Vos P (1987). In vitro expression of a full-length DNA copy of cowpea mosaic virus B-RNA: identification of the B-RNA encoded 24 Kd protein as a viral protease. EMBO J 6:549.
19. Garcia JA, Schrijvers L, Tan A, Vos P, Wellink J, Goldbach R (1987). Proteolytic activity of the CPMV-encoded 24-kilodalton protein synthesized in Escherichia coli. Virology 159:67.
20. Wellink, J, Jaegle M, Prinz H, Van Kammen A, Goldbach R (1987). Expression of the middle component RNA of cowpea mosaic virus in vivo. J gen Virol 6:2577.
21. Franssen H, Goldbach R, Van Kammen A (1984). Translation of bottom component RNA of cowpea mosaic virus in reticulocyte lysate: faithful proteolytic processing of the primary translation product. Virus Research 1:39.

Molecular Biology of Plant-Pathogen Interactions, pages 153-165

THE FIRST THOUSAND AND ONE NUCLEOTIDES OF GENOMIC CaMV RNA.

T.Hohn, JM.Bonneville, J.Fütterer, K.Gordon, B.Pisan, H.Sanfaçon, M.Schultze and J.Jiricny
Friedrich-Miescher-Inst., CH-4002 Basel, Switzerland.

ABSTRACT Reporter genes attached to Cauliflower Mosaic Virus (CaMV) control regions were introduced into plant protoplasts by electroporation and the activity of the reporters (CAT and GUS) assayed after an incubation period. Results show that:
1) The 600 nt leader of CaMV 35-S RNA contains some sequences that enhance and others that inhibit expression of downstream genes.
2) Transcriptional polyadenylation signals of CaMV are recognized differently by protoplasts from different plants and tissues.
3) Polycistronic translation of CaMV constructs is possible, but requires a novel type of transactivation.
4) In contrast to traditional retroviruses, the CaMV *gag* and *pol* genes are expressed individually.

INTRODUCTION

Cauliflower mosaic virus, although containing double stranded DNA, can be viewed as a retrovirus, since its genome is replicated by reverse transcriptase and one of its genomic forms, the 35S RNA, is terminally redundant as is retrovirus genomic RNA. Accordingly the CaMV ORFs IV, V, and VI resemble the standard retrovirus *gag*, *pol*, and *env* genes (1). In addition to these genes CaMV contains sequences, that might code for functions specific to plant viruses, e.g. systemic spreading, a possible function for ORF I (2), and aphid transmissibility, the function of ORF II. The 35S RNA is thought to be a polycistronic messenger for all CaMV open reading frames (ORFs) with the exception of ORF VI, which has its own (19S) messenger RNA.

Amazingly, the first 950 nucleotides of 35S RNA do not include any major coding sequences, although they contain a number of elements, some certainly, some probably, playing important roles in virus replication (Fig.1). These include

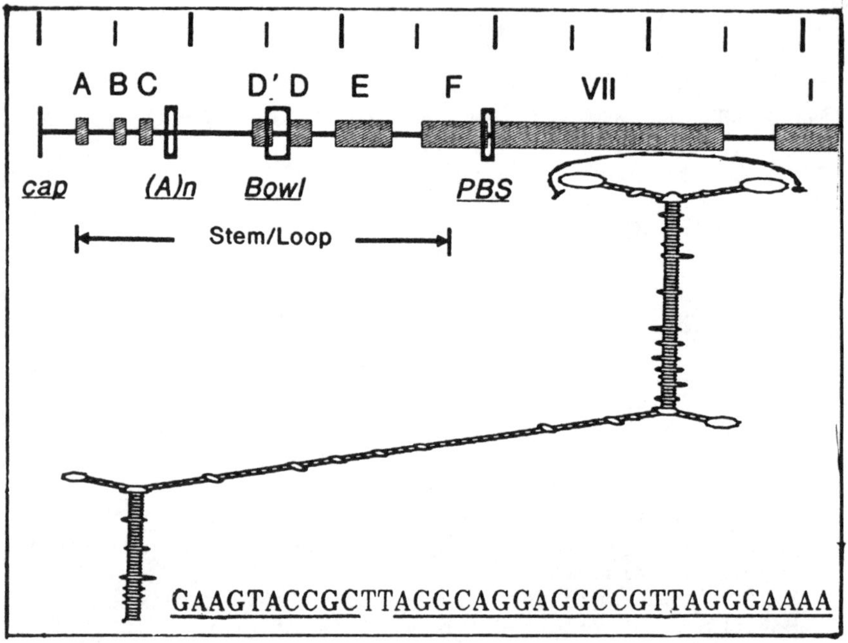

FIGURE 1. **Graphic representation of the first 1000 nucleotides of CaMV 35S RNA.** Positions of the sORFs and of the cap-site, polyadenylation signal and bowl sequence are shown. The location and size of a large stem/loop structure (goblet) is given and its SQUIGGLES outprint (3) is shown below. The bowl sequence is shown at the bottom, with the nts conserved in three sequenced caulimoviruses underlined.

the capping site, the facultative polyadenylation signal (its original bypass creates the terminal redundancy of CaMV 35S RNA) and the primer binding site (the origin of (-) DNA replication). The first 600 nucleotides (the region between the cap- and primer binding sites) contain 3 very small (2-4 codons) and 3 or 4 small (up to 34 codons) open reading frames (sORFs). The region thereafter, just following the primer binding site, comprises the 100 codon ORF VII. This ORF is not essential, but is likely to be translated, since certain frameshift mutants of it have polar effects (4). We define the region between the cap-site and ORF VII as the "leader". As in retroviruses we also refer to the region between cap-site and polyadenylation site as "R" and from thereon to the first larger coding region (ORF VII) as "U5."

MOST OF THE CaMV LEADER CAN BE FOLDED INTO A LARGE HAIRPIN STRUCTURE

The CaMV 35S RNA was folded in 1200 nt portions with 400 nt overlaps using the FOLD program (5). Fig.2 shows the secondary structure of the first 1200 nts in the "CIRCLES" graphical presentation. "CIRCLES" arranges the sequence counterclockwise starting at "3h" and connects pairing bases by arcs. A large series of such arcs can be discerned connecting the stretch of nucleotides 52 to 280 with 346 to 572. This corresponds to a large stem interrupted by minor and major loopouts (seen in the SQUIGGLES outprint; Fig.1; CaMV START). The arcs flank a "pair of eyes", corresponding to two short branches and loops. These we name here "bowl" and the total structure "goblet". No other structures with so large a stem were found in the remainder of the RNA, as exemplified by the output received for the 3′ terminal sequences (CaMV END in the Figure) (6).

The leaders of the two other caulimoviruses, whose sequence have been published (CERV [7]; FMV [8]), can also be folded into "goblet" like structures carrying "bowls" on their top (Fig.2; FMV START and CERV START). The first 50 to 80 nt of the leader have in all three cases little secondary structure. The stem has a varying number of short side branches, zero for CERV, one for FMV and two for CaMV. Free minimal energies for the goblets are -116 (FMV), -120 (CERV) and -144 (CaMV) kCal/Mol. In all cases the ascending arm of the stem contains the polyadenylation signal and the descending arm terminates ahead of the primer-binding site and before the first major ORF begins. In CERV a second (smaller) stem/loop structure is located between the large stem and the first ORF (Fig. 2b). Although the structures presented have not been confirmed experimentally (e.g. according to 9), the similarity of folds for the three caulimoviruses is remarkable and probably reflects important biological function.

The three caulimoviruses have considerable sequence homology in the region encoding ORFs I - VI (7,8), but little outside this region. Dot matrices of the non-coding regions, i.e. mainly the leaders, show that the only conserved sequences are the TATA box, the polyadenylation signal, the primer binding site, a (TC)n-rich region near the 5′ end and, most remarkably, a stretch of 36 nts of unknown function (Fig.1; also observed in ref. 8). Interestingly in all 3 cases this sequence is located in the bowl (Fig.2). Thus the goblet consists of a central

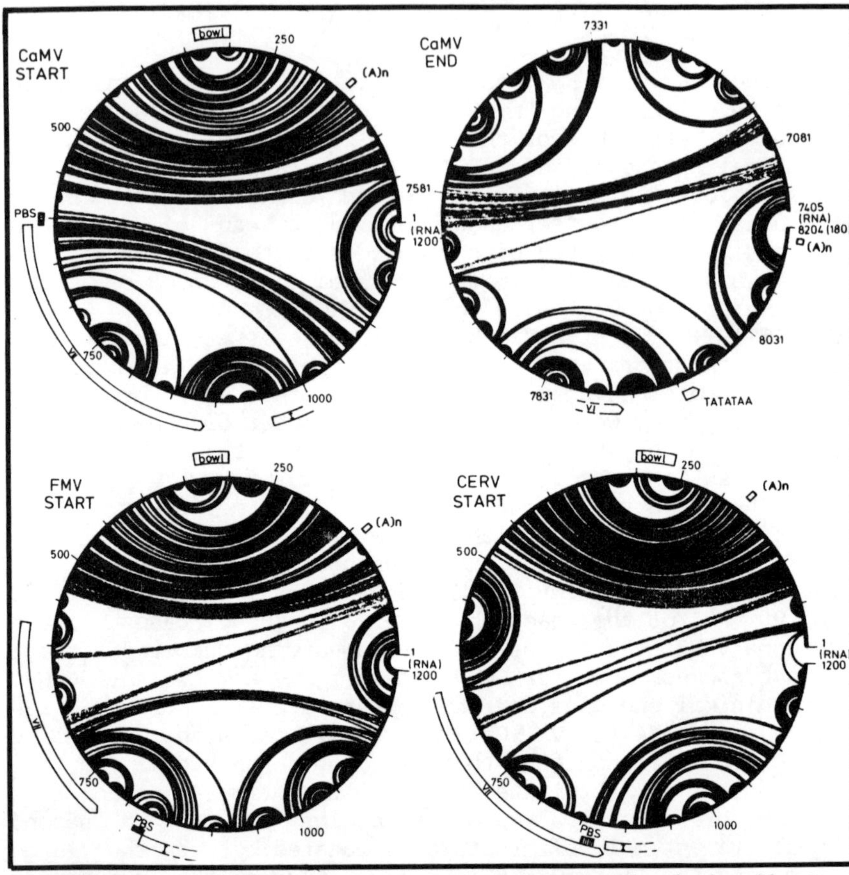

FIGURE 2). Graphical presentation (CIRCLES) of the first 1200 nts of the caulimoviruses. The sequences of CaMV, CERV and FMV were folded using the FOLD computer program (Zuker & Stiegler, 1981). For CaMV the last 1200 nts. of the RNA are also shown. The positions of the polyadenylation sites [(A)n], bowl sequences, primer binding sites (PBS) and major ORFs are indicated.

portion with conserved primary sequence ("bowl-sequence") embedded in flanking portions with conserved secondary structure (the stem). This conservation of secondary structure, despite the lack of primary sequence conservation, is probably indicative of some important function(s). Deletion of the bowl sequence and adjacent nucleotides in CaMV causes a dramatic increase in the latency period, from the normal 2 to 12 weeks (5).

TRANSLATION OF CaMV ORFs AND INFLUENCE OF THE LEADER

All larger ORFs of CaMV, including ORF VII, have been translated *in vitro* from artificial monocistronic RNA (10) and products of ORFs I to VI were detected in infected plants. Translation of RNA isolated from infected plants, however, yields as the only CaMV protein the ORF VI product, which is synthesized from the subgenomic 19S RNA (review: 11). *In vitro* produced 35S RNA can be translated *in vitro*, although inefficiently. This inefficient translation is probably due to the long leader sequence with its sORFs and to the polycistronic nature of the RNA.

To study the influence of the leader on expression *in vivo* and to test whether translation from the ORF VII start site is also possible in plant cells, we have fused the chloramphenicol acetyl transferase gene (CAT) without its own ATG to the first codon of ORF VII. A plasmid (pCaLC20) was prepared containing the CaMV 35S promoter region, all of the viral sequences from there to ORF VII, the fused ORF VII/CAT coding region and then the polyA signal. After introduction of pCaLC20 into plant protoplasts by electroporation (12), CAT was expressed (Fig.3-1).

Fusions of CAT to the third codons of sORFs D and E, respectively, in the leader also induced CAT activity in transfected protoplasts (Fig.3). This proves that the AUGs of these sORFs are in a context that allows efficient initiation of translation. It is therefore likely that peptides are produced from these sORFs. A comparison of efficiency of translation initiation at the AUG start codons of ORF D and E is not possible since the resulting CAT proteins differ by the amino acid that is encoded by the second codon (this codon stems from the respective sORF and was left in the respective fusion construct to conserve the natural sequence context of the AUGs). Such alterations may change the enzyme activity or stability.

If the CaMV leader was deleted from pCaLC20, the yield of CAT activity increased 3 - 10 fold in transfected *Crucifer* protoplasts (Fig. 3-2). A similar effect was achieved if only the 3′ proximal half of the leader with sORFs D′ - F was deleted (Fig.3-3). Deletion of the 5′ half, in contrast, led to a drastic reduction of CAT expression (Fig.3-4). Since similar effects were observed in experiments using *in vitro* translation of *in vitro* produced RNA (not shown), they can at least in part be attributed to properties of the translational machinery.

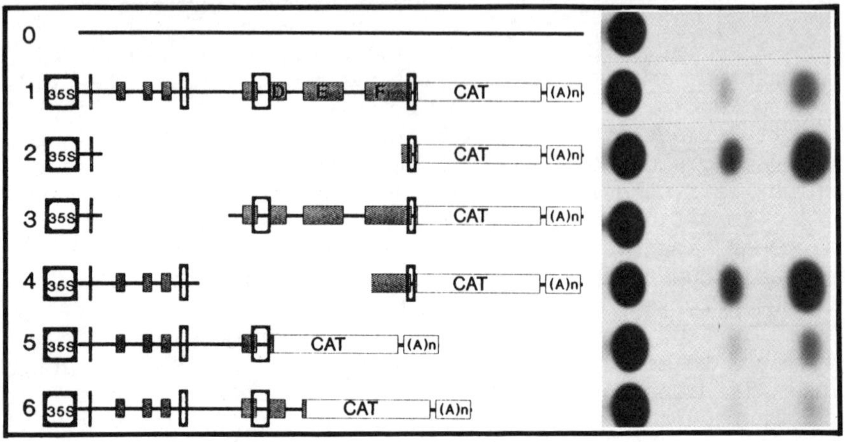

FIGURE 3. **Influence of the CaMV 35S RNA leader sequence on expression of a downstream gene.** Construct 1, (CaLC20) is pDW2 (13) with the CaMV leader inserted between the 35S promoter and the polyA signal. Constructs 2, 3 and 4 were derived from pCaLC20 by deletion of a HphI/ClaI, HphI/BglII and, respectively, a BglII/ClaI restriction fragment, and joining the scars with polynucleotide linkers. Constructs 5 and 6 were derived from pCaLC20 by oligonucleotide directed mutagenesis. 15 μg plasmid DNA was transfected by electroporation into protoplasts from a suspension cell culture of Orychophragmus violaceus (14) according to (12) and CAT activity was assayed after 18-24h. Soluble extracts were prepared by 3 cycles of freeze-thaw, 20 min incubation at 68 °C and centrifugation. Protein concentrations were determined in the supernatants and identical amounts were reacted in each CAT assay. Experiments were performed several times and representative results are shown. The exact sequences of the plasmids used are available on computerdisks upon request.

STUDIES ON THE POLYADENYLATION SIGNAL

The polyadenylation signal of CaMV, as of retroviruses, is of particular interest: it appears twice on the 35S RNA, within the leader and in the 3'-terminal portion of the RNA, as part of the terminal repeat (R). How the bypass of the upstream signal is achieved is still unknown.

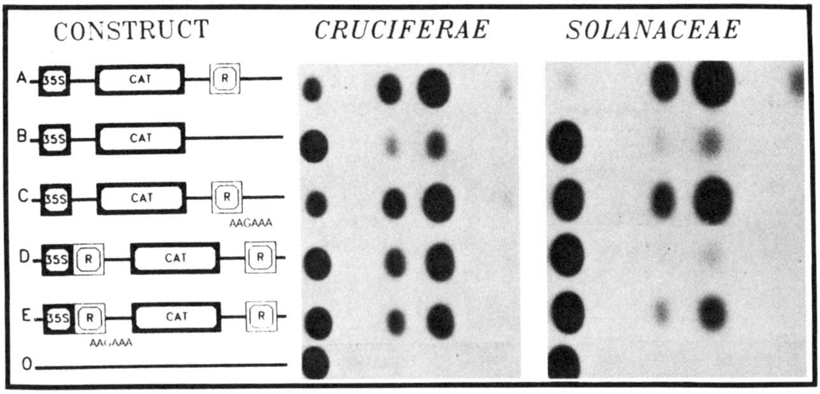

FIGURE 4. **Effect of the polyadenylation signal on gene expression in Solanaceae and Cruciferae** A, pDW2; B, the R region was removed as a PstI/HindIII restriction fragments and the ends joined by a linker; C, a derivative of pDW2 obtained by oligonucleotide directed mutagenesis; D, pCaLC20 as in Fig.3; E, point mutation of pCaLC20 obtained as for C. Transformations of plant protoplasts were as in Fig. 3. As an example for Solanaceae, Nicotiana tabaccum is shown and as an example for Cruciferae, Orychophragmus violaceus, but similar experiments were obtained with Hyoscyamus muticus (Solanaceae) and Brassica rapa (Cruciferae).

To determine the requirements for efficient polyadenylation, plasmid pDW2 was used in its original and modified forms. In this plasmid the polyadenylation signal after the CAT coding sequence is provided by a 180 nucleotide leader fragment corresponding to "R". Strong CAT activities were obtained from an extract of plant protoplasts 48 hrs after introduction of this DNA into Orychophragmus violaceus or Nicotiana tabacum protoplasts by electroporation (Fig.4-A). If the R fragment was deleted, the absence of a polyA signal caused a dramatic decrease of CAT activities (Fig.4-B), probably by preventing maturation of the primary transcript.

In animal genes polyadenylation signals comprise a highly conserved AATAAA sequence; a point mutation, e.g. T -> G, causes a dramatic decrease in mRNA-processing and usage. In contrast, introduction of this mutation into the

3′ terminal R fragment of CaMV RNA caused only a moderate decrease of CAT activity in *Nicotiana tabacum* and nearly no decrease in *Orychophragmus violaceus* (Fig. 4-C). It is therefore very likely that other sequences are also necessary for an optimum processing signal in plants.

To study the bypass of this signal at the 5′ end of the 35S RNA, pCaLC20 was used. In this plasmid the leader and therefore "R" is included upstream the CAT coding region, thus providing an upstream polyadenylation signal, that, if used, would prevent expression of the CAT gene. With this plasmid strong CAT activities were obtained in *Cruciferae* (*Orychophragmus violaceus* [Fig.4-D]; *Brassica rapa*), showing that the signal was bypassed. However in *Solanaceae* (*Nicotiana tabacum* [Fig.4-D], *Hyoscyamus muticus*) only weak CAT activities could be detected. To test whether the inhibitory effect in *Solanaceae* cells could at least partly be explained by the recognition of the polyA signal in the leader, the AAGAAA mutation was introduced at this position. In *Solanaceae*, but not in *Cruciferae*, an increase of CAT gene activity was observed (Fig.4-E). Based on these results we propose that the specificity of the polyA signal bypass is one of the factors limiting the CaMV host range.

TRANSACTIVATION

As a first step in studying translation of downstream genes on the polycistronic CaMV RNA the CAT reporter gene was fused to the 16 first codons of ORF I with ORF VII being retained upstream. When transfected alone into protoplasts such a plasmid directed only very little synthesis of the reporter protein. However, if transfected together with CaMV DNA, much higher CAT activities were obtained.

Search for the transactivating sequences on the CaMV genome defined the 19S transcription unit, coding for the inclusion body matrix protein (ORF VI product), as the entity both necessary and sufficient to enhance ORF I fusion expression (Fig.5). If the 19S promoter in front of ORF VI is replaced by the 35S promoter, the enhancement of ORF I fused activity becomes even more drastic (Fig.5, columns 7,8,9). Thus the coding region of the 19S transcription unit must contain the transactivator and the change to the stronger promoter would provide more copies of it.

Due to the sORFs it contains within the leader, the transcript from pCaLC20, the construct with CAT fused to ORF VII, can also be considered as polycistronic RNA. It was interesting to investigate whether also this construct could

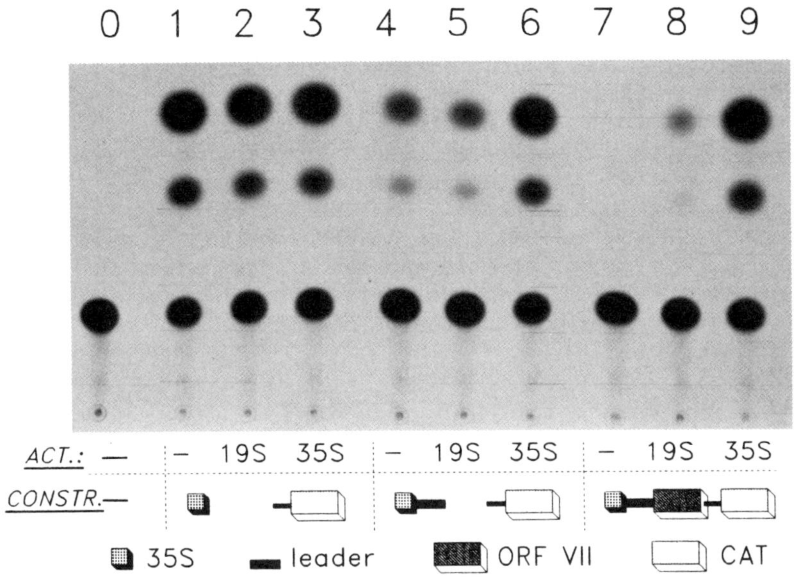

FIGURE 5. **Transactivator strength.** Samples of O. violaceus protoplasts were transfected with combinations of reporter- and transactivator plasmids in 20μg quantities. Reporter plasmids (drawings in line "constr"[uctions]) were: pCa74-7-B [columns 7,8,9], which contains the 35S enhancer, promoter and leader, ORF VII and the 16 first codons of ORF I fused in frame to the CAT reporter; pCaLC20 (Fig.3) [c.4,5,6]; pCaLN-1-CAT [c.1,2,3], which is pCa74-7-B with the leader and ORF VII deleted and lacks any ATG between transcription start and ORF I. Transactivator plasmids ("19S" and "35S" in line "act.") are: p19S [c.2,5,8], complete 19S operon cloned as SalI/ClaI fragment of pCa422 (15*) into pTZ19; p35S/VI [c.3,6,9], the EcoRV restriction fragment of pCa422, containing ORF VI including 80 bp upstream of it with the TATA-box, cloned into the SmaI site of pDH51, providing the 35S enhancer and promoter (13). Controls [c.1,4,7]: calf thymus DNA instead of transactivator plasmid; double controls [c.0] are mock transformations with calf thymus DNA. Assays were performed as in Fig.3.

be transactivated. In fact, the basal level of expression of pCaLC20 was also upgraded in presence of the 35S/ORF VI transactivator plasmid, although the 19S version was not sufficient (Fig.5, columns 4,5,6). This result shows that the ORF VII product is neither in _cis_ nor in _trans_ required to activate downstream gene expression and that transactivation can take place on at least two templates that differ in sequence. On the other hand, neither transactivating plasmid could enhance the already high expression of monocistronic and leaderless constructs (Fig. 5, columns 1,2,3), which argues in favor of transactivation taking place at a posttranscriptional step.

CONCLUSIONS

Transient expression of a reporter gene in protoplasts represents a powerfull tool for the study of not only promoters and upstream sequences involved in regulation of transcription, but also of 5′ untranslated leaders on the transcript. The 600 nts (bp) of CaMV sequence between capping site and ORF VII represents a most interesting example of such a leader, containing conserved secondary structure, conserved stretches of sequence, small ORFs, a facultative polyadenylation signal, a primer binding site and possibly other features, whose functions are not yet understood. These features may be involved in the regulation of the virus life cycle, allowing the virus to optimally exploit the specific developmental state or condition of the host cell, overcome defence reactions and coordinate RNA usage for either reverse transcription or translation. We show here that this leader sequence containes in fact elements that influence expression of a downstream gene at the level of transcript maturation and transcript usage.

Further we provide substantial evidence, that expression of ORFs downstream of ORF VII requires a novel type of transactivation. This does not only apply to ORF I expression, as shown here, but also to the expression of the 5th and 6th ORF (IV=_gag_; V=_pol_) (newer evidence, in prep.). In contrast to retroviruses _gag/pol_ fusion is not required as a means to express _pol_ (M.S. and J.J., unpublished). Comparing all these cases we could not deduce a simple consensus sequence required for transactivation in _cis_.

This novel transactivation activity allows use of most of the ORFs on 35S RNA and can be traced to the second (19S)

CaMV operon. There it relies on its coding region, ORF VI, since the promoter can be exchanged. Preliminary experiments show that frameshift mutations in this ORF abolish the activity and this makes it likely that the protein product, rather than the RNA, is the active agent.

We can presently only speculate, on how an ORF VI encoded protein, which is also the major component of the viral inclusion body, would act as transactivator. Since expression from monocistronic mRNA is not activated, it most likely acts on a posttranscriptional level.

Significant splicing consensus sequences (16) are not found in CaMV RNA, however an involvement in some type of splicing or RNA processing might still be possible. Plant et al. (17) have infered a minor RNA species specifically coding for ORF V, however they can not exclude that this species was created upon isolation- and enrichment-procedures by break down. When total CaMV RNA from infected plants is translated *in vitro* the only detectable product is that of ORF VI.

A further - and more probable - possibility is that the transactivator might modulate the translation machinery to facilitate reinitiation of translation. Usage of the 35S RNA as polycistronic messenger was proposed earlier as "relay race" model and arguments in its favour were provided (4,18). An ORF VI derived protein may directly interact with the ribosomes or translation factors from the cell or from prokaryotik-like chloroplasts. Interactions of protein VI with chloroplasts are indicated by the observation, that this protein causes symptoms in transgenic plants (19,20).

Another possibility would be that the inclusion body itself is responsible for the effect by providing a special environment (organelle), within wich properties of the translational machinery are modified to cope with polycistronic translation.

ACKOWLEDGEMENTS

We highly appreciate the gifts of *Orychophragmus* cell cultures and procedures to handle them by C.Matsui, and of cell cultures of *Nicotiana* (Nia) by Ion Negrutiu and *Hyoscyamus* by Dirk Inzé and by Pat King. The expert technical assistance of Hanny Schmid in providing constructs and Matthias Müller in handling the cell cultures is greatly acknowledged. We thank W.Zürcher very much for providing oligonucleotides for *in vitro* mutagenesis.

REFERENCES

1. Fütterer J, Hohn T (1987). Involvement of nucleocapsids in reverse transcription - a general phenomenon? TIBS 12:92
2. Hull R, Covey , (1985). CaMV: pathways of infection. Bioessays 3:160.
3. Caballero L, Devereux J, Karp Y, Marquess P, Smith M, Winsborough W (1987). Sequence analysis software package, vers.5. University of Wisconsin Genetics Computer Group.
4. Dixon L, Hohn T, (1984). Initiation of translation of the CaMV genome from a polycistronic mRNA. EMBO J. 3:2731
5. Zucker M, Stiegler P (1981). Optimal computer folding of large RNA sequences using thermodynamics and auxiliary information. Nucleic Acids Research 9:133.
6. Hohn T, Fütterer J, Pisan B, Penswick J, Gordon K (1988). in prep.
7. Hull R, Sadler J, Longstaff M (1986). The sequence of carnation etched ring virus DNA: comparison with CaMV and retroviruses. EMBO J. 12:3083.
8. Richins RD, Scholthof HB, Shepherd RJ (1987). Sequence of figwort mosaic virus DNA (caulimovirus group). Nucleic Acids Research 15:8451.
9. Ehresmann C, Baudin F, Mougel M, Romby P, Ebel JP, Ehresmann B. (1987). Probing the structure of RNAs in solution. Nucleic Acids Research 15:9109.
10. Gordon K, Pfeiffer P, 8). In vitro expression of CaMV genes. EMBO J. 7:309.
11. Pfeiffer P, Gordon K, Fütterer J, Hohn T, (1987). The life cycle of CaMV. **PLANT MOL. BIOL.** (Wettstein D, Chua NH, eds.) pp.443.
12. Fromm ME, Taylor LP, Walbot V (1986). Stable transformation of maize after gene transfer by electroporation. Nature 319:791.
13. Pietrzak M, Shilito RD, Potrykus I, Hohn T (1986). Nucleic Acids Research 14:5857.
14. Matsui C (1985) Doctoral Thesis. Nagoya University, Japan.
15. Penswick J, Hübler R, Hohn T (1988). A viable muation in CaMV, a retrovirus like plant virus separates its capsid protein and polymerase genes. J.Virol. 62:1460.

16. Wiebauer K,Herrero JJ, Filipowicz W (1988) Nuclear pre-mRNA processing in plants: distinct modes of3'-splice-site selection in plants and animals. Mol.Cell.Biol. 8:in press.
17. Plant AL, Covey SL, Grierson D (1985). Detection of a subgenomic mRNA for gene V, the putative reverse transcriptase gene of CaMV. Nucleic Acids Research 13:8305.
18. Sieg K, Gronenborn B (1982). Evidence for polycistronic messenger RNA encodeed by CaMV. Abstract NATO Advanced Studies Inst. p. 184.
19. Baugman GA, Jacobs JD, Howell SH (1988). CaMV gene VI produces a symptomatic phenotype in transgenic tobacco plants. Proc.Natl.Acad.Sci.(USA) 85:733.
20. Gowda S, Shepherd R, this conference.

Molecular Biology of Plant-Pathogen Interactions, pages 167-183

MOLECULAR GENETICS OF MAIZE STREAK VIRUS[1]

Sondra G. Lazarowitz and Allison J. Pinder

Department of Embryology, Carnegie Institution of Washington
Baltimore, MD 21210

ABSTRACT Mutational analysis has been used to functionally dissect the genome of the single component geminivirus maize streak (MSV). Using a unique approach to generate gene replacement mutants by homologous recombination within gene coding sequences following their introduction into maize plants, we have shown that unlike the bipartite geminiviruses the capsid of MSV is essential for systemic spread and symptom development. The "+" strand ORF located immediately upstream from the capsid gene and encoding a 10.9 kd protein was found to be essential for viability, and all of the information required for double-stranded DNA synthesis resides in that part of the genome which contains the two viral intergenic regions and two overlapping "-" strand ORFs homologous to AL1 in the bipartite viruses.

BACKGROUND

The geminiviruses are small single-stranded (ss)DNA-containing plant viruses which are transmitted either by whiteflies or by leafhoppers (1,2). The designation "gemini" derives from their double-icosahedral capsid structure (3,4). While the whitefly- and leafhopper-transmitted virions are morphologically indistinguishable and clearly members of the same group based on cytopathology and the diseases they cause, cloning and sequence analyses have shown that these two subgroups of geminiviruses are

---

[1] This work was supported by NSF grant PCM8216268, and funds from the Carnegie Institution and the Monsanto Company.

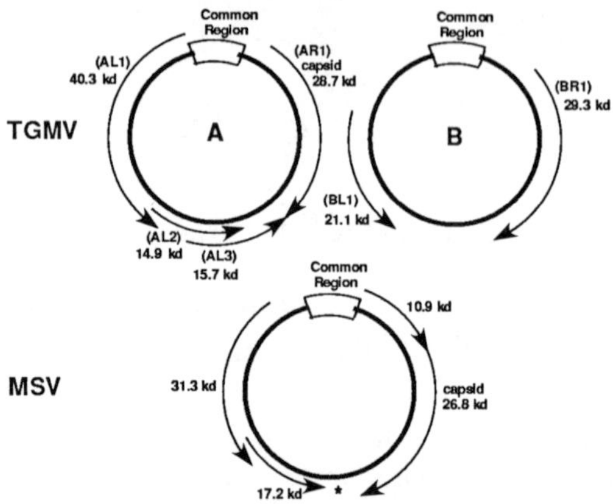

Fig. 1. Genomic organization of TGMV and MSV. Shown are ORFs and potential intergenic regions (5,12). Sizes and direction of translation of the predicted protein products are indicated in kd and shown as arrows. Common Region is shown as an open box. * shows position of primer DNA found on virion strand of MSV.

different in their genomic organization (fig. 1). The former are bipartite and contain two distinct circular genomic components (A and B) of ~2.7 kb each (5-7) while the latter contain only a single circular genomic component of ~2.7-2.9 kb (8-12). The study of beet curly top virus demonstrates that this difference in genomic organization is truly a leafhopper vs. whitefly distinction and not a difference between the monocot and dicot viruses in the group (11). Analysis of transgenic plants and transfected protoplasts has shown that the A component of the bipartite viruses is capable of autonomous replication, and provides functions in *trans* required for the replication of B (13,14). B encoded functions are required for systemic spread and subsequent symptom development in the infected plant (13).

Based on sequence analysis, the genomic organization of the single component viruses closely resembles that of the A component of the bipartite viruses. Thus, for example, comparing the genome of MSV with the A component of tomato golden mosaic virus (TGMV) (fig. 1), the capsid gene on the virion "+" strand and the two overlapping "-" strand ORFs homologous to AL1 are located in equivalent positions, and there is a viral intergenic region which by the presence of a conserved ~30 base geminivirus sequence element and its position between divergent ORFs is analogous to the bipartite virus Common Region (2,12). Analyzed in this manner, the essential difference between a single component virus such as MSV and the bipartite geminiviruses is that the former can successfully execute all of the same functions as the latter without the requirement for a separate B component to provide functions in *trans* for systemic spread and symptom development.

Mutational analysis of TGMV has delineated the functions encoded by the A component (15,16; Rogers et al., this volume). AL1 is essential for autonomous replication of A and in *trans* for the replication of B (16). AL2 encodes a function required for systemic spread and symptom development. However, encapsidation is not essential for systemic spread. Mutants lacking the capsid subunit do spread systemically, causing disease symptoms that are attenuated but clearly present (15). A mutation in AL3 also results in attenuated symptoms, and is also not essential for viability (Rogers et al., this volume).

In order to define the functional domains of the single component geminiviruses, we have begun a mutational analysis of the cloned genomic component of a South African isolate of MSV (MSV-S) (12). Using agroinoculation (17-19) of maize seedlings to analyze deletion, gene replacement, and point mutants, we find that the capsid is essential for systemic spread and the development of classic disease symptoms and that the bacterial chloramphenicol transferase (CAT) gene can be expressed in maize from an MSV promoter. Our results further demonstrate that the virion "+" strand ORF predicted to encode a 10.9 kd protein is essential for viability, and that all of the information required for viral dsDNA replication is located within that region of the genome containing the two viral intergenic regions and the two overlapping "-" strand ORFs which are homologous to AL1 (fig. 1).

STRUCTURAL ORGANIZATION OF THE MSV GENOME

The organization of the infectious genome of a South African isolate MSV-S (2) is illustrated in fig. 1. Based on sequence analysis of the viral DNA, cloned from dsDNA found in extracts from infected maize, there are five potential ORFs, two located on the virion "+" strand and three on the complementary "-" strand, separated by two apparent viral intergenic regions (Table 1). The two "+" strand ORFs encode the 26.8 kd capsid subunit (21) and a hypothetical 10.9 kd protein. The functional existence of this latter ORF has not been demonstrated. Primer extension and S1 analyses have identified two transcripts from this region (21). The major transcript maps in the middle of the upstream ORF with its 5′-end at position 163, 152

TABLE 1
PREDICTED OPEN READING FRAMES OF MSV-S

Translation Frame	TATA[a]	Start Codon[b]	Stop Codon	$^{A}_{G}$ATAA[c]	Protein (daltons)
2+	2659	2689	302[d]	(300)[f]	10,893
3+	2659	315	1047[d]	1052	26,778
2-	2480	2377	1561[e]	1538	31,294
3-	2140	1664	1220[d]	1072	17,194
2-	1075	505	250[d]	160	9,685

[a]Most likely TATA box for consensus sequence $T^{C}_{G}TATA^{T}_{A}A_{1-3}$ (42)
[b]AUG
[c]Most likely polyadenylation signal (20)
[d]UAA
[e]UAG
[f]A large transcript containing this ORF has been identified in MSV-N (21). This transcript maps between positions 2682 and 1114 (equivalent to positions 2686 and 1115 in MSV-S).

nucleotides upstream of the ATG start codon for the capsid subunit, and terminates at position 1114 as one might predict. A second less abundant transcript includes both "+" strand ORFs, and maps with its 5'-end only four nucleotides before the start codon of the 10.9 kd protein and its 3'-end co-terminal with the more abundant transcript. Whether both of these transcripts can function in the synthesis of the capsid subunit is not known.

Taken together, the proteins predicted to be encoded by the two overlapping "-" strand ORFs are homologous to the amino- and carboxy-terminus, respectively, of the predicted product of AL1 in the bipartite viruses (fig. 1) (22). Conservation of sequence varies, but there are several protein domains which are strictly conserved among all of the geminiviruses. Evidence from transcript mapping is consistent with these two ORFs being processed into a single transcript of ~1.2 kb from this region (21). The third "-" strand ORF potentially encoding a 9.7 kd protein (not shown) probably does not exist based on strain differences which

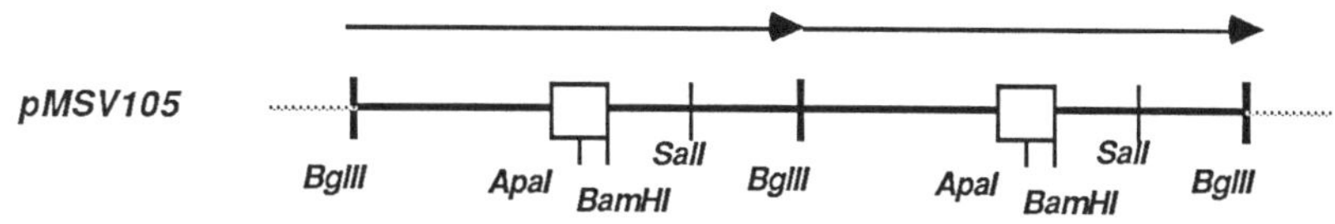

Fig. 2. Dimeric construct of MSV-S cloned as a direct repeat into *pMON505* (12). Arrows delimit one genomic copy.

drastically alter the predicted protein (12). A transcript corresponding to this ORF has not been detected (21).

That this single ~2.7 kb circular DNA represents the entire genome of MSV, being necessary and sufficient for infectivity, was shown by infectivity studies using agroinoculation (12,17). To do this a dimeric insert of MSV-S was cloned into pMON505, a Ti plasmid-derived binary vector (*pMSV105*) (12) (fig. 2), and introduced into *Agrobacterium tumefaciens* carrying a disarmed Ti plasmid (TiT37*SE*) (strain *ASE*) by the triparental mating procedure (23). 8-to-10 day old maize seedlings injected in the meristematic region at the coleoptile node with *MSV105(ASE)*

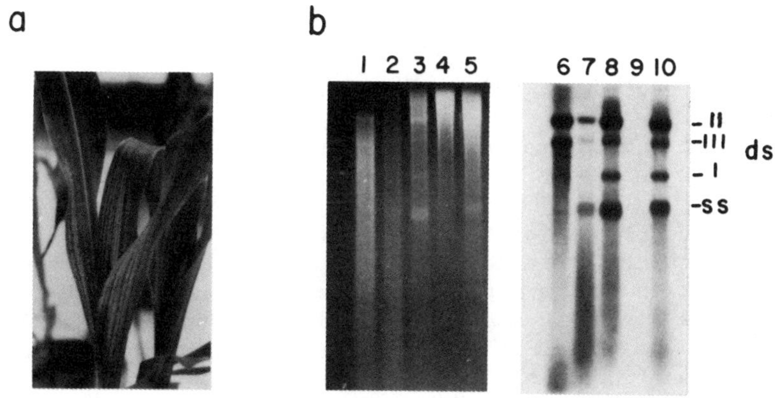

Fig. 3. (a) Maize plant agroinoculated with *MSV105(ASE)*. (b) Stained gel and blot from (1,2) leafhopper-inoculated, (3,5) agroinoculated, and (4) uninfected maize plants. Probe was MSV DNA. (Reprinted from NUCLEIC ACIDS RES (12) with permission of IRL Press.)

developed classic disease symptoms between 5 and 18 days postinoculation (fig. 3). Extracts from these symptomatic plants were found to contain abundant amounts of monomer-sized MSV circular ssDNA and dsDNA precisely co-migrating with the forms found in plants inoculated using viriliferous leafhoppers (fig. 3). No bacterial sequences were detected in the freely replicating and spreading MSV DNA. Maize streak disease was transmitted by leafhoppers fed on these agroinoculated plants, fulfilling Koch's postulates (12).

Thus, following introduction into the plant, the MSV DNA has excised from the binary plasmid by homologous recombination, generating freely replicating viral circular genomic DNA and initiating a normal infection. Success of this procedure is dependent on the presence of flanking homologous sequences (see below). These can be present as either viral DNA sequences (12,17) (fig. 2) or repeats of nonviral DNA sequences (24) (see below). The procedure is also dependent on the *A. tumefaciens* and the site of injection (12,17). A nopaline strain of *A. tumefaciens* is required (S.G. Lazarowitz, unpublished) and injection must be into the meristematic tissue within ~1 cm of the coleoptile. Injection or abrasion of *MSV105(ASE)* in any other part of the plant gives no infectivity. Similarly, injection of the MSV dimeric construct into the meristematic tissue as free DNA does not result in infection of the plant (12).

FUNCTIONAL ORGANIZATION OF THE MSV GENOME

While mutagenesis has been used to delineate the functions encoded on the A component of the bipartite geminivirus TGMV (15,16; Rogers et al., this volume), this has not been done for the single component geminiviruses. Of particular interest, given the similarities in structural organization of the single component genomes and the bipartite virus A component (fig. 1), is whether, as found in TGMV, the capsid is not essential for systemic spread and what viral functions, if any, may substitute for the B encoded function(s) and be involved in systemic spread. To address these questions, we have used site-directed mutagenesis employing synthetic oligonucleotides (25,26) to introduce point mutations, deletions, and gene substitutions into the genome of MSV-S (24), concentrating on the two virion "+" strand ORFs for the capsid subunit and the 10.9 kd protein (see fig. 1).

Deletion and Gene Substitution Mutants.

MSV deletion mutants lacking either the capsid coding sequences alone (*MSV31*) or in combination with those for the 10.9 kd protein (*MSV34*) were constructed. To delete only the capsid coding sequences, the unique BamHI site at position 1 which is part of the start codon for the 10.9 kd protein (fig. 1) was eliminated by a single base mutation, changing ATGGA<u>T</u>CC to ATGGA<u>C</u>CC. This third position codon change (GAT/GAC) retained the Asp in the predicted sequence of the 10.9 kd protein. This was a true silent mutation, with the resulting point mutant being indistinguishable in its biological properties from wildtype MSV-S (24). A new unique BamHI site was then introduced at position 306 between the coding sequences for the 10.9 kd and capsid proteins (fig. 4b), and the capsid coding sequences deleted by digestion with BamHI+NcoI, the 5'-protruding ends being filled-in before ligation to retain the unique BamHI and NcoI sites (figs. 1 and 4b). This mutant, *MSV31*, retains only the last 13 amino acids of the capsid subunit, and the relevant promoter and polyadenylation signals inferred to exist based on the sequence analyses and transcript mapping.

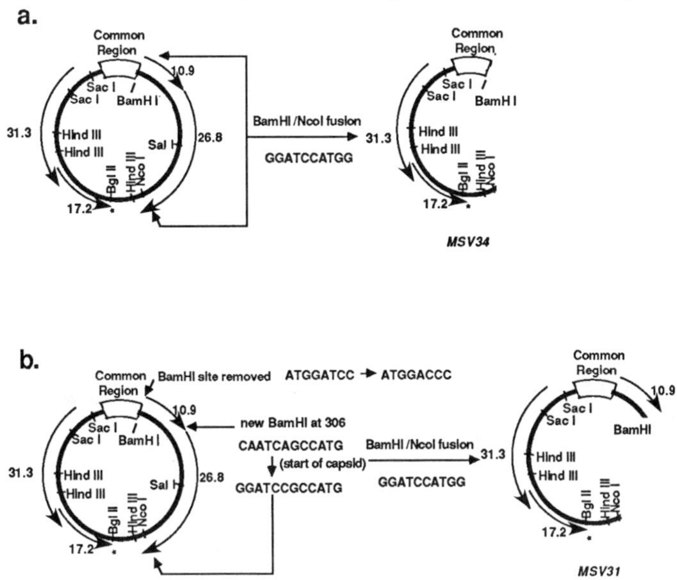

Fig. 4. Construction of MSV deletion mutants (a) *MSV34*, which lacks both "+" strand ORFs and (b) *MSV31*, which is missing the capsid coding sequences. See text for details.

Both "+" strand ORFs were deleted from MSV-S by digestion with BamHI+NcoI, followed by filling-in of the protruding 5′-ends and blunt-end ligation to retain both unique restriction sites (figs. 1 and 4a) as described above for *MSV31*. The BamHI site in MSV-S is part of the start codon for the 10.9 kd protein. Thus, to eliminate possible interference by what would be an upstream AUG in gene replacement constructs, a second BamHI site was introduced just upstream of the original BamHI site, and this ATG was eliminated by digestion with BamHI followed by ligation. This deleted 10 bases, recreating the cap site sequence two nucleotides closer to the potential TATA consensus sequence at +26 (24). Thus, deletion mutant *MSV34* lacks both "+" strand ORFs from the start codon for the 10.9 kd protein to the sequences encoding the last 13 amino acids of the capsid subunit, but retains possible MSV promoter and polyadenylation sites (fig. 4a).

To construct gene replacement mutants of MSV, we used a unique approach designed to investigate the sequence requirements for excision in the agroinoculation procedure, as well as to facilitate the introduction of a reporter gene sequence at any position in the viral genome. The method

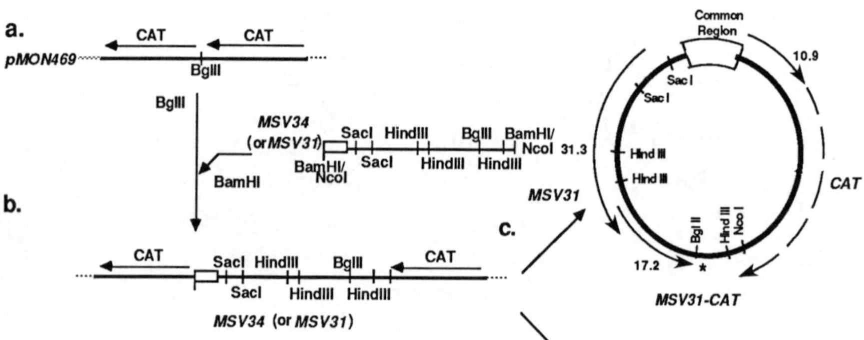

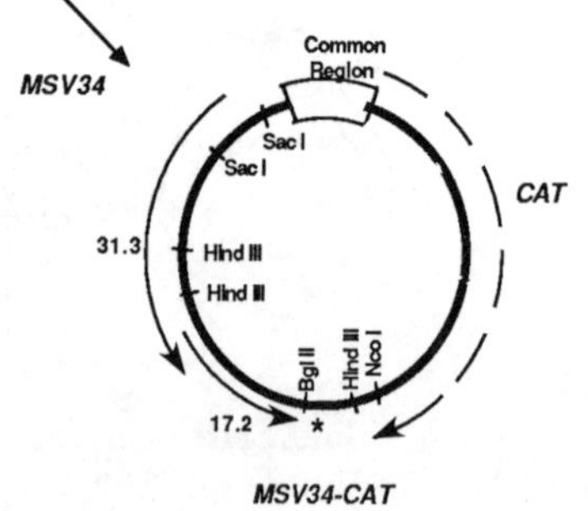

Fig. 5. Scheme for generating gene replacement mutants from *MSV31* and *MSV34*. (a) MSV BamHI linear cloned into pMON469 containing a direct repeat of CAT coding sequences. (b) MSV deletion mutant inserted in correct orientation is detected by restriction digests. (c) Inside the plant, CAT substituted mutants of MSV are generated by recombination within the flanking CAT sequences.

utilized a binary vector containing a direct repeat of two copies of the reporter gene separated by a unique restriction site into which MSV deletion mutants could be cloned. To substitute the bacterial chloramphenicol acetyltransferase (CAT) coding sequences for those of the capsid or both "+" strand viral ORFs, mutants *MSV31* and *MSV34* were cloned into the binary plasmid *pMON469* which contains two copies of the CAT coding sequences separated by a unique BglII site (24) (fig. 5). Following agroinoculation of maize plants, gene replacement mutants of MSV would be excised from the vector through homologous recombination within the flanking CAT sequences (fig. 5). By this approach, CAT gene substitutions corresponding to both deletion mutants *MSV31* and *MSV34* were obtained which had the CAT sequences inserted in correct (fig. 5) and reverse orientation relative to the direction of viral transcription.

Maize seedlings agroinoculated with *ASE* containing deletion mutants *MSV31* or *MSV34* as dimeric constructs cloned into *pMON505* did not develop disease symptoms (24). Replication of these deleted MSV genomes could not be detected, either in inoculated leaves (those leaves existing at the time of injection and which had needle marks on their

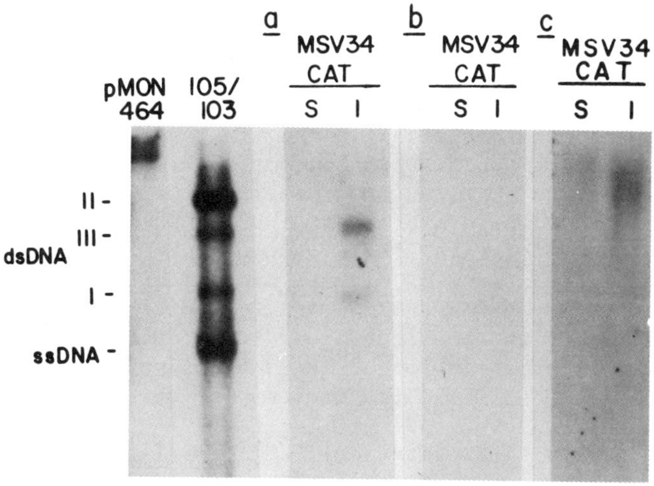

Fig. 6. Replication of *MSV34-CAT* in maize plants. Viral DNA was detected in inoculated (I) but not systemic (S) leaves. Probes are (a) Large MSV BglII-BamHI fragment; (b) Small MSV BamHI-SalI fragment; (c)binary vector excluding CAT sequences. See text for details.

expanded surfaces) or in subsequently developing "systemic leaves". However, restoration of the viral DNA to ~2.5 - ~2.8 kb by insertion of CAT sequences in either orientation restored the ability to replicate, with freely replicating gene substituted MSV DNA of the expected size being detected in extracts from inoculated leaves (24), but not systemically. This is shown in fig. 6 for the gene replacement mutant *MSV34-CAT*, where the expected ~2.5 kb dsDNA forms were detected in inoculated leaves and found to hybridize with the appropriate MSV fragments. This *MSV34-CAT* DNA did not hybridize with bacterial vector sequences besides the CAT sequences or with MSV sequences deleted from *MSV34*, and it was confined to the inoculated leaves, not being detected systemically (fig. 6). Upon long exposures a small amount of ssDNA was sometimes detected.

The same results were obtained for gene substituted *MSV31-CAT*, and for *MSV34-CAT'* and *MSV31-CAT'* containing the CAT sequences inserted in inverted orientation. Gene substituted MSV DNA of the expected size was found freely replicating in inoculated leaves, but not systemically. Using this approach, mutants containing the bacterial hygromycin coding sequences substituted for those of the capsid subunit or for both virion "+" strand ORFs have also been obtained (24). Thus, it appears that in the agroinoculation procedure repeats of any nonviral DNA can substitute for viral sequences and function in the excision of the viral DNA from the binary plasmid. This provides a convenient method for the insertion of a reporter gene sequence at different sites in the viral genome. Using this method, the gene substitution mutants *MSV31-CAT* and *MSV31-CAT'* demonstrate that, unlike the situation in the bipartite TGMV (15), the capsid protein of MSV is essential for systemic spread of this single component geminivirus and for subsequent development of disease symptoms (Table 2). The results with *MSV34-CAT* and *MSV34-CAT'*, while not addressing the function of the predicted 10.9 kd protein, do show that all of the information for at least viral dsDNA replication is located in the 1.7 kb fragment of the viral genome which contains the two overlapping "-" strand ORFs homologous to AL1 and the two viral intergenic regions (fig.1, Table 2). Finally, we found that MSV deletion mutants DNA ≤2. kb in size did not replicate. This could be due to torsional constraints in a molecule this small in size, or the result of the deletions bringing the two viral intergenic regions or other sequences which may interfere with replication in close juxtaposition.

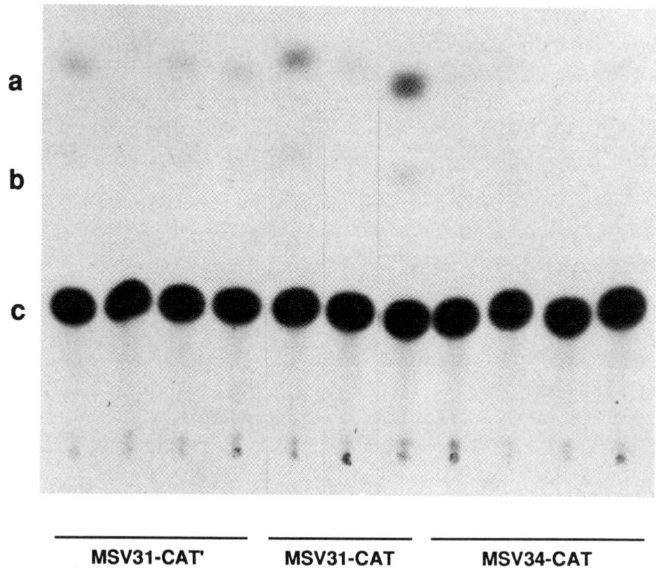

Fig. 7. CAT assays on inoculated leaf extracts from plants agroinoculated with *MSV31-CAT*, *MSV31-CAT'*, and *MSV34-CAT*. Middle *MSV31-CAT* extract contained no detectable *MSV31-CAT* DNA. All *MSV31-CAT'* and *MSV34-CAT* extracts contained amounts of viral DNA equal to or greater than those detected in the 2 positive *MSV31-CAT* samples. (a)di-acetylated, (b) mono-acetylated, and (c) unreacted chloramphenicol.

Expression of CAT Activity by Gene Substitution Mutants.

Extracts from inoculated leaves containing *MSV31-CAT* or *MSV34-CAT* were tested for bacterial CAT activity (27). Enzymatic activity was detected above background levels in leaves containing *MSV31-CAT* (24) (fig. 7). That this indeed was expression of the CAT gene from the mutant *MSV31-CAT* DNA in maize cells rather than from *A. tumefaciens* persisting in the plants was confirmed by testing extracts from inoculated leaves containing *MSV31-CAT'* which has the CAT sequences in inverted orientation. These latter extracts did not express CAT activity above background levels (fig. 7). Thus, the excised freely replicating *MSV31-CAT* which contains the CAT coding sequences inserted between viral promoter and polyadenylation signals is expressing bacterial CAT activity.

In contrast, *MSV34-CAT* did not express enzymatic activity (24) (fig. 7). This could be because the amount of transcript is too low, the transcript is unstable, or the mutant as constructed is not transcriptionally active. Thus, to directly test the existence and function of the hypothetical 10.9 kd protein, point mutations were introduced into MSV-S which eliminated what would be the start codon for this protein.

Function of the 10.9 kd Protein.

To address the functional existence of the predicted 10.9 kd protein, the sequence at the beginning of the ORF was mutated from TTCATG to TTAGTG, thus changing the ATG start codon to a GTG with an overlapping stop codon (24). The next ATG in the sequence is that for the capsid subunit. Hence, this mutation should only exert its effect on the synthesis of the hypothetical 10.9 kd protein. This mutant, *MSV273*, was not infectious for maize, suggesting that the 10.9 kd protein exists and does provide an essential function. These results, combined with the gene replacement mutants of *MSV34*, further suggest that this essential function is likely to be involved in systemic movement of the virus. Genetic complementation studies in progress will verify this result and directly demonstrate whether there is a 10.9 kd protein which functions in *trans*.

The predicted functions encoded in the MSV genome, inferred from the analysis of the deletion, gene substituted, and point mutants are summarized in Table 2.

CONCLUSIONS

Mutational analysis of the single component genome of MSV has begun to define viral encoded functions important in systemic movement of the virus and viral replication, demonstrating both similarities to and differences from the bipartite geminiviruses. In contrast to TGMV, the capsid of MSV is essential for movement and hence does not solely function in a protective capacity. However, like the bipartite geminiviruses where AL2 and at least one of the two ORFs on B both provide essential functions for movement, MSV may also have two genes essential for movement, namely the capsid and the 10.9 kd protein. Finally, all of the information required for at least dsDNA replication is

TABLE 2
PREDICTED FUNCTIONAL DOMAINS OF THE MSV GENOME

ORF[a]	Protein (kd)	Function	Mutants
2+	10.9	movement	*MSV273*
3+	26.8 capsid	encapsidation, movement	*MSV31* gene substitutions
2-[b]	31.3	replication?	*MSV34* gene substitutions[d]
3-[c]	17.2	replication?	*MSV34* gene substitutions[d]

[a] see Table 1
[b] predicted encoded protein homologous to amino-terminal domains of AL1 in the bipartite geminiviruses
[c] predicted encoded protein homologous to carboxy-terminal domains of AL1 in the bipartite geminiviruses
[d] Based on these mutants, all of the information for at least viral dsDNA is located within the region which includes the two overlapping "-" strand ORFs homologous to AL1 and the two viral intergenic regions. Mutational analysis of the Common Region has yet to be done. However, deletion of the primer shows this to be essential for infectivity (S.G. Lazarowitz, unpublished) and *in vitro* studies suggest that this functions in the synthesis of dsDNA from the virion ssDNA (8,12,28).

---

contained in that part of the MSV genome which contains the two overlapping "-" strand ORFs homologous to AL1 in the bipartite viruses, and the two viral intergenic regions. Further mutational analyses will directly demonstrate whether, as has been shown for AL1 in TGMV (16), a product(s) encoded by these ORFs is essential for replication, as well as define the roles of the two viral intergenic regions.

The ability to express a reporter gene such as CAT under the control of an MSV promoter should facilitate the identification of viral *cis-acting* sequence elements important in replication and transcription. Complementation studies under way to investigate the possible *trans-acting* nature of the 10.9 kd protein will demonstrate whether in the MSV system one component can function to move another component through the plant, thus in a sense creating a bipartite virus from a single component virus. Should this prove successful, it will amplify the low level of CAT activity detected in the present studies and greatly enhance the utility of the system described here in the analysis of viral sequence elements important in the regulation of gene expression. Finally, future progress in the study of these viruses will also begin to focus on defining the biochemical nature of the viral and host proteins involved in executing these processes.

ACKNOWLEDGMENTS

The authors thank Drs. Vernon M. Damsteegt and Adriana Hewings for generously making available the quarantine greenhouse facilities of the USDA Foreign Disease-Weed Science Research Unit, Ft. Detrick, MD, as well for providing leafhopper-inoculated tissue, encouragement and advice. We also thank Ms. Leslie Brand for providing the pMON469 binary plasmid and Dr. Stephen G. Rogers for many helpful discussions and advice.

REFERENCES

1. Goodman, R.M. (1981). Geminiviruses. J. Gen. Virol. 54:9.

2. Lazarowitz, S.G. (1987). The molecular characterization of geminiviruses. Plant Mol. Biol. Rep.4:177.

3. Hatta, T. and R.I.B. Francki (1979). The fine structure of chloris striate mosaic virus. Virology 92:428.

4. Francki, R.I.B., T. Hatta, G. Boccardo and J.W. Randles (1980). The composition of chloris striate mosaic virus, a geminivirus. Virology 101:233.

5. Hamilton, W.D.O., D.M. Bisaro, R.H.A. Coutts and K.W. Buck (1983). Demonstration of the bipartite nature of the genome of a single-stranded DNA plant virus by infection with the cloned DNA components. Nucl. Acids Res. 11:7387.

6. Stanley, J. and M.R. Gay (1982). The nucleotide sequence of cassava latent virus DNA. Nature 301:260.

7. Howarth, A.J., J. Caton, M. Bossert and R.M. Goodman (1985). Nucleotide sequence of bean golden mosaic virus and a model for gene regulation in geminiviruses. Proc. Natl. Acad. Sci. USA 82:3572.

8. Howell, S.H. (1984). Physical structure and genetic organisation of the genome of maize streak virus (Kenyan isolate). Nucl. Acids Res. 12:7359.

9. Mullineaux, P.M., J. Donson, B.A.M. Morris-Krsinich, M.I. Boulton and J.W. Davies (1984). The nucleotide sequence of maize streak virus DNA. EMBO J. 3:3063.

10. MacDowell, S.W., H. Macdonald, W.D.O. Hamilton, R.H.A. Coutts and K.W. Buck (1985). The nucleotide sequence of cloned wheat dwarf virus DNA. EMBO J. 4:2173.

11. Stanley, J., P.G. Markham, R.J. Callis and M.S. Pinner (1986). The nucleotide sequence of an infectious clone of the geminivirus beet curly top. EMBO J. 5:1761.

12. Lazarowitz, S.G. (1988). Infectivity and complete nucleotide sequence of the genome of a South African isolate of maize streak virus. Nucl. Acids Res. 16:229.

13. Rogers, S.G., D.M. Bisaro, R.B. Horsch, R.T. Fraley, N.L. Hoffman, L. Brand, J.S. Elmer and A.M. Lloyd (1986). Tomato golden mosaic virus A component DNA replicates autonomously in transgenic plants. Cell 45:593.

14. Townsend, R., J. Watts and J. Stanley (1986). Synthesis of viral DNA forms in *Nicotiana plumbaginifolia* protoplasts inoculated with cassava latent virus (CLV): evidence for the independent regulation of one component of the CLV genome. Nucl. Acids Res. 14:1253.

15. Gardiner, W.E., G. Sunter, L. Brand, J.S. Elmer, S.G. Rogers and D.M. Bisaro (1988). Genetic analysis of tomato golden mosaic virus: the coat protein is not required for systemic spread or symptom development. EMBO J. 7:899.

16. Elmer, J.S., L. Brand, G. Sunter, W.E. Gardiner, D.M. Bisaro and S.G. Rogers (1988). Genetic analysis of the tomato golden mosaic virus: the conserved AL1 ORF product is essential for replication. Nucl. Acids Res., in press.

17. Grimsley, N., T. Hohn and B. Hohn (1987). *Agrobacterium*-mediated delivery of infectious maize streak virus into maize plants. Nature 325:177.

18. Grimsley, N. and D.M. Bisaro (1987). Agroinfection. In Hohn, T., Schell, J. (eds.): "Plant DNA Infectious Agents," Vienna: Springer-Verlag, p 87.

19. Elmer, J.S., L. Brand, G. Sunter, W.E. Gardiner, C.K. Browning, D.M. Bisaro and S.G. Rogers (1987). Agrobacterium-mediated inoculation of plants with tomato golden mosaic virus DNAs. Plant Mol. Biol. 10:225.

20. Messing, J., D. Geraghty, G. Heidecker, N. Hu, J. Kridl and I Rubenstein (1983). In Kosuge, T., Meredith, C.P.,Hollaender, A. (eds.): "Genetic Engineering of Plants," New York: Plenum Press, p 211.

21. Morris-Krsinich, B.A.M., P.M. Mullineaux, J. Donson, M.I. Boulton, P.G. Markham, M.N. Short and J.W. Davies (1985). Bidirectional transcription of maize streak virus DNA and identification of the coat protein gene. Nucl. Acids Res. 13:7237.

22. Mullineaux, P.M., J. Donson, J. Stanley, M.I. Boulton, B.A.M. Morris-Krsinich, P.G. Markham and J.W. Davies (1985). Computer analysis identifies sequence homologies between potential gene products of maize streak virus and those of cassava latent virus and tomato golden mosaic virus. Plant Mol. Biol. 5:125.

23. Rogers, S.G., R.B. Horsch and R.T. Fraley (1986). Gene transfer in plants: production of transformed plants using Ti plasmid vectors. Meth. Enzymol. 118:627.

24. Lazarowitz, S.G., A.J. Pinder, V.M. Damsteegt, L. Brand and S.G. Rogers (1988): Genetic analysis of maize streak virus: Identification of viral functions essential for systemic spread and symptom development. Submitted for publication.

25. Smith, M. and S. Gillam (1981). In Setlow, J.K.,Hollaender, A. (eds.): "Genetic Engineering: Principles and Methods," New York: Plenum Press, p 1.

26. Kunkel, T. (1985). Rapid and efficient site-specific mutagenesis without phenotypic selection. Proc. Natl. Acad. Sci. USA 82:488.

27. Canon, F.C., J.R. Postgate and S.B. Primrose (1974). Chromosomal integration of Klebsiella nitrogen fixation genes in *E. coli*. J. Gen. Micro. 80:227.

28. Donson, J., B.A.M. Morris-Krsinich, P.M. Mullineaux, M.I. Boulton and J.W. Davies (1984). A putative primer for second-strand synthesis of maize streak virus is virion-associated. EMBO J. 3:3069.

Molecular Biology of Plant–Pathogen Interactions, pages 185–197

DEFECTIVE INTERFERING RNAs OF A PLANT VIRUS[1]

T. Jack Morris and Bradley I. Hillman[2]

Department of Plant Pathology, University of California, Berkeley, California, 94720

ABSTRACT Low molecular weight symptom modulating RNAs have been identified in association with a strain of tomato bushy stunt virus (TBSV). The 4.8 kb ssRNA viral genome, when inoculated alone, induces a lethal systemic necrosis in tobacco plants. The presence of linear ssRNAs of less than 1 kb in the inoculum results in symptom attenuation, plant survival and concommitant reduction of viral synthesis. Cloning and nucleotide sequence analysis of several of the small RNAs has revealed that they consist of sequences derived from 5', 3', and internal segments of the parent virus genome. These co-linear deletion mutants have all of the properties necessary to be considered the first defective interfering RNAs of a small RNA plant virus. They are analogous to the DI RNAs most commonly associated with the majority of animal virus infections. The origin of these DI RNAs from the parent viral genome has been demonstrated in a high multiplicity passage experiment. The cloning and sequencing of these *de novo* generated DI RNAs is currently in progress.

---

[1]This research was supported in part by USDA Competitive Grant #83-CRCR-1-1227 and a Campus Biomedical Research Support Grant.

[2]Present Address: Roche Institute of Molecular Biology, Nutley, 07110.

INTRODUCTION

We have recently discovered a unique class of symptom modulating RNAs which are associated with infection of plants by the cherry strain of tomato bushy stunt virus (TBSV), a small ssRNA virus of the Tombusvirus group. One of the symptom modulating RNAs has been molecularly characterized and demonstrated to have many properties in common with the defective interfering RNAs (DIs) commonly associated with animal virus infections. These TBSV-associated RNAs are DI-like in that they are deletion mutants of the helper virus genome that do not code for translation products but which have retained sequences necessary for replication and encapsidation (1,2). In addition, these DIs prevent the development of a lethal necrotic disease normally caused by the parent virus by interfering with normal virus replication (3). Defective viral genomes of this type have not been previously reported in association with small RNA plant virus infections (4).

Defective interfering virus particles have long been recognized as major controlling elements of animal virus replication. Indeed, DIs have been observed in virtually every critically analyzed animal virus system including both RNA and DNA viruses. The origin of the DI genomes has been attributed to aberrant replicative events which produce internally deleted genomes that are likely generated by template "hopping" or "switching" by the viral RNA polymerase (the copy-choice mechanism). The DIs interfere with the replication and spread of the parent virus because they become predominant in the virion RNA population due to their competitive advantage during replication and encapsidation. Such animal virus DIs have become increasingly useful models for the study of many important virological phenomena and their ubiquity in association with RNA viruses of animal systems suggests their existence may be a general virological rule. The fact that there has been no definitive documentation for their existence in association with the multitude of ssRNA plant viruses that have been described to-date is somewhat perplexing. Perhaps it reflects a fundamental difference between animal and plant virus infections such as the general tendency for animal viruses to induce cell death. Besides the TBSV-DI system which we describe here, there have only been reports of DI-like particles associated with plant rhabdoviruses (7) and the description of deletion mutants of the bipartite genome of soil-borne wheat mosaic virus (8). On the other hand, the existence of symptom-modulating satellite RNAs in association with plant virus infections is a well established phenomenon (4).

PROPERTIES OF TOMBUSVIRUSES

Tomato bushy stunt virus (TBSV) is the type member of the Tombusvirus group of plant viruses which comprises some 12 different serologically related viruses responsible for causing a number of serious virus disease problems worldwide (9). Tombusviruses consist of 30nm spherical particles composed of 180 subunits of 40kd coat protein and one molecule of ssRNA of 4800 nucleotides. TBSV was the first icosahedral virus to be crystallized and it represents one of the best studied of all viruses from a structural perspective. Tombusviruses are physicochemically related to a larger group of structurally similar viruses which includes turnip crinkle virus (TCV) and carnation mottle virus (CarMV) which we have recently proposed be included in a new group of Carmoviruses (10). The elucidation of the sequence and genomic organization of two Carmoviruses has been recently accomplished in our laboratory (11,12). These studies have clearly established a distinctive genome organization for these viruses because the sizes of subgenomic RNAs produced in vivo are different from those produced by Tombusviruses (13). In contrast, there have been few previous studies on the organization of a legitimate Tombusvirus genome such as that of TBSV. Progress in this area has been slow and the published information on the number and size of viral specific RNA species produced in infected hosts has been both conflicting and confusing. Because of the necessity of defining the origin of TBSV DI-RNA sequences, we initially focused our cloning and sequencing efforts on the ends of the genomic RNA. We have now sequenced about 80% of the TBSV genome and the combination of sequence data and northern blot analyses of viral specific RNAs produced in infected hosts has permitted us to more clearly define the general features of the genome organization of the TBSV strain under study in our laboratory (13). Our results show that three major viral specific ssRNAs are produced in infected plants. These include the 4.8 kb genomic RNA and two 3'-coterminal subgenomic RNAs of 2.2 and 1.0 kb as depicted by the diagram in Fig. 1. The genomic RNA encodes a long ORF which initiates at nucleotide 165 from the 5'-end to encode a polypeptide of 33 kd. Read-through of the UAG codon would result in a large polypeptide with sequence similarity to the polymerases of other RNA viruses. The 3'-proximal domain of the TBSV genome is organized differently than most small RNA plant viral genomes in that the coat protein ORF is not the most 3' proximal. The coat protein cistron is translated from the 2.2 kb subgenomic RNA while the 1.0 kb subgenomic RNA potentially encodes two polypeptides of 19 and 21 kd from two overlapping ORFs. The internal location of the coat protein gene is unique among monopartite RNA plant viruses and contrasts with the more typical gene order of the structurally similar Carmoviruses.

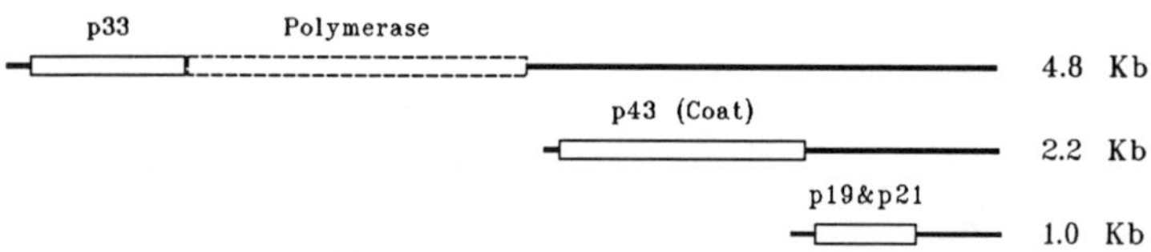

FIGURE 1. Genomic organization of Tombusviruses. The lines indicate scaled positions of the viral-specific RNAs. The open boxes indicate potentially expressed ORFs and the dashed box represents a region of incomplete sequence.

PROPERTIES OF SYMPTOM MODULATING RNAs

Low molecular weight RNA species have been reported in association with Tombusvirus infections in addition to the genomic and subgenomic RNA species described above. These include two classes of symptom modulating RNAs encapsidated in virus particles (Fig. 2): a 0.7 kb satellite RNA (14,15) and a group of DI-RNAs of about 0.4 kb (2,3). Our studies have primarily involved the smaller DI RNA species which we discovered in association with a necrosis inducing Tombusvirus originally described as the cherry strain of TBSV which is synonomous with the cherry isolate of petunia asteroid mosaic virus (10). We became interested in this particular Tombusvirus isolate because it caused an unusually severe and often lethal necrosis in systemic host plants. In addition, we noted a very dramatic symptom attenuation effect associated with the presence of low molecular RNAs in the virus inoculum. The presence of the RNAs conferred protection from what would have otherwise resulted in a rapid necrosis-induced wilting of the plants (3).

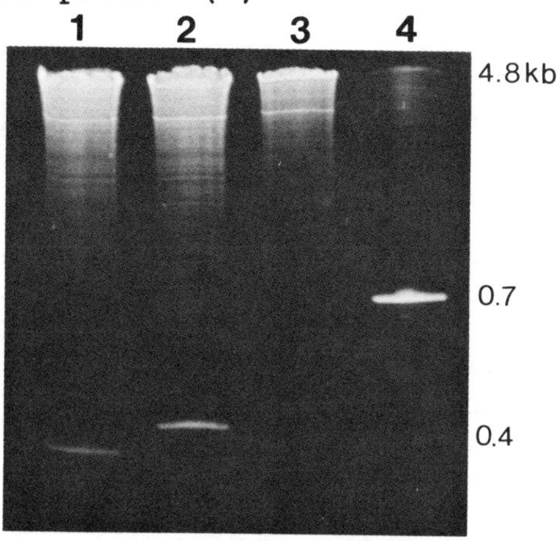

Figure 2. Formamide denatured virion RNAs separated on a 4.5% acrylamide/urea gel in TBE. Lanes contain RNAs from infections inoculated with genomic TBSV RNA plus (from left to right) 1) DI-1; 2) DI-2; 3) no other RNA; 4) Sat RNA.

Unexpectedly, all of our hybridization experiments performed at the time suggested that the small ssRNAs, which accumulated to high titer in the infected plants, shared sequence homology with the genomic RNA of the helper virus. These properties were consistent with the hypothesis that the small RNAs were defective interfering RNAs that had been previously described in association with only animal virus infections. Physical separation and biological passage experiments permitted the isolation of different sized isolates of the DI RNAs depicted in Fig 2. Using these isolates, it was possible to demonstrate that different sized DI species effected differing degrees of symptom attenuation. The largest of the DI RNAs was the most effective at preventing the lethal necrotic syndrome in _Nicotiana clevelandii_. We have also compared the biological effects of the presence of different DI isolates and the 0.7 kb satellite RNA on the replication and encapsidation of the genomic RNA of the helper TBSV strain (14). Several important properties characteristic of many of the animal virus DIs could be interpreted from these studies: i) Infectivity dilution studies clearly suggested that DI and genomic RNA are encapsidated in separate virion populations; ii) DI and satellite RNAs both markedly interfered with the level of accumulation of full-length genomic viral RNA in infected plants. The proportion of viral specific sequences present as low molecular weight RNA approached 90% on a molar basis for DI infections and 75% for satellite RNA infection; iii) However, the DI RNAs were much less efficiently encapsidated, approaching only 30% of the total encapsidated RNA on a molar basis. In contrast, the encapsidation of satellite RNA exceeded 50% on a molar basis with respect to genomic RNA.

These studies provided important clues suggesting that the mechanism of symptom modulation could not be explained by simple competition at either the replication or encapsidation stages. Indeed, although satellite RNA was the most efficiently encapsidated, it was the least effective at symptom attenuation and at reducing the level of accumulated helper virus RNA. These results also suggested that specific sequence differences among the DI RNAs may be important in effecting the symptom attenuation and that the mechanism of interference is different for the satellite and DI RNAs. Indeed, the possibility that complementary DI sequences may interfere with the normal replication of the helper virus and, in this way, modulate symptoms is suggested from previous studies on animal virus DIs (5).

MOLECULAR CHARACTERIZATION OF DI RNAs

The characterization of the molecular structure of one of the DI RNAs has been accomplished (2). The procedures used for the purification and analysis of the viral RNAs and for cDNA cloning and sequencing of the ssRNA viral genomes have been described in detail previously (1,2,11,12). The purification of DI RNA was best accomplished from infected plant tissue, as opposed to purified virion preparations, because of the greater relative abundance of DI in the plant extracts. The protocol involves phenol-chloroform extraction of infected tissue and fractionation in 2-4M lithium chloride. The ssRNA and dsRNA forms of the DI RNA remain soluble at high salt and are separated from the bulk of the viral and host ssRNAs (1).

The construction and characterization of recombinant plasmids of TBSV genomic cDNA provided 3'-terminal clones from which sequence was derived. These studies permitted the construction of oligonucleotide primers which would prime first strand cDNA synthesis on DI RNA template and the subsequent cDNA cloning from a purified DI RNA fraction. The nucleotide sequence of the DI RNA was determined by chemical degradation of cDNA clones and dideoxynucleoside chain termination of cDNA extensions that were primed with the specific oligonucleotides. The sequence analysis revealed a consensus sequence representative of the DI RNAs (Fig. 3) and several important features pertaining to the regions of the viral genome from which the DI RNAs were derived (Fig. 4).

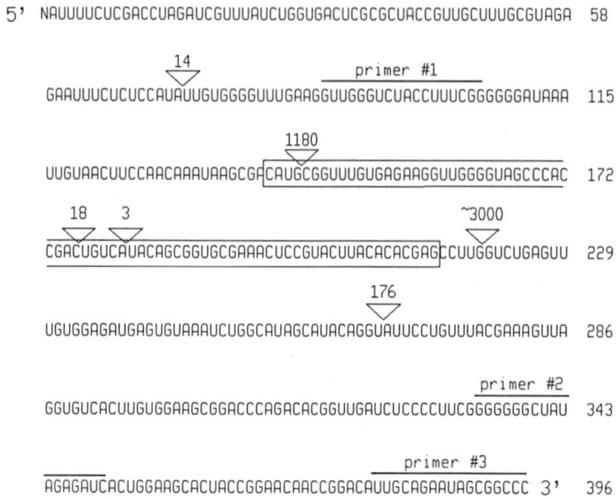

Figure 3. Composite sequence of a DI RNA. Triangles represent regions of deleted sequence. The box depicts the tandem direct repeat region.

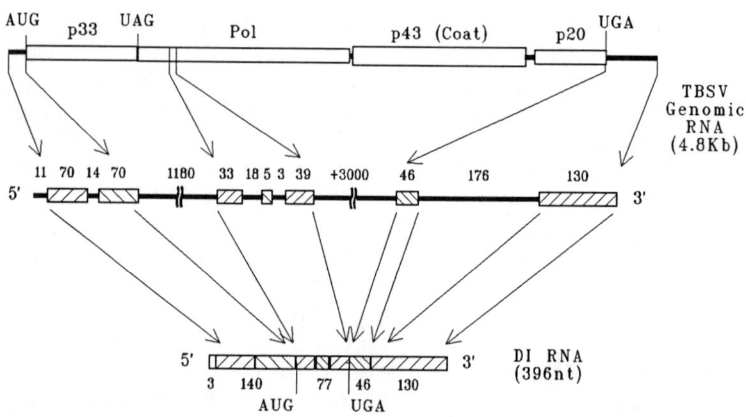

Figure 4. Alignment of the TBSV genomic (top diagram) and DI RNA (bottom diagram) sequences. The middle diagram shows the size (nts) and position of the regions of genomic sequence deleted to produce the DI RNA species.

Virtually the entire sequence of the DI, including a 130 nucleotide portion of the exact 3'-end and all but 3 nucleotides of the extreme 5'-end, was derived from the TBSV genomic RNA. The DI is a composed of a complex mosaic of sequences derived from various regions of the parent helper virus genome. Almost all of the coding sequences have been deleted in the DI RNAs. The only coding regions included in the DI RNA are the first AUG codon which opens the most 5' proximal ORF, 77 nucleotides of the polymerase gene and the last codon before termination of the overlapping p20 ORFs. Sequence heterogeneity in the DI RNA population was also evident from analysis of several clones. The consensus sequence in Fig. 3 includes a repeated block of internal sequence present in one of the clones which contains most of the 77 nucleotides derived from the polymerase coding region. It is possible that this duplication accounts for the size difference noted among different DI RNA isolates (see Fig. 2) and may be the region responsible for conferring the greater degree of symptom modulation noted for this larger DI species.

ORIGIN AND EVOLUTION OF DI RNAs

The experimental approach used to address the origin of animal virus DIs has involved cell culture passaging at high multiplicity (m.o.i.) of a clonally pure virus inoculum which had originally been derived from a single plaque. It is generally accepted that size and sequence heterogeneity in the DI populations resulting from such experiments reflect <u>de novo</u> generation of DIs from the helper virus genome rather than selection of pre-existing DI molecules. We initiated an analogous experiment to address the origin of the TBSV DI RNAs. A DI-free preparation of TBSV RNA was inoculated to the local host <u>Nicotiana glutinosa</u> and 12 single lesion isolates were selected and passed on either of two systemic hosts, <u>N. clevelandii</u> and <u>N.benthamiana</u>. Six of the single lesion isolates maintained in each host were serially passed without dilution (high m.o.i.) and two were passed at a sap dilution of 1/200 (low m.o.i.) at weekly intervals. Symptom attenuation was evident in the high m.o.i. inoculations as early as passage 3 and all such isolates eventually developed attenuated disease expression. None of the 4 low m.o.i. passage isolates displayed reduced virulence by passage 12 when the experiment was terminated. In all cases, the appearance of symptom attenuation was coincident with the appearance of DI RNA molecules in the plants as monitored by northern blot analysis.

The appearance and evolution of one such DI RNA generated by high m.o.i. passage of one of the local lesion isolates through N. benthamiana is presented here. Northern blot analysis of the 3M lithium chloride soluble RNA fraction isolated from infected tissue at each passage is depicted in Fig. 5A. The spontaneous appearance of a complex population of viral-specific RNAs of about 700-1000 nucleotides at passage 3 coincided with the absence of the normal lethal necrotic response caused by DI-free virus. Further high m.o.i. passage selected for more pronounced symptom attenuation and predominance of a single major DI RNA species of about 700 nucleotides which was encapsidated in virions purified from the infected plants at passage 10 and which hybridized strongly to a probe derived from a 3' terminal genomic RNA clone (Fig. 5B). DI RNAs of this size were absent in virus isolated from plants infected with a comparable isolate maintained through the same number of low m.o.i. passages. Each of the 12 de novo DI RNAs generated by high m.o.i. passage hybridized to probes containing both 5' and 3' genomic RNA sequences and each possessed a distinctively different electrophoretic mobility in denaturing gels. Different degrees of symptom attenuation were also evident for different isolates. The likelihood that there was a preferred sequence motif selected in the high multiplicity passage experiment is suggested from the fact that all of generated DI RNAs were larger than those previously characterized and they were also much more efficiently encapsidated. Cloning and sequence analysis is currently in progress.

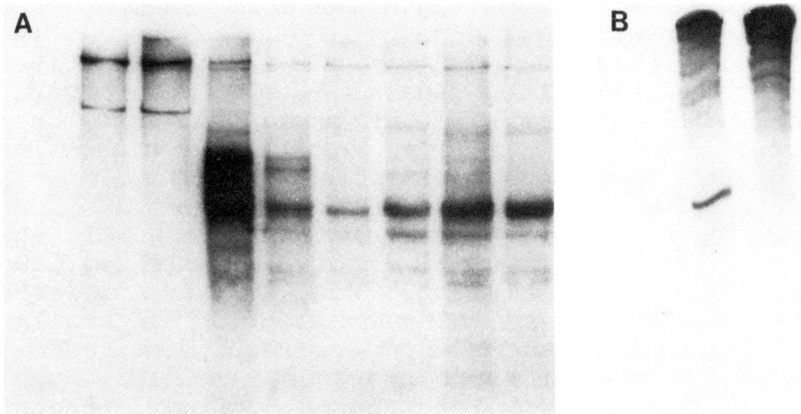

Figure 5. A) Northern blot hybridization of 3M lithium chloride soluble RNA fractions isolated from <u>N. benthamiana</u> after serial high m.o.i. passage of a DI-free isolate of TBSV. Lane 1 contains RNA from a healthy plant and the remaining lanes contain RNA isolated from plants at each successive high m.o.i. passage of the same local lesion isolate. B) RNAs isolated from virus particles purified from infected <u>N. benthamiana</u> after 10 successive high m.o.i. (left lane) or low m.o.i. (right lane) passages. The RNAs were separated on a 5% acrylamide gel, electrotransferred to nylon membrane and developed with a nick translated clone of the 3'-end of the viral genome.

DISCUSSION

The TBSV DI RNAs described here have many features in common with animal virus DIs in general and more specifically with the DI RNAs of alphaviruses which, like TBSV, have positive-sense ssRNA genomes. Mosaic-type DI RNAs have been reported for both positive and negative--sense animal virus infections with one of the more interesting described for Semliki Forest virus (5,6). In a striking parallel with the TBSV system, undiluted passage of the SFV DI resulted in a progressive increase in size due to duplication of internal blocks of sequence. Other similarities include rigid conservation of 3'-end sequences and divergence of 5'-end sequences. The DIs of alphaviruses have been well characterized and some information regarding sequences required for both replication and packaging have been obtained using complete recombinant clones to produce infectious transcripts of the DIs in vitro (16). Similar studies with the TBSV DIs should prove as informative in view of the extensive knowledge we have regarding the structure of this plant virus. In addition, the TBSV system offers the advantage of a smaller helper virus genome than corresponding animal virus systems and hence provides a valuable model system for studying both the helper and dependent components of the system using cloned inoculum. In addition, these DI RNAs may prove useful tools for exploring the molecular basis of symptom suppression which may lead to novel approaches for genetically engineering plants with virus disease resistance.

ACKNOWLEDGEMENTS

We thank Drs. A.O. Jackson, Louis Heaton, and David Knorr for helpful discussions and Patrick Hearne and Ruth Mullin for providing invaluable technical assistance.

REFERENCES

1. Hillman BI (1986). Genome organization, replication and defective RNAs of tomato bushy stunt virus. Ph.D Thesis, Univ California, Berkeley, CA.
2. Hillman BI, Carrington JC, Morris TJ (1987). A defective interfering RNA that contains a mosaic of a plant virus genome. Cell 51:427.
3. Hillman B I, Schlegel DE, Morris TJ (1985). Effects of low molecular weight RNA and temperature on tomato bushy stunt virus. Phytopathology 75:361.
4. Francki RIB, (1985). Plant virus satellites. Ann Rev Microbiol 39:151.
5. Holland JJ (1986). Generation and replication of defective viral genomes. In Fields BN,

Knipe DM (eds): "Fundamental Virology." New York: Raven Press, 768 pp.
6. Barrett ADT, Dimmock NJ (1986). Defective interfering viruses and infections of animals. Curr Top Microb Immunol 128:55.
7. Adam G, Gaedigk K, Mundry KW (1983). Alterations of a plant rhabdovirus during successive mechanical transfers. Z Pflanzenkr Pflanzensch 90:28.
8. Hsu YH, Brakke M (1985). Cell-free translation of soil-borne wheat mosaic virus RNAs. Virology 143:272.
9. Martelli GP, Gallitelli D, Russo M (1988). Tombusviruses. In Koenig R (eds): "The Plant Viruses, Vol. 3". New York: Plenum, p13.
10. Morris TJ, Carrington JC (1988). Carnation mottle virus and viruses with similar properties. In Koenig R (eds): "The Plant Viruses, Vol. 3". New York: Plenum, p73.
11. Guilley H, Carrington JC, Balazs E, Jorand G, Richards K, Morris TJ (1985). Nucleotide sequence and genome organization of carnation mottle virus RNA. Nucleic Acids Res. 13:6663.
12. Carrington JC, Morris TJ, Stockley PG, Harrison SC (1987). Structure and assembly of turnip crinkle virus. IV: Analysis of the coat protein gene and implications of the subunit primary structure. J Mol Biol 194:265.
13. Hillman BI, Hearne P, Rochon D, Morris TJ (1988). Characterization of the coat protein gene of tomato bushy stunt virus. In prep.
14. Hillman BI, Morris TJ (1988) Comparison of a Satellite and two defective interfering RNAs associated with tombusviruses. In prep.
15. Gallitelli D, Hull R (1985). Characterization of satellite RNAs associated with tomato bushy stunt virus and five other defintive tombusviruses. J Gen Virol 66:1533.
16. Levis R, Weiss BG, Tsiang M, Huang H, Schlesinger S (1986). Deletion mapping of Sinbis virus DI RNAs derives from cDNAs defines the sequences essential for replication and packaging. Cell 44:137.

Molecular Biology of Plant-Pathogen Interactions, pages 199-215

MOLECULAR GENETICS OF TOMATO GOLDEN MOSAIC VIRUS

S.G.Rogers, J.S.Elmer, G.Sunter[1], W.E.Gardiner[1], L.Brand, C.K.Browning[1], and D.M.Bisaro[1]

Plant Molecular Biology, Biological Sciences
Monsanto Company, 700 Chesterfield Village Pkwy
St. Louis, MO 63198
and
[1]Department of Molecular Genetics and Ohio State Biotechnology Center, Rightmire Hall
Ohio State University
Columbus, OH 43210

ABSTRACT Progress in defining the functions of the proteins encoded by open reading frames (ORFs) of the tomato golden mosaic virus (TGMV) is reviewed. Mutations in the TGMV ORFs have been produced and their effects on infectivity and replication investigated following agroinoculation. Deletion of the coat protein ORF does not abolish systemic spread but symptom severity is decreased. Deletion of the C-terminal portion of the AL3 ORF results in attenuation of symptoms and vein clearing. Disruption of the TGMV B ORFs,the AL1 or AL2 ORF leads to loss of infectivity. Mutations in the AL1 ORF, alone, totally abolish DNA replication. We have also developed a vector for expression of foreign proteins in infected plants by replacing the coat protein ORF with the *E. coli* chloramphenicol acetyltransferase (CAT) coding sequence. The modified TGMV shows delay and attenuation of symptoms

---

[1]DMB, WEG, CKB AND GS were supported in part by USDA grant no. 87-CRCR-1254, NSF grant DMB-8796326 and by a grant from the Monsanto Company.

similar to those for the coat protein deletion. Most importantly, the DNAs produced in the systemically infected leaves are identical to the predicted CAT replacement DNAs and high levels of CAT activity are present in extracts of these leaves. This result demonstrates that TGMV can be adapted as a vector that stably replicates and expresses foreign proteins in systemically infected plants.

During the past five years, our knowledge concerning geminivirus genome structure and organization as inferred from sequence data has rapidly increased. There are a number of excellent review articles (1-3) that cover the pathology, systematics and structural aspects of the viruses and their genomes. Although this review will briefly cover these areas, it will concentrate on the available information concerning genetic analysis of the functions essential to the geminiviruses including replication and systemic movement. Since this review is based mainly on results from our laboratories, these topics will be covered primarily for the group of geminiviruses whose genetic information is split between two single-stranded circular DNAs. Similar information on the single component genome geminiviruses can be found in the paper by Lazarowitz (this volume). Functions for the products of the ORFs known at the time this review was prepared and educated conjectures as to possible functions are discussed. We also report data on expression of a foreign gene during infection that show TGMV can be adapted for use as a vector.

The Geminiviruses

The geminiviruses are named for their particle morphology which consists of twinned icosahedra. They are separated into two major subgroups based on their genome structure and the insect vector that transmits them. One subgroup has members that infect a wide range of either dicot or monocot hosts, are transmitted by leafhoppers and have a genome consisting of one single-stranded circle of

DNA about 2.8 to 3.0 kilobases (kb) in size. This group is represented by beet curly top virus (BCTV; 4) and maize streak virus (MSV; 5-7), both of which have been cloned and their genomes sequenced. The other major group of geminviruses has members that each infect a narrow range of dicot hosts, are transmitted by whiteflies and have a genome split between two single-stranded circular DNAs each 2.5 to 2.7 kb in size. This subgroup is represented by cassava latent virus (CLV, also known as ACMV: african cassava mosaic virus;8), bean golden mosaic virus (BGMV;9), squash leaf curl virus (SqCLV;3) and tomato golden mosaic virus (TGMV; 10). The genomes of all of these have been cloned and the sequences of both components determined. The members of this class are readily transmitted mechanically as virus particles, viral DNAs or as cloned DNAs released from the cloning vector. In the latter case, both genome components are essential for infection (11,12). The ease of mechanical inoculation with cloned DNAs is the reason that genetic studies have proceeded the furthest with members of this subgroup.

Genome Structure of TGMV

A map showing the structure and organization of the double-stranded forms of the tomato golden mosaic virus genome appears in Figure 1. The organization is typical of a split-genome geminivirus. The A and B genome components are 2588 and 2508 nucleotides in size, respectively (10), and share 230 nucleotides of nearly identical sequence referred to as the Common Region (CR). Since the CR is the only region of extensive homology in the two components, it is thought to contain an origin of replication for the two DNAs or perhaps an origin of assembly for their encapsidation (1). The CRs of other two component genome geminviruses and the large intergenic regions of the one component genome geminiviruses all contain a stem and loop structure. The sequence of the loop is conserved in all geminiviruses (3) and a sequence within the loop is highly homologous to the cleavage site for the ϕX174 gene A protein (13). Cleavage at this site is essential for the synthesis of the single-stranded(ss) form from the φX double-strand (ds) replicative form I (RFI) DNA.

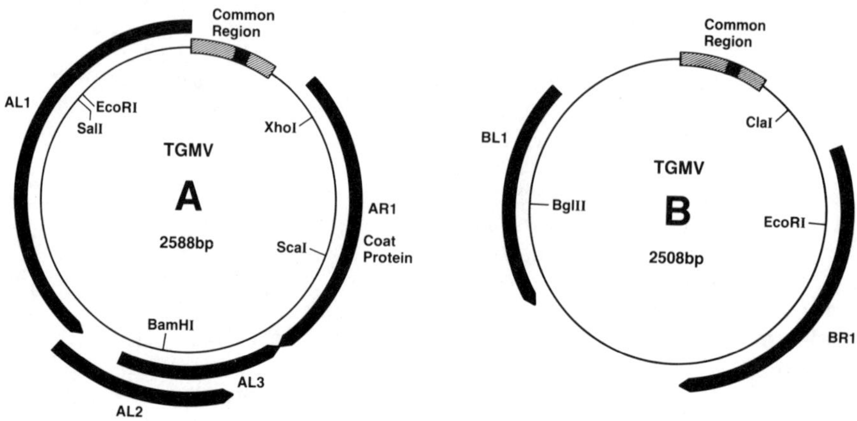

Figure 1. Maps of the double-stranded forms of the TGMV A and B DNAs. The open reading frames (ORFs) are labeled according to their position on the standard map (10). The sizes and direction of translation of the potential proteins encoded by each of the ORFs are shown as solid arrows. The Common Region is shown as a shaded block and the solid block represents the conserved stem and loop found in all geminivirus DNAs. The restriction endonuclease cleavage sites shown in each component are unique.

Comparison of the computer-identified open reading frames (ORFs) of the geminiviruses show that they are encoded by both strands of the viral DNA with initiation of translation being CR proximal. The ORFs encode proteins that are highly homologous and similarly organized among the various two component geminiviruses (14,15). This organization is illustrated by the TGMV A component which encodes five ORFs that could produce proteins larger than 10 kD, four of which are shown in Figure 1. The fifth ORF, AL4, is contained entirely within the N-terminal portion of AL1 and could encode a protein of 11 kD. The TGMV B component could encode at least two proteins.

Townsend and colleagues (16) have shown that the poly-adenylated RNAs produced during CLV infection are transcribed from both strands of the two components, in agreement with the orientation of the ORFs. The most abundant is the coat protein transcript. The transcripts from the left side of CLV 1 component (which is homologous to the TGMV A component) initiate near the common region or in a region 5' to the AL2 ORF homologue and both leftward transcripts terminate at the point where the AL3 and coat protein homologue ORFs overlap. Transcripts for the rightward and leftward ORFs of the CLV2 component were also identified. The precise endpoints of the CLV transcripts were not mapped thus no information concerning precise promoter locations or processing of the geminivirus RNAs is available.

Replication of Geminivirus DNA

TGMV replication only occurs in cells that are in S phase and actively synthesizing their own DNA (17). This is consistent with the close association of most geminiviruses with the phloem and the metabolically active phloem companion cells in infected plants. Like other geminiviruses (1), TGMV replicates in the nucleus of the infected cell and the nucleus eventually becomes filled with arrays of the geminate particles (18). There is one reported study of geminivirus DNA synthesis in nuclei isolated from infected plants (19). TGMV DNA replication was not sensitive to aphidicolin, an inhibitor of DNA polymerase alpha, the polymerase active in replication of nuclear DNA. This surprising result suggests that possibly the beta, gamma or a new uncharacterized DNA polymerase is involved in TGMV DNA synthesis, but further work using fractionated cellular extracts will be needed to conclusively identify the host and viral proteins responsible for viral replication.

A recent report showed that *Abutilon* mosaic virus (AbMV) single-stranded DNA is found in the chloroplasts of infected cells (20). Whether the chloroplast is the site of replication or the particles or DNAs are transported to and accumulate in the plastid is not clear at this time. Perhaps the AbMV virus represents a new group of geminiviruses with an alternate strategy for replication.

DNAs prepared from infected plants show predominantly monomeric single- and double-stranded circular forms. Multimeric forms are also present in lower amounts (21,22) and their roles as replication intermediates remains to be defined. It is not known at this time if these forms consist exclusively of one component or are mixed multimers containing both of the genome components.

Functions Encoded by the TGMV ORFs

The AR1 ORF encodes the viral coat protein (16). The coat protein is nonessential for infectivity in CLV (23). Deletion of nearly the entire TGMV coat protein ORF results in attenuated symptom development and delayed systemic spread of the virus but, likewise, does not affect replication (24).

No functions have been proposed for the AL2, AL3 and AL4 ORFs. The product of the AL1 ORF is remarkably homologous to two ORFs of the single component geminiviruses. This sequence conservation has led to speculation that AL1 encodes a replication protein with a highly conserved essential function. Initial support for this hypothesis came from the work of Townsend et al.(17) who demonstrated by transfection of tobacco protoplasts with cloned DNAs that the CLV 1 component contains all the information necessary for its own DNA replication. Similar findings have been obtained by Rogers et al.(13), who showed that transgenic petunia plants containing integrated dimers of the TGMV A component produce free, autonomously replicating TGMV A DNAs. Both of these studies clearly show that component A, which encodes the highly conserved AL1 ORF, produces all the virally-encoded factors necessary for its own replication. It is also clear that this factor is likely to be a protein since it acts in *trans* to promote replication of TGMV B. Proof that AL1 is a replication factor is discussed below.

The transgenic plants that contain tandem repeats of the TGMV A or B DNAs integrated into their chromosomes are normal in appearance. However, one-quarter of the progeny produced by crossing an A plant with a B plant show virus symptoms and contain infectious virus particles (25). These results show that the integrated tandem copies of the TGMV DNAs are functional and maintain their ability to produce infectious virus when genetically combined in the same cell. Furthermore, these results also show that one or both of the two TGMV B component ORFs encode a function or functions essential for systemic movement and symptom production.

Creation and Analysis of Mutations in the TGMV ORFs

Mutational analysis of the TGMV ORFs has been conducted to investigate the role that each predicted protein plays during infection.

The cloned DNAs of the TGMV components are infectious when delivered either as a linear molecules after release from the cloning vector by cleavage with the restriction endonuclease used for cloning (11,12) or as uncut plasmid DNAs when the component is present as a tandem dimer (26). The efficiency of free DNA inoculation with linear molecules is poor but the use of the multimeric clones can give routine frequencies of infection as high as 85% when both component DNAs are present as multimers in the same clone (26). However, this method is difficult to apply to mutational analysis of these DNAs because of the problems in constructing plasmids that contain dimers of both component DNAs. When creating and assaying mutations in the cloned DNAs, it is essential to use a method that allows easy construction of variants so that many mutants can be made and gives high rates of infection so that a large number of inoculated host plants can be obtained.

Fortunately, a more efficient method for virus DNA delivery called "agroinfection" was described by Grimsley et al.(27-29) and adapted for use with TGMV by Elmer et al. (30). This procedure uses the T-DNA transfer system of *Agrobacterium* to inoculate susceptible host plant cells with T-DNAs that contain partial tandem duplications of virus DNAs. The procedure works not only for TGMV on dicotyledonous hosts but can also be used to inoculate MSV into maize thus overcoming the difficulties of mechanical transmission mentioned above (7,28). The efficiency of infection following coinoculation of *Nicotiana benthamiana* with two strains of *Agrobacterium* each carrying tandem duplications of either the A or B component is over 80%. A further increase in the efficiency of inoculation can be obtained by agroinoculation of transgenic *N. benthamiana* plants that carry tandem repeats of the TGMV B component DNA integrated into their chromosomes. Following agroinoculation of these B plants with *Agrobacterium* carrying tandem duplications of the A component, greater than 97% of the plants become infected (30). The time of appearance and degree of symptoms are uniform and similar to those obtained following inoculation with crude virus.

Mutants have been created in all of the ORFs of TGMV using clones of the component DNAs by insertion of linkers(31), by repair and rejoining DNA ends created by restriction endonuclease cleavage (24,30,32), and by site-directed mutagenesis (24,32). The mutated component DNAs have been inserted into a plasmid or T-DNA vector as multimers and the undigested plasmid DNA introduced mechanically or by agroinoculation onto host plants. In our studies (24,32), TGMV A mutations were assayed by agroinoculation of transgenic *N. benthamiana* B plants and TGMV B mutations were assayed by coinoculation of nontransgenic *N. benthamiana* plants with *Agrobacterium* containing wild-type TGMV A multimers. The results of assays of mutants in each of the TGMV ORFs appear in Table 1 and are summarized below.

The AR1 ORF (coat protein) is not essential and may be completely deleted (24). Coat protein deletions still produce systemic infection but have attenuated, delayed symptoms on *N. benthamiana* plants. The coat protein deletion mutant produces the ss and ds DNA forms associated with TGMV infection but the forms are only 1.9 kb in size, rather than the 2.6 kb wild type size. It should be noted that this result contrasts with the findings of Brough et al.(31) who reported that small deletions (28 bp) of the coat protein ORF were infectious with delayed symptoms but that larger deletions (178 or 603 bp) were not infectious. The difference in these results is not due to our use of agroinoculation as opposed to free DNA inoculation since we find the same result after coinoculation of nontransgenic hosts. At this time, we cannot explain Brough et al.'s failure to obtain infectious large deletions.

Table 1 Predicted Products of the TGMV ORFs and Functions Assigned from Mutant Studies

ORF	Size kD	Symptoms	Replication plants	Replication discs	Function
AR1	29	atten,del	ss,ds	ss,ds	coat protein
AL1	40	none	none	none	replication
AL2	15	none	none	ss,ds	movement?
AL3	16	atten,del	ss,ds	ss,ds	morphogenesis?
AL4	11	normal	ss,ds	ss,ds	?
BR1	29	none	none	ND	movement?
BL1	21	none	none	ND	movement?

atten,del- attenuated, delayed symptoms with less chlorosis and leaf rugation
ND - not done.

An amber mutation in the AL4 ORF (not shown in Fig. 1) which is completely contained within N-terminal region of the AL1 ORF and translated in the same direction, shows no reduction in symptom severity or delay in appearance (32). The amounts of ss and ds DNAs are the same as with normal TGMV infection. Since we find no phenotype associated with an AL4 mutation, we believe that AL4 does not encode an function essential for infection and have omitted it from the TGMV map.

An 80 bp deletion of the 3' region of the AL3 ORF that does not overlap the AL2 ORF leads to delay in appearance and attenuation of symptoms. The infected leaves show little rugation and are characterized by chlorosis over the vascular tissue. The DNAs present in the infected plants show the ss and ds forms characteristic of TGMV.

Mutations in AL2 that do not also affect the AL1 or AL3 ORFs abolish symptom production and none of the DNAs produced during normal infection can be detected (32). Since Brough et al. (31) only created mutations that simultaneously affected the

AL2 and AL3 ORFs they were unable to determine the phenotypes of separate mutations in the AL2 or AL3 ORFs.

Mutations in the AL1 ORF abolish symptom production and none of the DNAs produced during normal infection can be detected (31,32).

Mutations in either the BL1 or BL2 ORFs abolish symptom production and none of the DNAs produced during normal infection can be detected in infected plants (31,33). This result extends earlier studies (13) that suggested that at least one of the B ORFs is required for systemic spread and movement of the virus in the infected plant. It appears that both of the B ORFs are necessary for systemic spread.

Replication of Mutants in Infected Cells

One advantage of the agroinoculation procedure can also be used to assay directly the replication of TGMV in leaf disc explants (32). DNA prepared from agroinoculated, nontransgenic petunia or *N. benthamiana* leaf discs show the ss and ds circular DNAs characteristic of TGMV infection as early as one day post-inoculation (32). This procedure permits rapid analysis of the replication capacity of mutants independent of systemic infection and is much easier to perform than protoplast infections. This assay was used to characterize the cellular replication of the TGMV mutants described above.

The AL2 mutants and a deletion mutant lacking the 400 bp portion of the AL2 and AL3 ORFs that does not overlap the AL1 ORF are all able to replicate in cells of leaf discs (32). All of the ss and ds forms were detected. These results combined with the inability of the AL2 mutations to produce infection suggest that the AL2 product is essential for systemic movement of TGMV. We have suggested the the AL2 protein may be a DNA binding protein but further study is required to firmly demonstrate this (32).

Mutants with lesions in AL1 show no replication in leaf discs (32). This result combined with those above shows that the product of AL1 is the only virally encoded protein essential for replication and is in agreement with the fact that AL1 is the most conserved ORF among the single and two component geminiviruses. The absence of all of the TGMV DNA forms shows that the AL1 is necessary for the synthesis of both ss and ds DNA forms. This suggests that the ss form is an obligatory precursor to the ds form and supports a model for TGMV replication in which there is no ds to ds replication. More work is necessary to demonstrate this model.

Prospects for Vector Development

Will the geminiviruses provide useful vectors for stable plant transformation or for the study of plant gene expression in transient assays? A great deal has been written about the theoretical adaptation of geminviruses as vectors (1,34) as well as a descriptive listing of several potential approaches (35). However, no report of the successful use of a geminivirus vector to express a heterologous protein has appeared in the scientific literature.

Is foreign DNA stably replicated and expressed during systemic infection? The finding that the coat protein may be deleted without loss of infectivity permitted us to perform the following experiment. We replaced the TGMV coat protein coding sequence from the XhoII site at bp 312 to the AsuII site at bp 1037 with a 750 bp DNA encoding the *E. coli* pBR325 (36) chloramphenicol acetyl transferase (CAT) gene from a newly introduced BglII site immediately 5' to the AUG initiation codon to an AsuII site located 3' to the coding sequence. The new construct was used to agroinoculate transgenic *N. benthamiana* plants carrying tandem copies of the TGMV B component in their genome. Control plants agroinoculated with TGMV A showed symptoms on average at 13 to 14 days post-inoculation. The TGMV A-CAT plants showed symptoms on average at 22 days post-inoculation. The attenuated symptoms were similar to those produced by the coat protein deletion but the delay in appearance was three days longer than for the deletion (24). Analysis of the DNAs in the symptomatic leaves showed that ss and ds DNAs of the predicted size for the TGMV A-CAT construct (2.6 kb) are present. The DNAs are uniform in size indicating no deletions had occurred. As shown in Figure 2, these DNA forms can be detected with either a probe homologous to the CAT gene (Lanes 1 and 2) or to TGMV A (Lane 3). Assays of CAT activity in extracts of the symptomatic leaves (Figure 3) showed that appreciable levels of the acetyltransferase are present in these leaves. This data provides a first demonstration that foreign coding sequences can be stably maintained and expressed during systemic infection when inserted in place of the coat protein ORF. We are currently extending these studies to determine if there are any limits on the size of insert that may be maintained and propagated.

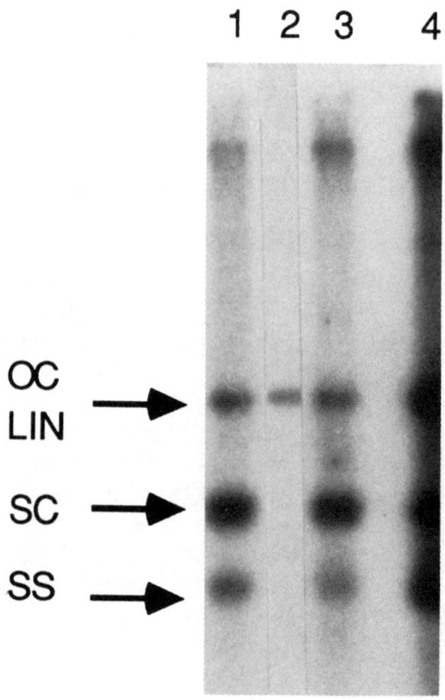

Figure 2. Southern blot analysis of TGMV A DNAs produced in leaves of transgenic B tobacco plants. Total DNA from leaves of inoculated plants was prepared and 2-5 ug were separated as described by Rogers et al (13). Lanes 1 and 3 contain undigested total leaf DNA from TGMVA-CAT agroinoculated transgenic B plants. Lane 2 contains the same DNA that was digested to completion with PvuII which does not cleave TGMV A DNA but cleaves once in the CAT coding sequence.

The loss of the ss form during the PvuII digestion may be accounted for by contaminating single-strand specific nuclease. Lane 4 contains undigested total leaf DNA from wild type TGMV A agroinoculated transgenic B plants. Hybridizations were carried out as described previously (13) using nick-translated CAT specific probe (Lanes 1 and 2) or a TGMV A component specific probe (Lanes 3 and 4). The autoradiogram was obtained from a one day exposure at room temperature. OC, LIN, SC and SS refer, respectively, to the open circular, linear, supercoiled and single-stranded forms of the DNAs.

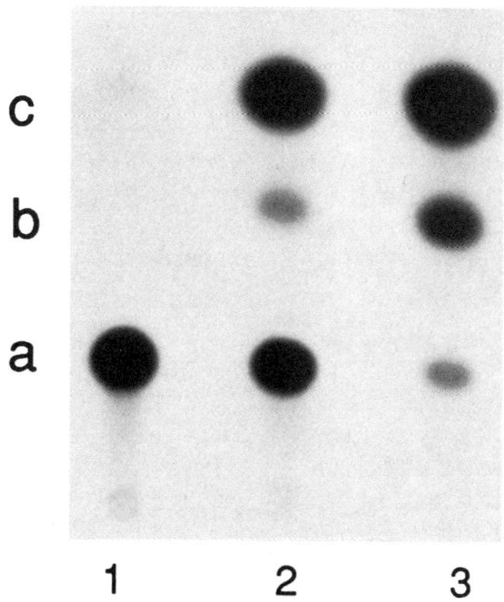

Figure 3. Autoradiogram of products of the chloramphenicol acetyl transferase assay. Extracts were prepared from leaves of agroinoculated plants and assayed for CAT activity as described by Canon et al.(37). The extracts were prepared from leaves of transgenic B plants agroinoculated with wild type TGMV A (Lane 1) or TGMV A-CAT (Lane 2). Lane 3 shows the reaction products from 0.5 units of CAT prepared from *E. coli* cells. a is the position of unreacted chloramphenicol, b is the position of the mono-acetylated chloramphenicol, and c is the position of the di-acetylated form.

Future Needs and Directions

One deficiency in our catalog of what is known about geminiviruses is in the area of viral transcription. The analysis of CLV transcripts by Townsend et al. (16) is the only description of transcription of a split-genome geminivirus. A complete, detailed transcriptional map of a geminivirus is needed to locate the promoter elements and to determine whether or not processing of primary transcripts occurs. Without a better knowledge of the RNAs produced, progress toward understanding the regulation of geminivirus gene expression and replication cannot be obtained.

The study of the geminiviruses has reached the stage where protein molecular biology and biochemistry are essential for further progress. The coat protein is the only geminivirus protein whose function has been identified (16). None of the products of the other geminvirus ORFs have been demonstrated to be the proteins predicted from sequence or mutational analysis. In order to identify and characterize these proteins in infected plants, the products of the different ORFs must be expressed in *E. coli* or any other appropriate host, purified and used to make poly- and monoclonal antibodies. These antibodies will permit us to determine the locations and associations of the proteins in infected hosts. The use of transgenic plants that produce the TMGV A and B DNAs or the proteins encoded by each of the component DNAs in combination with the available mutants will allow rapid progress on these biochemical studies.

ACKNOWLEDGEMENTS

The authors thank Dr. Linda Hanley-Bowdoin for assistance in editing this manuscript.

REFERENCES

1. Davies JW, Townsend R, Stanley J (1987). The structure, expression, functions and possible exploitation of geminivirus genomes. In Hohn T, Schell J (eds): "Plant Gene Research, Plant DNA Infectious Agents",Vienna: Springer-Verlag, p 31.

2. Harrison BD (1985). Advances in Geminivirus Research. Ann. Rev. Phytopathol. 23:55.
3. Lazarowitz SG (1987). Molecular characterization of geminiviruses. Plant Mol. Biol. Reporter 4:177.
4. Stanley J, Markham PG, Callis RJ, Pinner MS (1986). The nucleotide sequence of an infectious clone of the geminivirus beet curly top virus. EMBO J. 5:1761.
5. Mullineaux PM, Donson J, Morris-Krsinich BAM, Boulton MI, Davies JW (1984). The nucleotide sequence of maize streak virus DNA. EMBO J. 3:3063.
6. Howell SH (1984). Physical structure and genetic organization of the genome of maize streak virus (Kenyan isolate). Nucl. Acids Res. 12:7359.
7. Lazarowitz, SG (1988) Infectivity and complete nucleotide sequence of the genome of a South African isolate of maize streak virus. Nucleic Acids Res. 16:229.
8. Stanley J, Gay M (1983). The nucleotide sequence of cassava latent virus DNA. Nature 301:260.
9. Howarth AJ, Caton C Bossert M, Goodman RM (1985). Nucleotide sequence of bean golden mosaic virus and model for gene regulation in geminiviruses. Proc. Natl. Acad. Sci., USA 82:3572.
10. Hamilton WDO, Stein VE, Coutts RHA, Buck KW (1984). Complete nucleotide sequence of the infectious cloned DNA components of tomato golden mosaic virus: Potential coding regions and regulatory sequences. EMBO J. 3:2197.
11. Stanley J (1983) Infectivity of the cloned geminivirus genome requires sequences from both DNAs. Nature 305:643.
12. Hamilton WDO, Bisaro DM, Coutts RHA, Buck KW (1983). Demonstration of the bipartite nature of the genome of a single-stranded plant virus by infection with the cloned DNA components. Nucl. Acids Res. 11:7387.
13. Rogers SG, Bisaro DM, Horsch RB, Fraley RT, Hoffmann NL, Brand L, Elmer JS, Lloyd AM (1986). Tomato golden mosaic virus A component DNA replicates autonomously in transgenic plants. Cell 45: 593.
14. Mullineaux PM, Donson J, Stanley J, Boulton MI, Morris-Krsinich BAM, Markham PG, Davies J (1985). Computer analysis identifies sequence homologies between potential gene products of Maize

Streak Virus and those of Cassava Latent Virus and Tomato Golden Mosaic Virus. Plant Mol. Biol. 5:125.
15. MacDowell SW, Macdonald H, Hamilton WDO, Coutts RHA, Buck KW (1985). The nucleotide sequence of cloned wheat dwarf virus. EMBO J. 4:2173.
16. Townsend R, Stanley J, Curson SJ, Short MN (1985). Major polyadenylated transcripts of cassava latent virus and location of the gene encoding coat protein. EMBO J. 4:33.
17. Townsend R, Watts J, Stanley J (1986). Synthesis of viral DNA forms in *Nicotiana plumbaginifolia* protoplasts inoculated with cassava latent virus (CLV); evidence for the independent replication of one component of the CLV genome. Nucl. Acids Res. 14:1253.
18. Rushing AE, Sunter G, Gardiner WE, Dute RR, Bisaro DM (1987) Ultrastructural aspects of tomato golden mosaic virus infection in tobacco. Phytopathology 77: 1231.
19. Coutts RHA, Buck KW (1985). DNA and RNA polymerase activities of nuclei and hypotonic extracts of nuclei isolated from tomato golden mosaic virus infected tobacco leaves. Nucleic Acids Res. 13:7881.
20. Groning BR, Abouzid A, Jeske, H (1987). Single-stranded DNA from abutilon mosaic virus is present in the plastids of infected *Abutilon sellovianum*. Proc Natl Acad Sci, USA, 84:8996.
21. Hamilton WDO, Bisaro DM, Buck KW (1982). Identification of novel DNA forms in tomato golden mosaic virus infected tissue: evidence for a two component viral genome. Nucleic Acids Res. 10:4901.
22. Stanley J, Townsend R (1985). Characterization of DNA forms associated with cassava latent virus infection. Nucleic Acids Res.13:2189.
23. Stanley J, Townsend R (1986) Infectious mutants of cassava latent virus generated in vivo from intact recombinant DNA clones containing single copies of the genome. Nucl. Acids Res. 14:5981.
24. Gardiner WE, Sunter G, Brand L, Elmer JS, Rogers SG, Bisaro DM (1988). Genetic analysis of tomato golden mosaic virus: the coat protein is not required for systemic spread or symptom development. EMBO J. 7:899.
25. Sunter G, Gardiner WE, Rushing AE, Rogers SG, Bisaro DM (1987). Independent encapsidation of tomato golden mosaic virus A component DNA in transgenic plants. Plant Mol. Biol. 8:477.

26. Hayes RJ, Brough CL, Prince VE, Coutts RHA, Buck KW (1988). Infection of *Nicotiana benthamiana* with uncut cloned dimers of tomato golden mosaic virus DNA. J. Gen. Virol. 69:209.
27. Grimsley N, Hohn B, Hohn T, Walden R(1986). "Agroinfection," an alternative route for viral infection of plants by using Ti plasmid. Proc. Natl. Acad.Sci. USA 83:3282.
28. Grimsley N, Hohn T, Davies JW, Hohn B (1987). *Agrobacterium*-mediated delivery of infectious maize streak virus into maize plants. Nature 325:177.
29. Grimsley N, Bisaro, DM (1987). Agroinfection. In Advances in Plant Gene Research, Vol IV, Hohn T and Schell J, eds, Vienna: Springer-Verlag, p 87.
30. Elmer JS, Brand L, Sunter G, Gardiner W, Browning CK, Bisaro DM, Rogers SG (1987). Agrobacterium-mediated inoculation of plants with tomato golden mosaic virus DNAs. Plant Mol. Biol. 10:225.
31. Brough CL, Hayes RJ, Morgan AJ, Coutts RHA, Buck KW (1988). Effects of mutagenesis *in vitro* on the ability of cloned tomato golden mosaic virus DNA to infect *Nicotiana benthamiana* plants. J. Gen. Virol. 69:503.
32. Elmer JS, Brand L, Sunter G, Gardiner W, Bisaro DM, Rogers SG (1988). Genetic analysis of the tomato golden mosaic virus: the conserved AL1 ORF product is essential for replication. Nucleic Acids Res. In Press.
33. Browning CK, Bisaro DM, In preparation.
34. Buck KW, Coutts RHA (1983) The potential of geminiviruses in the construction of plant host vector systems. Plant Mol. Biol. 2:351.
35. Coutts RHA., Buck KW, Roberts EJF, Brough CL, Hayes RJ, Macdonald H, MacDowell SW, Petty ITD, Slomka MJ, Hamilton WDO, Bevan MW (1987). "Studies on the replication of tomato golden mosaic virus and the construction of gene vectors" in Molecular Strategies for Crop Protection, Arntzen, C Ryan, C, eds., New York: Alan R. Liss Inc., p 307.
36. Soberon X, Corvarrubias L, Bolivar F (1980). Construction and characterization of new cloning vehicles IV. Deletion derivatives of pBR322 and pBR325. Gene 9:287.
37. Canon FC, Postgate JR, Primrose SB (1974). Chromosomal integration of Klebsiella nitrogen fixation genes in E. coli. J. Gen. Micro. 80:227.

Molecular Biology of Plant–Pathogen Interactions, pages 217–227

TURNIP CRINKLE VIRUS SATELLITE DOMAINS INVOLVED IN VIRULENCE AND PROCESSING[1]

Anne E. Simon,[2] Henk Engel,[3] and Stephen H. Howell

Department of Biology C-013
University of California San Diego
La Jolla, California 92093

Clifford D. Carpenter

Department of Plant Pathology
University of Massachusetts
Amherst, MA 01003

ABSTRACT Turnip crinkle virus (TCV) supports the replication of a small family of satellite RNAs (RNAs C, D and F). RNA C is a virulent satellite, producing severe symptoms in host plants, while RNAs D and F are avirulent satellites. Using the techniques of *in vitro* mutagenesis combined with *in vitro* transcription of infectious satellite cRNA, we have identified regions of the TCV satellite RNA C involved in symptom production, monomeric satellite accumulation, and infectivity. RNA C, unlike many other small infectious RNAs, can tolerate large insertions and deletions throughout the mid section of the molecule. Based on the results of insertion and deletion mutagenesis, and results of inoculations with a chimeric satellite constructed

---

[1]This work was supported by NSF award DMB-8704124 and NIH postdoctoral fellowship to A.E.S. and NSF award DM84-17352 to S.H.H.
[2]Present address: Department of Plant Pathology, University of Massachusetts, Amherst, MA 01002
[3]Present address: Department of Biochemistry, University of Groningen, 9747 AG Groningen, The Netherlands

between virulent RNA C and avirulent RNA F, we have generated a functional map of RNA C.

INTRODUCTION

Viruses produce a variety of disease symptoms in host plants including stunting, crinkling, chlorosis and vein clearing. Although the symptoms which appear in many virus-host plant combinations are well described in the literature, the menas by which viruses produce symptoms are poorly understood. Our work focuses on a small, virus-associated satellite RNA which determines the expression of symptoms produced by the helper virus in infected plants. Small pathogenic RNAs such as viroids and satellites are small (190-400 b), single stranded, and not thought to encode proteins. Satellites, unlike viroids, are only infectious when inoculated with a specific helper virus. Satellites do not, in general, have any sequence homology with their helper virus (1).

Several satellites, such as non-necrotic strains of cucumber mosaic virus (CMV) sat-RNA or the satellite associated with tobacco ringspot virus, are known to reduce the severe symptoms of their helper virus when co-inoculated on some plants (2,3). Symptom amelioration is sometimes, but not always, accompanied by a reduction in the accumulation of helper virus in the infected plant (4). Other satellites, such as the virulent strains of CMV satellite (5) and turnip crinkle virus (TCV) satellite RNA C (6), intensify helper virus induced symptoms. The mechanism by which satellites increase or decrease symptoms of their helper virus is not presently understood.

The development of systems for the *in vitro* synthesis of infectious cRNA combined with *in vitro* mutagenesis has made possible the development of functional maps of satellite RNA. These functions include viral and/or plant RNA replicase recognition signals; sequences which may be involved in the intensification or amelioration of the symptoms associated with the helper virus; sequences required for encapsidation in virus particles; and processing signals which affect the accumulation of monomeric and multimeric forms. We have developed the TCV satellite system as a model to study how small pathogenic RNAs interact with their helper virus and the host plant to produce disease symptoms.

RESULTS

The TCV Satellite System.

TCV supports the replication of several related satellite RNAs, three of which have been characterized (6,7). The largest satellite, RNA C (355 b), intensifies the normally mild symptoms of its helper virus on turnip plants whereas the smaller satellites, RNA D (194 b) and RNA F (230 b), have no effect on symptoms. The satellites

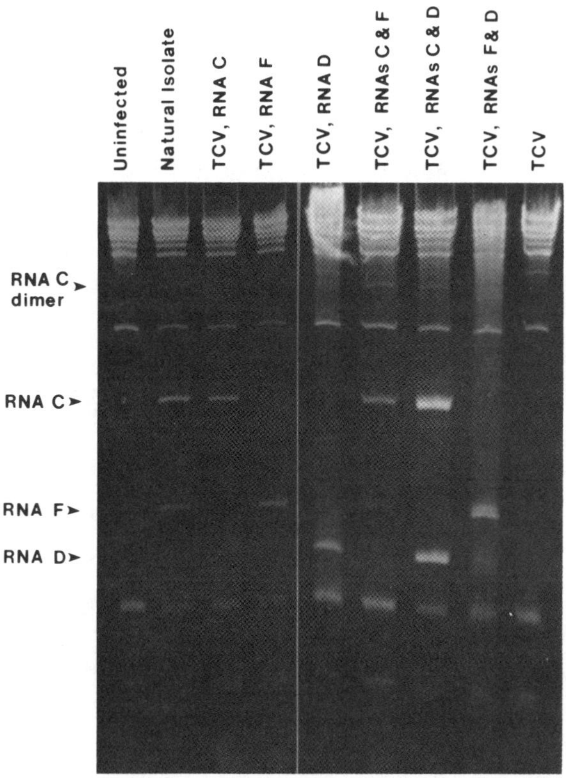

FIGURE 1. Family of satellite RNAs associated with TCV infection. Gel-purified TCV, RNAs C, D, and F were inoculated in various combinations on turnip. Total RNA was isolated 3 weeks post-inoculation and analyzed on 4% acrylamide, 50% urea gels stained with ethidium bromide.

can be inoculated separately or in various combinations along with TCV on turnip (Fig. 1). The accumulation of each satellite in turnip leaves varies depending on which other satellites are also present. For example, there is much more accumulation of RNA D if RNA F is not present. Likewise, the accumulation of RNA F is enhanced in the absence of RNA C.

Our primary focus is to understand how the TCV satellites replicate, accumulate in their final forms (i.e. monomeric and multimeric), and in the case of RNA C, intensify the symptoms of TCV. Towards this goal, we have cloned and sequenced all three satellites (7). A schematic representation of the homology among the satellites and the 3′ end of the helper virus genome (8) is shown in Figure 2. Surprisingly, the virulent satellite RNA C is composed of two domains, a 3′ domain (166 b) similar to two regions at the 3′ end of the helper virus TCV and a 5′ domain (189 b) similar to the entire sequence of the avirulent satellite RNA D. The other avirulent satellite, RNA F, differs from RNA D mainly by a 36 b insert near the 3′ end of RNA F. Because the 3′ domain of RNA C is unique among the satellites, we propose that the symptoms produced by RNA C may be due to some property of the 3′ domain. In order to test this hypothesis, we utilized a system for synthesizing *in vitro* infectious RNA copies from full length RNA C cDNA

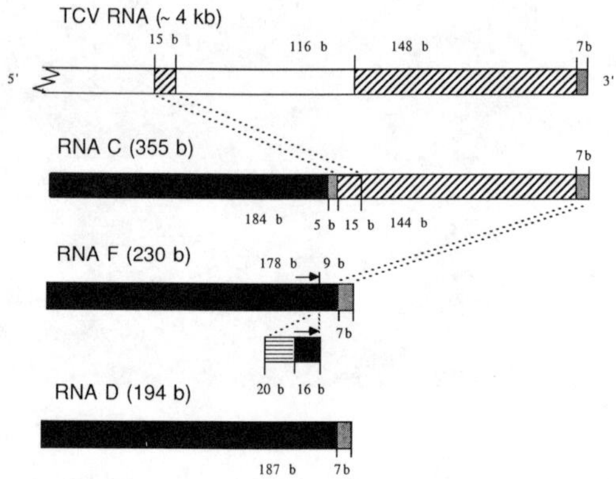

FIGURE 2. Comparison of the sequences of RNAs C, D, and F and the 3′ end of TCV (8). (Reprinted from EMBO J 5:13, 3423–3428 with permission of IRL Press.)

templates cloned into the *in vitro* transcription vector pPM1 (9). pPM1 contains the λp^r *E. coli* RNA polymerase promoter sequence (10) which permits synthesis of *in vitro* transcripts from satellite cDNA inserted downstream of the promoter to begin exactly at the satellite 5′ end. Both monomeric and multimeric transcript copies of RNA C were infectious when inoculated together with the helper virus.

The 3′ domain of RNA C determines virulence.

In order to determine whether the 3′ domain of RNA C is responsible for symptom intensification, chimeric satellite cDNA was constructed composed of 155 b at the 5′ end of the non-virulent satellite RNA F joined to 200 b from the 3′ end of RNA C. This 155 b segment of RNA F differs from the corresponding segment of RNA C by 12 nucleotides including 5 inserted bases and one deleted base. Plants inoculated with *in vitro* synthesized chimeric satellite cRNA along with the helper virus TCV showed severe symptoms typical of those produced by wild-type RNA C and clearly distinguishable from the symptoms produced by the helper virus alone (Simon et al., submitted). In order to confirm that plants were infected with the chimeric satellite and not with a wild-type RNA C contaminant or revertant, the relevant regions of the putative chimeric satellite which accumulated in non-inoculated leaves was sequenced. The sequence of RNA in the region analyzed (the 5′ one half of the molecule) corresponded exactly to the original chimeric transcript previously used to inoculate the plants. Therefore, we conclude that the severe symptoms produced by plants infected with the *in vitro* synthesized RNA F/C chimeric satellite resulted from the 200 b at the 3′ end of RNA C which is largely composed of the domain of homology with the 3′ end of the helper virus genome.

In vitro mutagenesis of RNA C.

Analysis of RNA C insertion mutants. We have created a series of mutations, both insertions and deletions, in a cloned monomeric copy of RNA C in order to identify other functional regions of the satellite. Mutated satellite RNA was transcribed *in vitro* and inoculated on turnip along with the helper virus. Despite numerous attempts at inoculating RNA C containing insertions in the 3′ region of the molecule, these were never infectious. However, insertions of up to 60 b in the midsection of RNA C resulted in infectious satellite which produced the characteristic intense symptoms on turnip (Fig. 3). We also attempted to insert 300, 800, or 1800 b into the SnaB I, Nco I and Dra I sites in order to determine if the satellite could accommodate even larger inserts. None of these larger inserts resulted in infectious satellite (Simon, unpublished results). This may be due to a size limitation in replication or packaging. In no case in our analysis of RNA C insertion mutants did we find a mutant satellite that retained infectivity but lost the ability to produce symptoms. However, mutations in the Sna BI site resulted in RNA C which produced more intense symptoms. Symptoms in these plants appeared about one week earlier and were more severe (greater stunting) than the symptoms produced by normal, unmodified satellite.

<u>Analysis of RNA C deletion mutants.</u> A number of

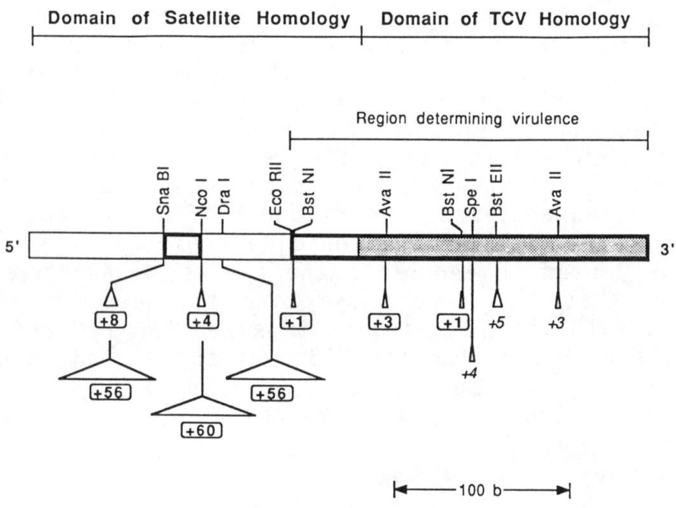

FIGURE 3. Map of the insertion mutations created in RNA C. Full length RNA C cDNA is shown. Sequences were inserted at various restriction sites using *E. coli* DNA polymerase I large fragment, or by insertion of the pUC 19 polylinker. Numbers represent the number of bases inserted. RNA C mutants which were infectious and produced severe symptoms are boxed.

deletion mutants were also created in RNA C (Fig. 4). Mutant satellite containing deletions in the 3′ region were not infectious. Some deletions in the midsection of the satellite did not destroy the infectivity of RNA C while others did. For example, deleting nucleotides 79 - 100 (Sna BI - Nco I) did not destroy the infectivity of RNA C, however an 18 b deletion from the Nco I site towards the 3′ end resulted in uninfectious satellite. Thus, although small insertions and internal deletions are tolerated in the midsection of RNA C, this region cannot be removed entirely. As noted with insertions in the Sna BI site, satellite containing deletions from the Sna BI site also produced more intense symptoms.

Sequences affecting the accumulation of monomeric RNA C. The most intriguing mutation constructed in RNA C was the 22 b deletion between the Sna BI and Nco I sites (see Fig. 4). Little or no RNA C monomers accumulated in plants previously inoculated with monomeric satellite transcripts containing this deletion. Instead, a new RNA species migrating slightly faster than normal RNA C dimers was found (Fig. 5). We demonstrated by

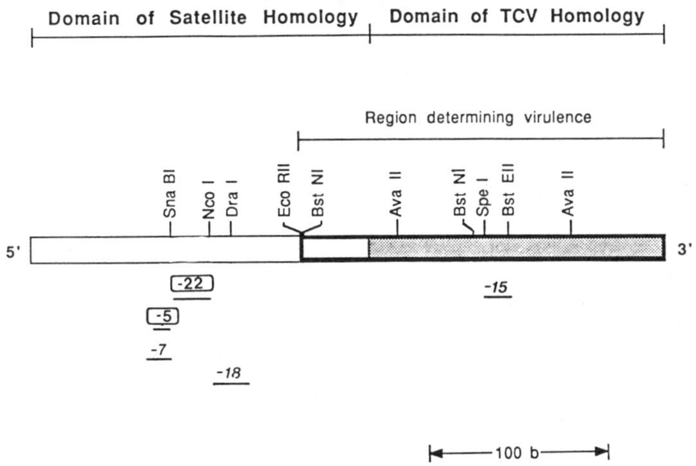

FIGURE 4. Map of deletion modifications in RNA C. Deletions were created between restriction sites or by using the enzyme Bal 31. Numbers represent the number of bases deleted. RNA C mutants which were infectious and produced severe symptoms are boxed.

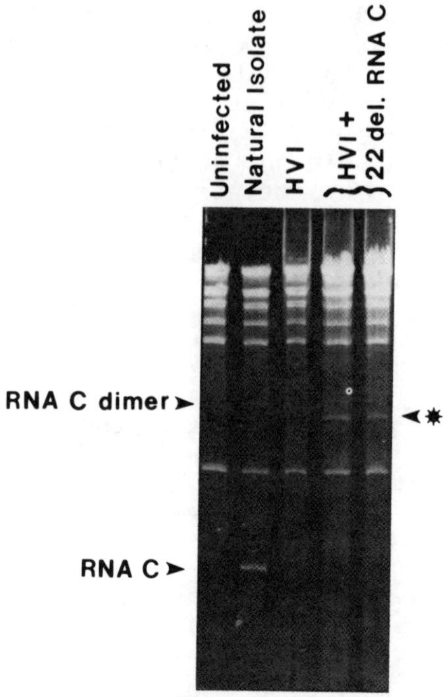

FIGURE 5. Gel pattern of total RNA isolated from turnip plants inoculated three weeks previously with RNAs as indicated. HVI; helper virus inoculum. Asterick (*) indicates position of dimeric RNA C containing the 22 b deletion.

sequencing that this new RNA was RNA C dimer (with deletions in both monomeric units). The block in the accumulation of RNA C monomers was unexpected since insertions of up to 60 b in either the Sna BI or Nco I sites had no effect on satellite accumulation.

In order to locate more precisely the sequence within the 22 b region which was responsible for preferential dimer accumulation, a series of converging Bal 31 deletions were constructed from the Sna BI site and Nco I sites (Fig. 6). Individual mutant satellite transcripts were synthesized *in vitro* and inoculated on turnip along with the helper virus. After three weeks, RNA was isolated from infected plants and the presence or

```
                                                                      Main Form of RNA C

   76                                                        105      Monomer    Multimer
       SnaB I                                          Nco I
...U A C G U A G C A G C C G G G G G G G U U U G A C C A U G G...     X
...U A C   U A G C A G C C G G G G G G G U U U G A C C A U G G...     X
...U A C     A G C A G C C G G G G G G G U U U G A C C A U G G...     X
...U A C       G C A G C C G G G G G G G U U U G A C C A U G G...     X
...U A C         C A G C C G G G G G G G U U U G A C C A U G G...     X
...U A C           A G C C G G G G G G G U U U G A C C A U G G...     X            X
...U A C             G C C G G G G G G G U U U G A C C A U G G...                  X
...U A C               C C G G G G G G G U U U G A C C A U G G...                  X
...U A C G U A G C A G C C G G G G G G G U U U G A   C A U G G...     X
...U A C G U A G C A G C C G G G G G G G U U U G     C A U G G...     X
...U A C G U A G C A G C C G G G G G                 C A U G G...     X
...U A C G U A G C A G C C G G                       C A U G G...                  X
...U A C G U A G                                     C A U G G...                  X
...U A                                               C A U G G...                  X

                   A G C C G G G G G
```

FIGURE 6. Stepwise deletion series generated in cloned RNA C to determine the sequence involved in monomeric satellite accumulation. Underlined sequence is the minimum involved in this phenomena.

absence of monomeric RNA C was determined by analyzing the RNA on denaturing polyacrylamide gels followed by ethidium bromide staining. A 6 b deletion from the Sna BI site or an 11 b deletion from the Nco I site was sufficient to eliminate the accumulation of RNA C monomers. Thus, it appears that the sequence AGCCGG(GGG) is essential for the normal accumulation pattern of RNA C.

DISCUSSION

The virulent TCV satellite, RNA C, is composed of two domains: a 5′ domain which is nearly identical to the avirulent satellite, RNA D, and a 3′ domain which shares 94% similarity with two sequences at the 3′ end of the helper virus TCV. Hence, RNA C is an intermediate between a true satellite which, by canonical definition, has no appreciable similarity to its helper virus genome (1) and a defective interfering (DI) RNA, which is entirely composed of discontinuous regions of helper virus genome. It is intriguing that the first plant virus DI RNA discovered is associated with tomato bushy stunt virus, a member of the same virus group (tombusvirus) as TCV. If the generation of DI RNAs occurs because of a viral polymerase's ability to detach from its template and rejoin it downstream (11) then this could be a natural attribute of other tombusvirus polymerases which may give an indication of the mechanism whereby RNA C was initially generated.

The virulent properties of the RNA F/RNA C chimeric satellite have confirmed our earlier hypothesis (7) that the ability of RNA C to intensify symptoms on turnip is vested in the 3′domain of the molecule. However, two insertions toward the 5′ end of this domain, a 3 b insertion at the Ava II site and a single base insertion at the Bst NI site, yielded infectious responsible for symptom intensification (the terminal 100 b at the 3′ end). So far we have been unable to introduce small insertions and deletions in this smaller region without destroying infectivity. We are currently involved in constructing single base mutations in the 3′ end of RNA C in an attempt to separate virulence-determining from infectivity- determining elements, but we cannot yet eliminate the possibility that the simple accumulation of RNA C in any replicating form will produce symptoms.

We have identified a specific region of RNA C which, when deleted, disrupts the normal accumulation of RNA C monomers. It is not known at this time if the lack of accumulation of satellite monomers is due to a defect in RNA C processing or whether deletion of these sequences results in a destabilization of the monomeric satellite. Little is known about how linear satellites are processed to yield the normal accumulation of monomeric and multimeric forms. Unlike the self-cleavage reaction which is responsible for processing circular satellites and some viroids (12,13), we have not observed self-processing of *in vitro* synthesized RNA C dimers under a variety of conditions (Simon and Klucher, unpublished results). A different mechanism may therefore be involved in processing linear satellite RNAs such as RNA C.

Finally, we have observed that disruption of the RNA C Sna BI site, 76 b from the 5′ end, results in a further intensification of symptoms. This was unexpected since this region lies well outside the 3′ virulence-determining domain. However, the effect of these mutations on virulence may be indirect, perhaps by altering the timing of symptom production. Plants inoculated with these mutants express symptoms earlier than those inoculated with normal RNA C. Thus, increased stunting may be a result of earlier symptom expression. Nonetheless, we have called this region near the Sna B1 site a virulence modulating region to distinguish it from the virulence determining region near the 3′ end.

REFERENCES

1. Francki RIB (1985). Plant virus satellites. Annu Rev Microbiol 39:151.
2. Waterworth HE, Kaper JM, Tousignant ME (1979). CARNA 5, the small cucumber mosaic virus-dependent replicating RNA, regulates disease expression. Science 204:845.
3. Schneider IR (1977). Defective plant viruses. In Romberger JA (ed): "Beltsville Symposia in Agricultural Research. I. Virology in Agriculture," New Jersey: Allenheld, Osmun, Montclair, p 201.
4. Harrison BD, Mayo MA, Baulcombe DC (1987). Virus resistance in transgenic plants that express cucumber mosaic virus satellite RNA. Nature 328:799.
5. Kaper JM and Waterworth HE (1977). Cucumber mosaic virus associated RNA 5: Causal agent for tomato necrosis. Science 196:429.
6. Altenbach SB and Howell SH (1981). Identification of a satellite RNA associated with turnip crinkle virus. Virology 112:25.
7. Simon AE, Howell SH (1986). The virulent satellite RNA of turnip crinkle virus has a major domain homologous to the 3′ end of the helper virus genome. EMBO J 5:3423.
8. Carrington JC, Morris TJ, Stockey PG, Harrison SC (1987). Structure and assembly of turnip crinkle virus IV. Analysis of the coat protein gene and implications of the subunit primary structure. J Mol Biol 194:265.
9. Simon AE, Howell SH (1987). Synthesis *in vitro* of infectious RNA copies of the virulent satellite of turnip crinkle virus. Virology 156:146.
10. Ahlquist P, Janda M (1984). cDNA cloning and *in vitro* transcription of the complete brome mosaic virus genome. Mol Cell Biol 4:2876.
11. Holland JJ, Kennedy IT, Semler, BL, Jones CL, Roux L, Grabau EA (1980). Defective interfering RNA viruses and the host-cell response. In Fraenkel-Conrat H, Wagner RR (eds): "Comprehensive Virology," Plenum Publishing Corporation, Vol 16 p 137.
12. Buzayan JM, Gerlach WL, Bruening G (1986). Non-enzymatic cleavage and ligation of RNAs complementary to a plant virus satellite RNA. Nature 323:349.
13. Forster AC, Symons RH (1987). Self-cleavage of plus and minus RNAs of a virusoid and a structural model for the active sites. Cell 49:211.

Molecular Biology of Plant-Pathogen Interactions, pages 229–243

PATHOGENESIS AND HOST RANGE DETERMINATION BY CAULIMOVIRUSES[1]

S. Gowda, K-B. Goldberg, J. Kiernan, J. Schoelz, M. Young, R. Richins, R. Shepherd

Department of Plant Pathology, University of Kentucky, Lexington, KY 40546-0091

ABSTRACT A single gene of the caulimoviruses appears to be largely responsible for the pathogenic effects of these viruses. This gene (gene VI) is the only one of six genes expressed as a separate RNA transcript. It specifies a protein (P62) that accumulates in infected plants and probably makes up a major component of virus inclusion bodies. Information from mutagenesis of gene VI and pathogenic analysis of hybrid virus strains of cauliflower mosaic virus (CaMV) indicate that gene VI is mainly responsible for disease induction. In addition, gene VI transformations (using a Ti plasmid-*Agrobacterium* system) have shown that gene VI expression is accompanied by chlorosis and mottling similar to virus infections. These experiments suggest that P62 perturbs some process in plants to cause disease.

It has also been found that gene VI determines the host response to infection (hypersensitive versus compatible reactions) and virus host range. Moreover, this gene appears to be the major factor in host adaption by these viruses as shown by recent experiments with figwort mosaic virus (FMV). When this virus was adapted to a new host it was found that a strain with a greatly modified form of gene VI predominated in the new host.

---

[1]This work was supported by USDA grants 86-CRCR-1-2261 and 87-CRCR-1-2528.

INTRODUCTION

The caulimoviruses have small circular DNA genomes of about 8000 base pairs. The genome is organized into six major genes common to all caulimoviruses plus one or more smaller open reading regions that are not conserved (9, 12, 14) (Fig. 1, Table 1). The functions of some genes have been identified. For example, the insect transmission gene, the coat protein, the reverse transcriptase and the inclusion body matrix protein have been identified as regions II, IV, V and VI, respectively (1, 4, 5, 6, 20, 21).

The caulimoviral genome is expressed as two sets of genes. The first five genes which are closely clustered in the genome, comprise one set. These are expressed by a single polycistronic transcript (35S RNA). The second set consists of a single gene, region VI, which is expressed as a monocistronic transcript (19S RNA) (Fig. 1). This transcript is translated to produce P62 a protein that accumulates in relatively large ammounts in virus infected plants. It probably is localized in cytoplasmic virus inclusion bodies where it may be a component of the electron-dense matrix. Reverse transcription and encapsidation of the virus genome appear to occur in these structures and P62 may participate in these processes. However, the specific function of gene VI is not known.

We have studied the biological effects associated with gene VI for the last several years. Its role in pathogenesis and host range will be briefly reviewed.

RESULTS

The naked DNA of caulimoviruses, including that cloned in bacteria, is infectious when rubbed over leaves of healthy plants with an abrasive. This is a great advantage for manipulating these viruses genetically. It allows convenient mutagenesis and restructuring of the viral genomes and the propagation of large amounts of native or mutant DNA, or non-infectious subgenomic pieces useful for modular construction of genomes. The latter is particularly useful in making artificial hybrids of viral genomes of different phenotype to associate disease or other biological properties with certain segments of the circular genome.

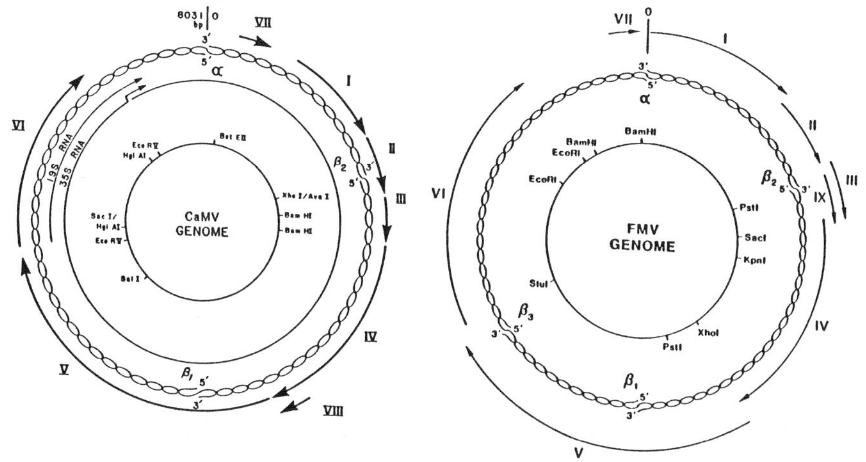

Figure 1. Physical maps of the cauliflower mosaic virus (CaMV) and figwort mosaic virus (FMV) genomes. The circular double-stranded DNAs of about 8000 bp in each case are indicated by the interwoven lines. Encapsidated DNA has 3-4 specifically located interruptions, one (designated α) in the transcribed or minus strand, and two or three (designated β_1, β_2 and β_3) in the complementary or plus strand. The heavy peripheral arrows indicate the location of the translational open reading regions (tentative genes) which occur in the full-length (35S) RNA transcript. The two main RNA transcripts, 19S and 35S RNA of CaMV, are indicated by the lighter inner lines in the diagram.

Disease Responses Associated with CaMV Gene VI

A series of mutagenesis experiments with a severe strain of CaMV provided the first suggestion that gene VI was mainly responsible for disease induction (7). A series of single, small, in-phase insertions, mostly of 12 bp, were made in cloned DNA of CaMV Cabb B-Davis followed by inoculation of the mutant DNA to turnip (Brassica campestris) in the greenhouse. Two of the mutants with insertions in gene VI were infectious. However, in each case the disease induced was milder than that of the wild-type strain. In fact one of the insertional mutants converted the severe wild-type strain to one that caused no stunting or necrosis. Only mild mottling symptoms without a noticeable reduction in growth was induced by this mutant (7).

Similar insertions in other open reading regions were inactivating, so the effect on disease could not be evaluated (7). However the marked reduction in disease by selective mutagenesis of region VI suggested that other regions of the genome may have only indirect roles in disease induction. This has been supported by other observations.

A second series of observations associating disease responses largely with region VI came from experiments with recombined genomes of CaMV (8, 15, 18). In this case strains of CaMV which differed in phenotype were recombined *in vitro* (as the cloned DNAs) to produce hybrid genomes. The only limitation on experiments of this sort are the variety of virus strains that are available and the necessity for having common restriction endonuclease cleavage sites for exchanging segments of the genome.

New recombinant strains have been constructed that induce less severe disease, or more severe disease, than either parent strain used in the exchanges, or than strains of CaMV encountered in nature (8, 17). For example, the CaMVH3 recombinant is more severe than its Cabb B parent which is the most severe naturally occurring strain we have observed.

When recombining parent strains that have virulent versions of gene VI, disease expression cannot be mapped to a single locus. Instead a broad spectrum of reactions are obtained suggesting that more than one locus may be involved in disease induction. However, we do not now believe that typical disease is multigenic in nature. When disease induction is mapped using the D4 strain (Datura strain), which has an avirulent gene VI, a single locus is evident. It now seems likely that disease expression is multigenic only to the extent that other regions of the genome affect the expression of gene VI or induce atypical effects. Since each of the major genes of CaMV except for the insect acquisition gene (region II) are essential for virus activity, we speculate that these other essential genes (I, III, IV and V) probably affect the level of virus multiplication, encapsidation, movement, etc. ...and in this indirect manner affect the level of expression of region VI.

The mapping of disease expression as a single locus

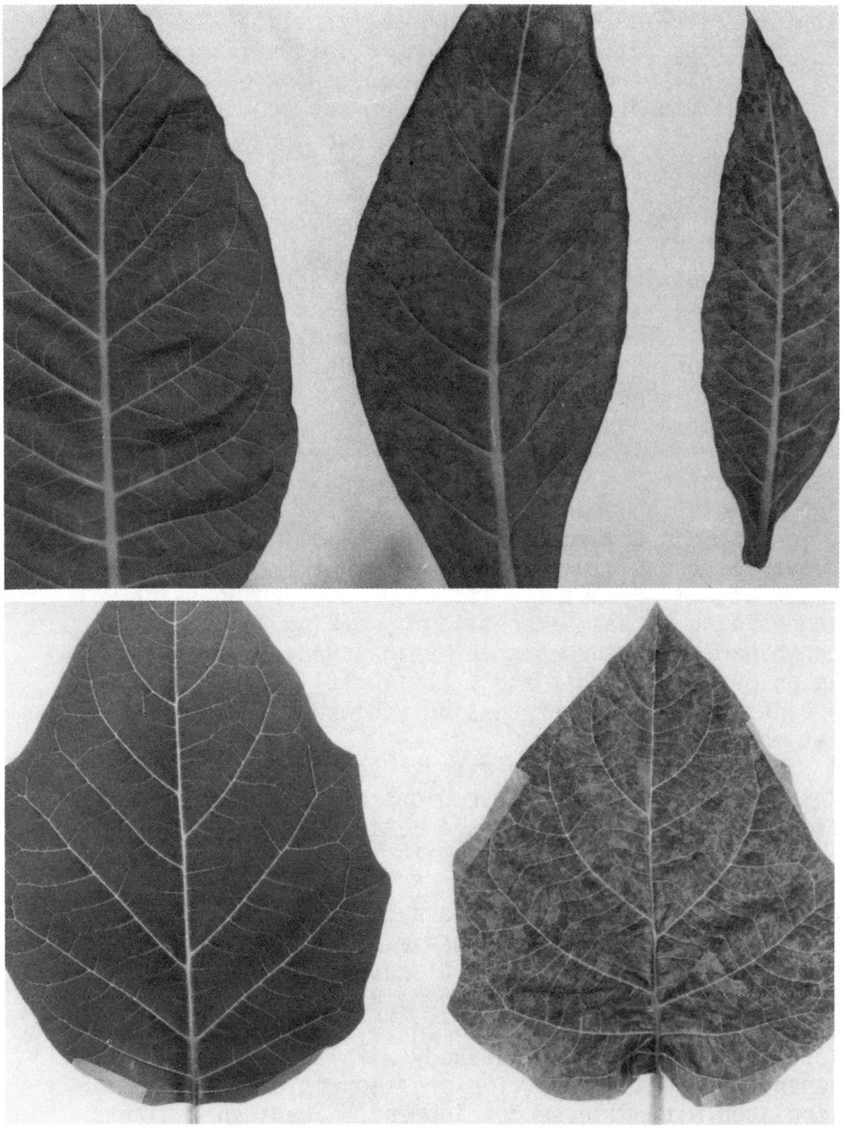

Figure 2. Symptoms induced on *Nicotiana tabacum* (above right) and *Datura innoxia* (below right) following transformation with gene VI of cauliflower mosaic virus strain CM1841. The leaves on the left in each case are healthy.

can be illustrated with various recombinant viruses made with CaMV strains CM1841 and D4 (8, 15, 17). Substitution of a DNA fragment containing gene VI of D4 into the normal position, with the remainder of the genome being derived from CM1841 to produce CaMVH7, leads to the attenuation of disease. Yet virus development appears to occur normally in symptomless plants. In fact, CaMVH7 is a particularly productive strain illustrating that high levels of virus with an avirulent gene VI is relatively harmless to the host plant (8, 18).

In discussing disease expression, with the caulimoviruses at least, it is important to distinguish conventional symptoms from other unusual manifestations of disease. For example, the single strain of CaMV that has an avirulent gene VI (strain D4) causes very unusual symptoms for a caulimovirus (16). The disease it induces does not resemble that of any other strain of CaMV. Where most strains cause mottling and chlorosis of plants this strain causes an unusual necrosis of the smallest veinlets of leaves. No chlorosis or mottling is induced and ordinarily one would never suspect that this virus was a strain of CaMV except for its occurrence on *Brassica*. When mapping disease expression by making artificial recombinants the induction of veinal necrosis maps to some region between genes I and V (15). It is only conventional disease expression (chlorosis and mottling) that maps to gene VI.

The third type of experiment used to associate disease expression with particular regions of the CaMV genome has developed from genetic transformation of plants with gene VI. When region VI of CaMV, with its homologous promoter, is integrated into the genome of tobacco (*Nicotiana tabacum*) or *Datura innoxia* via a Ti plasmid gene vector and *Agrobacterium*, the transgenic plants frequently develop a chlorotic mottling disease (Fig. 2). In these plants the level of P62, the gene VI protein, appears to be related to disease expression (3, 10). When western blots are done with P62 antibody with extracts of transgenic plants, gene VI expression is closely associated with disease development. Transgenic plants which show low levels of P62, or none at all, do not develop chlorotic mottling symptoms. In contrast, some transgenic plants which showed a more generalized yellowing contained high levels of P62. These experiments suggest that P62 may be the major virus induced component that perturbs plants to cause disease (10). Similar results have been reported by other laboratories (3).

Host Range Effects Associated with Gene VI

Several strains of CaMV show the unusual property of causing systemic infections in solanaceous plants in contrast to the usual strains which infect only cruciferous plants. The experimental approach to identify regions which determine host range has been to make recombinant viruses by exchanging DNA segments between cloned genomes of host range variants that have common restriction cleavage sites. The hybrid genomes were then tested for host range differences on both cruciferous and solanaceous plants (8).

Our initial experiments suggested that a single host range determinant existed in the CaMV genome that mapped to gene VI. In fact, the first half of gene VI appeared to contain the domain controlling host range (15). However, later studies showed that host range control was more complex than originally proposed with the whole of gene VI and at least one other locus being involved (18). However, the number of host range determinant loci in these experiments seemed to be related to the particular strains of CaMV being used as if different segments of the genome or their gene products were interacting to determine whether a particular host became systemically infected. The success of interactions by various components appeared to vary with the origin of the different virus strains. We concluded that gene VI was probably the major host range determinant of CaMV, but that this region must be combined with compatible versions of genes I-V in order to function well in new hosts (18).

Interactions between gene VI and other coding regions of the genome probably occur during the course of viral DNA replication and virion assembly. Much evidence has accumulated recently that these processes take place in viral inclusion bodies. P62, the gene product of region VI, appears to be a major constituent of these structures. In addition, the proteins of regions I, III, IV, and V appear in these bodies and these are all products of essential virus genes. Hence, it seems likely that these may act in concert with P62 during viral DNA replication and assembly. In fact, there is evidence that reverse transcription of CaMV DNA occurs in partially assembled virions, which would require the participation of the reverse transcriptase and coat protein in the course of viral DNA replication in inclusion bodies. If so, even subtle variations in the structure of these proteins might affect a tentative interaction with P62, the product of region VI, the major host range determinant.

It must also be pointed out that host range determination of CaMV may be related to the way plants react to initial infection, i.e. whether the initial host response is hypersensitivity or compatibility. This, again, is determined by gene VI as shown by a variety of hybrid viruses inoculated to _Datura stramonium_ or _Nicotiana edwardsonii_. The type of local response is determined by the strain which donates gene VI to the hybrid genome (8, 18). However, it must also be emphasized that systemic development of an infection from a hybrid genome is not wholly associated with the initial host response. Strains which cause non-hypersensitive infections, which are presumably compatible, do not necessarily develop systemically in that particular host.

Hypervariable versus Conserved Regions of Gene VI

Gene VI is the least conserved of the six major genes common to all caulimoviruses (14). This is true for the three strains of CaMV and the other caulimoviruses that have been sequenced. Different caulimoviruses with different host ranges show much less homology in gene VI than different strains of CaMV. For example, the amino acid sequence of region VI of FMV versus that of CaMV or carnation etched ring virus (CERV) shows the level of amino acid homology to be only 26% and 21%, respectively (Table 1). Comparisons of gene VI of CaMV versus CERV shows a higher level of relatedness (Table 1).

We have previously pointed out a hypervariable region in the first half of gene VI of CaMV which probably accounts for some of the host range and host response phenotypes of different strains (17). Other regions of gene VI of six strains of CaMV that have been sequenced show minor differences at the amino acid level.

The distribution of the homologies in the gene VI proteins of three different caulimoviruses are shown in a computer-generated graphical plot in Fig. 3. The relationships between conserved versus variable regions of these polypeptides for viruses with different host ranges is emphasized in these comparisons. Although short tracts

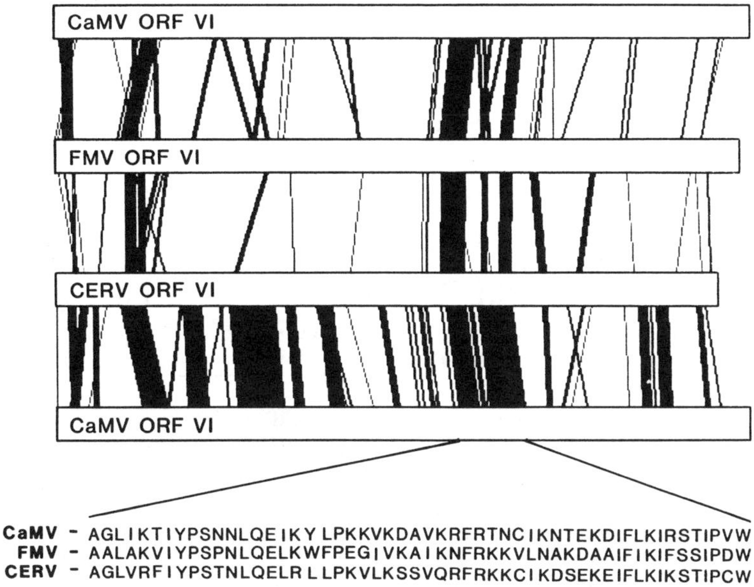

Figure 3. Amino acid homologies of gene VI proteins of three caulimoviruses. CaMV-cauliflower mosaic virus, FMV-figwort mosaic virus, CERV-carnation etched ring virus. Homologous regions between polypeptide chains are displayed as dark lines. A window of 8 amino acids is the unit of comparison with homologies exceeding 62% being scored positive (i.e., as a dark line in the graphical plot). Homologous sequences offset by more than 25 amino acid residues in either direction along the polypeptide chain were not recorded in the plot. The amino acid sequence of the central conserved region is indicated. Data is from Richins _et al_. (14). (Reprinted from NUCLEIC ACIDS RES 15:8451-8466 with permission of IRL Press.)

of homologous amino acid sequence occur near the N-terminus of each gene VI polypeptide, the most extensive region is near the center of the gene. A central conserved domain with a run of 47 amino acid residues, with 47% of the residues being identical between FMV and either CaMV or CERV, is identified (Fig. 3). This central conserved tract may be the region of the protein responsible for its molecular function. One can speculate that the more variable regions toward either end of the polypeptide may interact with the host in the establishment of a compatible interaction needed for optimum function of the gene.

Changes in Gene VI Associated with Host Adaption by Caulimoviruses

Sequence changes localized to region VI of FMV have been associated with adaption of the virus to a new host (19). In the particular experiment referred to, a cloned strain of FMV taken from its native host (*Scrophularia californica*) was transferred to *Datura innoxia*, a species that can be grown as a perennial in the greenhouse. During a two year period virus appeared to change to a form that caused less severe disease on related solanaceous plants (e.g. *Datura stramonium*) but reached much higher concentrations in these hosts. When restriction maps of adapted virus were compared to the original virus from *Scrophularia*, 10 restriction site changes were observed of which 8 were clustered in region VI (19).

We have recently sequenced the strain which seems to be adapted to solanaceous plants and compared gene VI with that of the original. Fig. 4 illustrates the differences in gene VI of the two strains. The N-terminal portion of the protein up to amino acid residue 136 had only a single exchange. The next segment of the protein (residue 136 to residue 267) was markedly different with only 29% of the amino acid residues being the same. A region through the center of the protein (residues 267 to 402) were much more similar (83% homology). This subregion of the protein was followed by another extensive region that deviated markedly in the two strains. Less than half the amino acids of residues 402 to 503 were the same (Fig. 4). At this point 25 amino acids were deleted from the strain adapted to solanaceous plants. The extreme C-terminal 21 amino acids were the same in the two strains.

These sequence differences may account for the different levels of productivity of the two strains in solanaceous plants and for the differences in virulence. However, gene VI exchanges would have to be made between the two strains followed by evaluation of disease and level of replication to show that these sequence

TABLE 1. PROTEIN CODING REGIONS OF THE CaMV, CERV AND FMV GENOMES.

Coding region	Protein molecular weights and amino acid homologies		
	CaMV	CERV	FMV
I	328 (36,825)[a]	319(36,531)[a] 48.3%[b]	323(36,957) 54%, 49%[c]
II	159 (17,878)	168(18,799) 53.6%	164(18,934) 42%, 38%
III	129 (14,136)	128(14,232) 41.4%	115(12,659) 37%, 31%
IV	488 (56,614)	494(56,888) 41.3%	489(57,346) 38%, 33%
V	678 (78,698)	659(76,518) 66.9%	666(76,938) 64%, 64%
VI	520 (57,833)	496(56,423) 33.1%	512(58,133) 26%, 21%
VII	11,398[d]	10,301[d]	7,447
VIII	12,430	----	----
IX	----	----	11,924

[a]Assuming that translation begins with the first ATG and ends with the first stop codon within each open reading frame. The first figure gives the number of amino acid residues followed by the molecular weight in parentheses and percent amino acid homology.

[b]These numbers are the percent direct homology of the amino acid sequences in each putative coding region.

[c]The first percentage given is the homology of FMV versus CaMV, the second gives the homology of FMV versus CERV.

[d]The homologies between region VII were so low that a reliable degree of homology could not be determined.

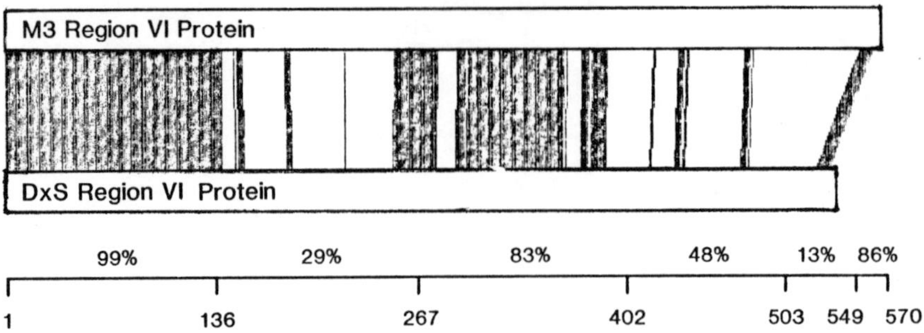

Figure 4. Amino acid homology of gene VI proteins of native figwort mosaic virus (M3 strain) and a variant (DxS strain) adapted to solanaceous hosts. The top diagram is a computer-generated plot in which a line is drawn whenever 5 of 8 successive amino acids are the same. Homologous sequences offset more than 25 amino acid residues (the size of the deletion near the C-terminal end) in either direction along the polypeptide chain were not recorded in the plot. The lower portion of the figure shows the percent amino acid homology for each sub-region of the gene (along the top of the diagram) and the amino acid boundaries of each sub-region (along the bottom of the diagram).

---

differences accounted for the biological differences in the two forms of FMV.

DISCUSSION

The molecular function for gene VI of the caulimoviruses has not been identified. Its role in mediating the virus-host interaction, however, is starting to emerge. It clearly has a major role in the initial reaction of the host to virus infection, i.e. whether the host response is hypersensitive or compatible, and systemic development of the virus. In addition to host response and host range determination, gene VI appears to be a major determinant of disease development. Perhaps all three of these phenomena are manifestations of its molecular function.

Gene VI is the only region set off from the rest of the genome by a separate promoter and a separate RNA transcript (Fig. 1). This suggests that it has some function needed very early in infection. Hence, one can speculate what this function might be. One suggestion is that P62 is needed for efficient translation of genes I through V aligned on the polycistronic 35S transcript (J.M. Bonneville - paper presented at Amer. Soc. Virology, June 1988, Austin, Texas).

The mechanism of translation of genes I through V of caulimoviruses has been the subject of much speculation. No subgenomic forms of these genes (except for gene V) have been found as RNA transcripts. If readily translatable forms of these genes occurred one might expect to find RNA transcripts with these genes in 5'-proximal positions. However, with the exception of 22S RNA which has been translated to give the gene V product (13), no subgenomic mRNA of the closely packed genes I-V have been found in previous investigations of CaMV RNA. If promoters other than the 19S promoter, leading to the production of subgenomic transcripts of CaMV occur, it seems that these RNAs would have been found. Consequently, doubt has been placed on whether these occur in infected plants and the origin of 22S RNA has not been satisfactorily explained.

The structure of the CaMV genome and its retro-transcriptional mode of replication argue against the likelihood of RNA processing to give rise to subgenomic RNAs. Processing of 35S RNA seems unlikely because of the lack of RNA splicing signals in suitable positions and the observations that intervening sequences of other genes, when inserted into the non-essential gene II position of the genome, are spliced out of the viral genome during the course of its multiplication in plants (11). This observation emphasizes the unlikely chance that a full length RNA could serve as both replicative intermediate and mRNA if it contained splicing signals for RNA processing. Reverse transcription and mRNA function, at least if the latter requires splicing, would appear to be mutually incompatible. Consequently, it seems likely that 35S RNA serves as mRNA for genes I through V and that it is translated as a polycistronic messenger. If so, perhaps P62 has some role in the efficiency of translation of this polycistronic messenger RNA. Consequently, knowledge of the specific nature of this function may provide an important clue as to how P62 perturbs host cells to cause disease.

ACKNOWLEDGEMENTS

We are grateful to the University of Kentucky for facilities and support and to Gynheung An of Washington State University, Pullman, for the pGA472 gene vector (2) used for plant transformation.

LITERATURE CITED

1. Al-Ani R, Pfeiffer P, Whitechurch O, Lesot A, Lebeurier G, Hirth L (1980). A virus specified protein produced upon infection by cauliflower mosaic virus. Ann Virol (Inst Pasteur) 131E:33-53.
2. An G, Watson BD, Stachel S, Gordon MP, Nester EW (1985). New cloning vehicles for transformation of higher plants. EMBO J 4:277-284.
3. Baughman GA, Jacobs JD, Howell SH (1988). Cauliflower mosaic virus gene VI produces a symptomatic phenotype in transgenic tobacco plants. Proc Natl Acad Sci 85:733-737.
4. Armour SL, Melcher U, Pirone TP, Lyttle DJ, Essenberg RC (1983). Helper component for aphid transmission encoded by region II of cauliflower mosaic virus DNA. Virology 129:25-30.
5. Covey SN, Hull R (1981). Transcription of cauliflower mosaic virus DNA. Detection of transcripts, properties, and location of gene encoding the virus inclusion body protein. Virology 111:463-474.
6. Daubert SD, Richins R, Shepherd RJ, Gardner R (1982). Mapping of the coat protein gene of cauliflower mosaic virus by its expression in a procaryotic system. Virology 122:444-447.
7. Daubert SD, Shepherd RJ, Gardner R (1983). Insertional mutagenesis of the cauliflower mosaic virus genome. Gene 25:201-208.
8. Daubert SD, Schoelz JE, Shepherd RJ (1984). Expression of disease symptoms of cauliflower mosaic virus genomic hybrids. Jour Mol Appl Genet 2:537-547.

9. Gardner RC, Howarth A, Hahn P, Brown-Leudi M, Shepherd RJ, Messing J (1981). The complete nucleotide sequence of an infectious clone of cauliflower mosaic virus by M13mp7 shotgun sequencing. Nucleic Acids Res 9:2871-2888.
10. Goldberg KB, Young MJ, Schoelz JE, Kiernan JM, Shepherd RJ (1987). Single gene of CaMV induces disease. Phytopathology 77:1704.
11. Hohn B, Balazs, Ruegg D, Hohn T (1986). Splicing of an intervening sequence from hybrid cauliflower mosaic virus RNA. EMBO Jour 5:2759-2762.
12. Hull R, Sadler J, Longstaff (1986). The sequence of carnation etched ring virus DNA: comparison with cauliflower mosaic virus and retroviruses. EMBO J 5:3083-3090.
13. Plant AL, Covey SN, Grierson D (1985). Detection of a subgenomic mRNA for gene V, the putative reverse transcriptase gene of cauliflower mosaic virus. Nucleic Acid Research 13:8305-8321.
14. Richins RD, Scholthof HB, Shepherd RJ (1987). Sequence of figwort mosaic virus DNA (caulimovirus group). Nucleic Acids Res 15:8451-8466.
15. Schoelz J, Shepherd RJ, Daubert SD (1986). Region VI of cauliflower mosaic virus encodes a host range determinant. Mol Cell Biol 6:2632-2637.
16. Schoelz JE, Shepherd RJ, Richins RD (1986). Properties of an unusual strain of cauliflower mosaic virus. Phytopathology 76:451-454.
17. Schoelz JE, Shepherd RJ, Daubert SD (1987). Host response to cauliflower mosaic virus (CaMV) in solanaceous plants is determined by a 496 bp DNA sequence within gene VI. In Arntzen CJ, Ryan CA (eds): "Molecular Strategies for Crop Protection" New York: Alan R. Liss, pp 253-265.
18. Schoelz JE, Shepherd RJ (1988). Host range control of cauliflower mosaic virus. Virology 162:33-42.
19. Shepherd RJ, Richins RD, Duffus JE, Handley MK (1987). Figwort mosaic virus: properties of the virus and its adaption to a new host. Phytopathology 77:1668-1673.
20. Toh H, Hayashida H, Miyata T (1983). Sequence homology between retroviral transcriptase and putative polymerases of hepatitis B virus and cauliflower mosaic virus. Nature (London) 305:827-829.
21. Volovitch M, Modjtahedi N, Yot P, Brun G (1984). RNA-dependent DNA polymerase activity in cauliflower mosaic virus-infected plant leaves. EMBO J 3:309-314.

V. IDENTIFICATION OF GENES FOR PLANT DISEASE RESISTANCE

Molecular Biology of Plant-Pathogen Interactions, pages 247-254

PLANT DEFENSE GENES INDUCED BY VIRUS INFECTION

John F. Bol,[1] Jan A.L. van Kan[1], and Ben J.C. Cornelissen[2]

[1]Department of Biochemistry, Leiden University Wassenaarseweg 64, 2333 AL Leiden, The Netherlands

[2]MOGEN International N.V., Einsteinweg 97, 2333 CB Leiden, The Netherlands

ABSTRACT cDNA clones to seven classes of mRNAs, which are induced in Samsun NN tobacco after infection with tobacco mosaic virus (TMV), were used to isolate corresponding genes from a genomic library. Five classes of clones were found to correspond to known acidic pathogenesis-related (PR) proteins or their basic homologues. Another class corresponds to genes encoding a glycine-rich protein (GRP). An analysis of the clones revealed that PR- and GRP-proteins are encoded by small multigene families some of which contain silent genes. The upstream sequences of the genes show limited homologies that may reflect cis-acting elements involved in the coordinate induction of the genes by TMV infection. Knowledge about the function of the TMV-induced tobacco proteins supports their putative role in various defense mechanisms.

INTRODUCTION

The hypersensitive response of plants to infection with viruses, fungi or bacteria induces a resistance of the plants to further infection by these pathogens and results in the *de novo* synthesis of several classes of proteins (for recent reviews see 1, 2 and 3). At least three different classes of induced proteins may be distinguished. One class of cytoplasmic proteins consist of enzymes involved in the biosynthesis of aromatic compounds such as lignin precursors or the antimicrobial phytoalexins. Another class is represented by hydroxyproline-rich glycoproteins (HRGP) of different molecular weights, that become incorporated in the plant cell walls. The HRGP or extensin molecules serve as a matrix for the attachment of the lignin network and this lignification process probably plays an important role in attempts of the plant to prevent systemic spread of a pathogen by surrounding the site of infection by an impermeable wall. The third class of proteins consists of the "pathogenesis-related" (PR) proteins that are excreted by the plant cells into the intercellular space of the leaf or accumulate in vacuoles. Such PR proteins have been observed in over 20 different plant species. We are investigating the genes encoding the PR proteins that are induced in Samsun NN tobacco by infection with tobacco mosaic virus.

PROPERTIES OF TMV-INDUCIBLE TOBACCO PROTEINS

Infection of Samsun NN tobacco with TMV induces the synthesis of at least ten acidic PR proteins which have been classified into five different groups (4). Basic homologues to at least three of these groups have been identified thus far. The molecular weights and other known properties of these proteins are listed in Table 1. The homology between the acidic proteins 1a, 1b and 1c is over 90%; they show a 65% amino acid homology to their basic counterparts (5). The higher mwt. of the basic isoform is due to a C-terminal extension of 37 amino acids. The function of PR-1 proteins is not known. PR proteins 2, N and O were recently shown to be β-1.3-glucanases; they are serologically related to a basic tobacco glucanase (6). At the amino acid sequence level, the homology between the acidic chitinases P and Q and the basic tobacco chitinase is approximately 65%; the higher mwt. of the basic isozyme is caused by a N-terminal extension of 49 amino acids (7). Plant chitinases and glucanases are believed to be involved in an anti-fungal response (1,2,3).

The three groups of basic PR's are constitutively expressed in the roots of healthy tobacco plants whereas their acidic counterparts are not (8,9). Moreover, relatively small amounts of the basic PR's are found in the intracellular fluid of TMV-infected tobacco (L.C. van Loon, personal communication), suggesting that they accumulate in the

TABLE 1
PROPERTIES OF TOBACCO PROTEINS INDUCED BY TMV INFECTION

Acidic PR proteins		Basic PR's	
Name	Mw x 10^{-3}	Mw x 10^{-3}	Properties
1a,1b,1c	15	19	unknown
2,N,O	40	33	β-1.3-glucanases
P,Q	28/30	32/34	chitinases
R	13/15	-	unknown
S	23	-	amylase/protease inhibitor?
Non PR proteins		**Mw x 10^{-3}**	**Properties**
"A"		40	unknown
GRP		15	glycine-rich

vacuoles as has been shown for the basic chitinase of bean plants (10). The acidic proteins in the intercellular space of the leaf and the basic proteins in the vacuoles may represent first and second lines of defense of the plant, respectively. Basic homologues of PR's R and S have not yet been observed. PR-S is homologous to a maize inhibitor of α-amylase and protease that is implicated in a defense against insects (11).

We have isolated cDNA clones to mRNAs encoding acidic and basic PR-1 proteins, acidic and basic chitinases, and PR-S (7,12). In addition, cDNA was cloned to two TMV-induced mRNAs that do not encode known PR proteins (12,13). One was arbitrarily named "A"-mRNA, the other is called GRP-mRNA because the encoded protein contains 25% glycine residues (GRP: glycine-rich protein). Like the PR-1 proteins, GRP is strongly inducible by spraying tobacco with a solution of salicylic acid. As this treatment inhibits virus multiplication by a specific block of viral RNA replication, the salicylic acid inducible proteins may be involved in an anti-viral response (14).

COMPLEXITY OF TMV-INDUCIBLE TOBACCO GENES

The available cDNA clones have been used as probes to estimate the number of corresponding genes in the Samsun NN genome by Southern blot hybridization. Table 2 lists the results. The number of bands seen in the genomic blots

TABLE 2
ESTIMATED COPY NUMBER OF TMV-INDUCIBLE TOBACCO GENES

PR genes	Acidic	Basic
PR-1	8	8
Chitinases	2-4	2-4
PR-S	2-4	-
Non PR genes		
"A"	8	
GRP	8	

ranged from 2 to approximately 8; as far as they have been analysed, each hybridizing DNA fragment was found to contain a single TMV-inducible gene. Probably not all these genes are expressed after TMV-infection. For instance, only three acidic PR-1 proteins and mRNAs have been identified in infected plants, suggesting that five of the eight genes for acidic PR-1 proteins are pseudo-genes.

STRUCTURE OF TMV-INDUCIBLE TOBACCO GENES

The available cDNAs have been used as probes to screen a genomic library of Samsun NN tobacco. Clones corresponding to all seven gene families listed in table 2 were obtained. The complete nucleotide sequence of genes from three classes has been deduced; the structure of genes from other classes is under investigation.

The primary structure and flanking sequences of PR-1 (acidic) genes and GRP genes was determined to permit an identification of possible common cis-acting elements involved in the coordinated induction of these genes by TMV-infection and salicylic acid treatment. The sequence of the PR-1a gene and two putatively silent PR-1 genes showed that these genes do not contain introns (5). On the other hand, elucidation of the structure of two GRP genes (GRP-4 and GRP-8) showed that these genes do contain an intron (13). Evidence from S1 nuclease mapping studies indicated that GRP-8 is expressed after TMV-infection whereas GRP-4 is not. Fig. 1 (upper panel) shows a comparison of the upstream sequences of the PR-1a and GRP-4 genes. Limited homologies were detectable within the first 90 base pairs. Preliminary experiments indicate that in the GRP gene salicylic acid responsive elements are present in this part of the promoter region whereas enhancer elements are located further upstream (J.A.L. van Kan *et al.*, manuscript in preparation).

The upstream sequences of the PR-1 and GRP genes contain a number of direct and inverted repeats (5,13). Most prominent is a 64 bp inverted repeat in the GRP sequence between nucleotides -208 and -507. A comparison with known sequences of plant genes showed that a homologous 64 bp inverted repeat is present in the upstream sequence of the rubisco small subunit (rbcS) gene of tobacco (13) (see Fig. 1, lower panel). It has been shown that there is considerable similarity in the light dependence and organ specificity in the expression of the GRP and rbcS genes of tobacco (9). It remains to be determined whether or not the 64 bp inverted repeat reflects a common regulatory element.

Recently, two homologous PR-S genes and flanking regions were sequenced (J.A.L. van Kan *et al.*, manuscript in preparation). Like the PR-1 genes, these genes do not contain introns. A comparison of the upstream sequence of the PR-S genes with the GRP and PR-1a genes revealed limited homologies, similar to those shown in Fig. 1 (upper panel).

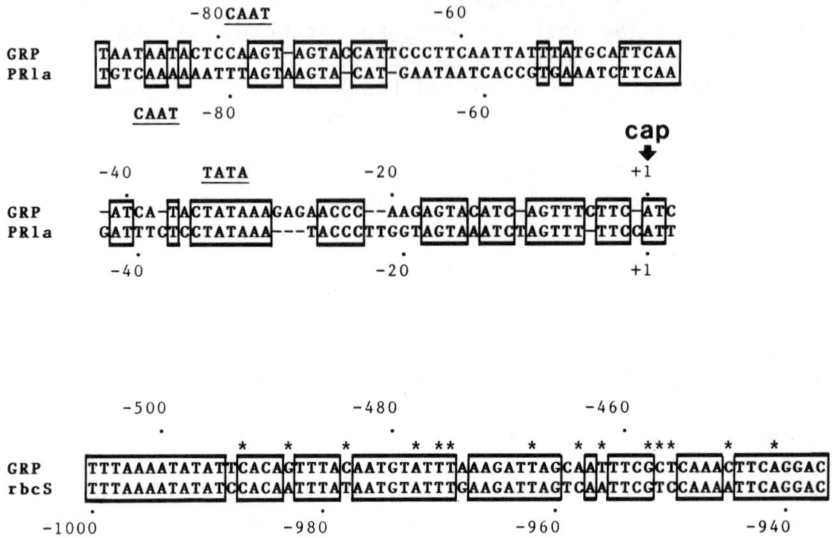

FIGURE 1. Comparison of the upstream sequence of the GRP gene with those of the tobacco PR-1a gene (upper panel) and the tobacco ribulose bisphosphate carboxylase small Subunit (rbcS) gene (lower panel). Identical nucleotides are boxed. The sequence shown in the lower panel represents a 64 bp inverted repeat occurring both in the GRP and rbcS gene. The asterisks show the mismatches in the 64 bp inverted repeat of the GRP gene. Reprinted, with permission from J.A.L. van Kan *et al.* (13).

CONCLUSIONS

The necrotic infection of plants by viruses, fungi or bacteria appears to result in the non-selective induction of a variety of defense mechanisms. The TMV-induced glucanases and chitinases are probably involved in defenses against fungi or bacteria (1,2,3,10), PR-S may be involved in an anti-insect response (11) and proteins with an antiviral function may be found among the PR's of which the function is not yet known. In tobacco, all PR's are systemically induced at places distant from the site of infection. It has been speculated that oligosaccharides, released from damaged plant cell walls by hydrolytic enzymes accumulating around the local lesions, are responsible for the systemic induction of PR genes (2). On the other hand, PR genes are differentially induced by chemicals like salicylic acid or ethylene (3), their induction is light-dependent and shows differences in organ-specificity (9). This indicates that the promoter regions of these genes must consist of a complex mosaic of different regulatory sequences. The cloning of these genes permits an analysis of the cis-acting elements and transacting factors involved in their expression under various stress-conditions.

ACKNOWLEDGEMENTS

This work was supported by the Netherlands Foundation for Chemical Research (SON) with financial aid from the Netherlands Organization for the Advancement of Pure Research (ZWO).

REFERENCES

1. Collinge DB, Slusarenko AJ (1987). Plant gene expression in response to pathogens. Plant Mol Biol 9:389.
2. Bol JF, Van Kan JAL (1988). The synthesis and possible functions of virus-induced proteins in plants. Microbiological Sciences 5:47.
3. Van Loon LC (1988). Stress proteins in infected plants. In Nester EW, Kosuge T (eds): "Plant-microbe interactions; molecular and genetic perspectives," New York: Macmillan Publ. Co., in press.
4. Van Loon LC, Gerritsen YAM, Ritter CE (1987). Identification, purification and characterization of pathogenesis-related proteins from virus-infected Samsun NN tobacco leaves. Plant Mol Biol 9:593.
5. Cornelissen BJC, Horowitz J, Van Kan JAL, Goldberg RB, Bol JF (1987). Structure of tobacco genes encoding pathogenesis-related proteins from the PR-1 group. Nucleic Acids Res 15:6799.
6. Kauffmann S, Legrand M., Geoffroy P, Fritig B (1987). Biological function of "pathogenesis-related" proteins. Four PR-proteins of tobacco have 1,3-β-glucanase activity. EMBO J 6:3209.
7. Hooft van Huijsduijnen RAM, Kauffmann S, Brederode FTh, Cornelissen BJC, Legrand M, Fritig B, Bol JF (1987) Homology between chitinases that are induced by TMV infection of tobacco. Plant Mol Biol 9:411.

8. Shinshi H, Mohnen D, Meins F (1987). Regulation of a plant pathogenesis-related enzyme: Inhibition of chitinase and chitinase mRNA accumulation in cultured tobacco tissues by auxin and cytokinin. Proc Natl Acad Sci USA 84:89.
9. Memelink J (1988). Altered gene expression in T-DNA transformed tobacco tissues. Thesis, Leiden University.
10. Boller T (1986). Hydrolytic enzymes in plant disease resistance. In Kosuge T, Nester EW (eds): "Plant-microbe interactions; Molecular and genetic perspectives," New York, MacMillan Publ Co, Vol 2, p 385.
11. Richardson M, Valdes-Rodriguez S, Blanco-Labra A (1987). A possible function for thaumatin and a TMV-induced protein suggested by homology to a maize inhibitor. Nature 327:432.
12. Hooft van Huijsduijnen RAM, Van Loon LC, Bol JF (1986). cDNA cloning of six mRNAs induced by TMV infection of tobacco and a characterization of their translation products. EMBO J 5: 2057.
13. Van Kan JAL, Cornelissen BJC, Bol JF (1988). A virus-inducible tobacco gene encoding a glycine-rich protein shares putative regulatory elements with the ribulose bisphosphate carboxylase small subunit gene. Mol Plant-Microbe Int, in press.
14. Hooft van Huijsduijnen RAM, Alblas SW, De Rijk RH, Bol JF (1986). Induction by salicylic acid of pathogenesis-related proteins and resistance to alfalfa mosaic virus infection in various plant species. J Gen Viol 67:2135.

VI. TRANSFORMATION OF PLANTS FOR EFFECTIVE VIRUS RESISTANCE

Molecular Biology of Plant–Pathogen Interactions, pages 257–267

CONTROL OF VIRAL INFECTION IN TRANSGENIC PLANTS BY EXPRESSION OF SATELLITE RNA OF CUCUMBER MOSAIC VIRUS[1]

David Baulcombe, Martine Devic, Martine Jaegle, and Bryan Harrison*

Institute of Plant Science Research (Cambridge Laboratory) Maris Lane, Trumpington, Cambridge CB2 2LQ, England

*Scottish Crop Research Institute Dundee DD2 5DA, Scotland

ABSTRACT Transgenic plants expressing multimers of benign forms of satellite RNA of cucumber mosaic cucumovirus (sat CMV) show resistance against CMV and tomato aspermy cucumovirus (TAV). The resistance has some useful attributes but is not yet ready for use in the field. Three features of sat CMV RNA have been identified which may be manipulated to improve the resistance in transgenic plants. The first is an affinity between the satellite and its helper strain which could be modified so that the satellite RNA will compete effectively against virulent strains of the satellite RNA. The second feature concerns virulence determining domains in the satellite RNA which may be modified to eliminate the possibility of releasing virulent satellites. The third feature is the low specific infectivity of the primary sat CMV transcripts in the transgenic plants. Analogy with the work on satellite RNA of tobacco ringspot virus (sat TobRSV) suggests that a transcript with high specific infectivity could arrest viral infection in the inoculated leaf.

[1]This work was supported by the Rockefeller Foundation and the Agricultural Genetics Company, Cambridge, U.K.

INTRODUCTION

Satellite RNA of cucumber mosaic cucumovirus (sat CMV) is a particularly unusual RNA molecule. Even in its largest known form (1,2) it is only 369 nucleotides long. Other forms are around 335 nucleotides in length (3,4,5,6,7). However, packed inside this short sequence is a surprising amount of functional information. Firstly, there must be sequences which are recognised by the viral RNA polymerase and which promote replication of the sat CMV. This recognition sequence is not a straightforward similarity with the viral genomic RNA, although there is some evidence for partial similarity between the viral genomic RNA and sat CMV (3). There must be, in addition, a sequence which allows sat CMV to be encapsidated in virions (8). More interestingly, however, there are functions of sat CMV which can modify the way in which the virus interacts with the host plant or which may even affect a host response directly. These interactions are seen as effects on the multiplication of the virus (9) and on symptom production (9). Some forms of sat CMV, which we designate benign satellites, cause the attenuation of CMV effects (5). Symptom expression may be reduced or eliminated as shown in Figure 1 and the amount of virus in the plant may also be reduced (9). It seemed likely therefore, if transgenic plants could be induced to express sat CMV constitutively, that the plants would resist the effects of CMV. This paper summarises our earlier work (10,11) which shows that, at least under experimental conditions, transgenic plants expressing sat CMV do resist CMV effects. It also describes newer work which is attempting to refine the resistance so that the satellite RNA strategy can be used in crop plants grown in the field.

SATELLITE RNA PRODUCED IN TRANSGENIC PLANTS IS BIOLOGICALLY ACTIVE

The general strategy for production of a new RNA in transgenic plants involves insertion of an appropriate DNA template into the expression cassette of a transformation vector. In our experiments to transform tobacco plants, the transformation vector was a binary plasmid system from *Agrobacterium tumefaciens* (12). The expression cassette comprised the 35S RNA promoter from cauliflower mosaic virus, a transcriptional terminator from the nopaline

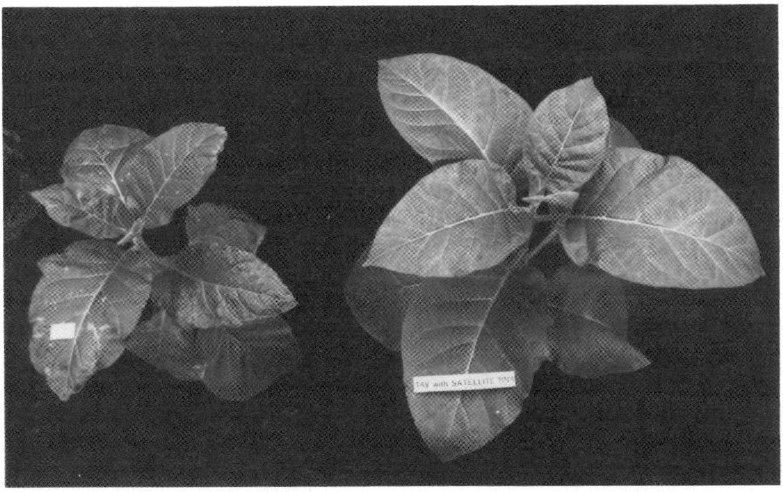

FIGURE 1. The effects of sat CMV on viral symptoms. The plant on the left was inoculated with TAV alone and the plant on the right with TAV and sat CMV.

synthase gene of <u>A. tumefaciens</u> T-DNA and various forms of cDNA of the satellite RNA of CMV (10). Two of these constructions contained complete cDNAs in head to tail multimer configurations of either 1.3 or 2.3 units. Multimeric forms of satellite RNA were used because Northern blot analysis had detected head to tail multimers of sat CMV in extracts of virus particles (Figure 2). By analogy with studies on viroids, it was considered possible that these multimers are an intermediate stage in the replication of sat CMV. If this were the situation, the multimers produced in transgenic plants would be a type of replication intermediate and would be an efficient source of biologically active satellite RNA.

Transformed plants having integrated each of these two different constructions into their nuclear DNA were tested

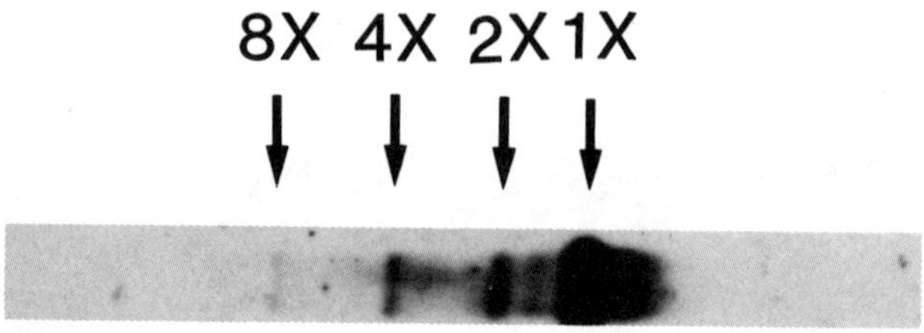

FIGURE 2. Multimers of CMV satellite RNA. A Northern blot analysis of RNA from purified virus particles with a single stranded cDNA probe of sat CMV. The monomer (1X), dimer (2X), tetramer (4X) and octamer (8X) length satellite RNAs are indicated. No hybridisation was observed with the complementary probe, confirming that these are head to tail multimers.

for production of satellite RNA, either in the absence or in the presence of CMV. In the absence of virus the satellite RNA was detected at a low level and in transcripts which corresponded to the length of cDNA which was inserted into the binary vector expression cassette. After viral infection, however, the satellite RNA was very abundant and predominantly in unit length form (10). As no satellite was detected in the non-transformed plants inoculated with CMV, it was clear that the transcribed satellite RNA in the transgenic plants was being replicated by the virus.

In all respects, this satellite RNA which was derived by replication from the primary transcripts appeared identical to natural satellite RNA. It was packaged into virions and could be spread in a secondary infection as part of the virus culture (10). Most importantly the ability to attenuate viral symptoms was also preserved and the transgenic plants showed reduced effects of CMV infection (11). As with the symptom attenuation produced when satellite RNA was included in the viral inoculum, the effect in the transgenic plants was most marked after the infection had spread into the first systemically invaded leaf. After this time, any evident symptoms faded and there was no further symptom development. A similar resistance was observed when the plants were inoculated with tomato aspermy cucumovirus (TAV), but there was no effect with other viruses either within or outside the cucumovirus group (11).

In many respects this resistance is particularly useful as, unlike resistance obtained through the expression of viral coat protein genes (13), it was not necessary to produce any foreign protein in the transgenic plants. The satellite transcripts were effective even from the lowest detectable level of expression. Presumably this is because the incoming virus amplifies the transcribed satellite RNA. This amplification may also account for our observations (11) that resistance was obtained irrespective of the amount of virus inoculated on plants.

However, the sat CMV also has features which preclude its use as part of a resistance strategy to be used in the field. These problem features arise because the resistant plants which are not showing viral symptoms may still contain substantial amounts of virus (11). This is a particular problem because not all satellite RNAs are benign on every host of CMV. For example, the satellite RNA which we have transferred to tobacco plants, from strain $I_{17}N$ (14) causes viral symptom attenuation on tobacco, but with CMV on tomato it triggers a lethal necrotic disease. A second type of satellite RNA, from the Y strain of CMV, has the same affect on CMV-infected tomato, but on tobacco induces a chlorotic symptom (15). There are satellites which are not known to cause symptom production on any plant (14), but in these instances the nucleotide sequences are similar to those of virulent satellites (2,3,4). It is possible therefore that a benign satellite in transgenic plants might mutate to a form which is virulent either on the transformed plant or on a species which could be secondarily infected from the transformed plant.

It is also possible that a strain of CMV containing a virulent satellite RNA would infect a transgenic plant and that the virulent satellite would out-compete the endogenous benign satellite. In this situation no viral attenuation would be observed. We are attempting to assess these difficulties and find solutions through an understanding of the basis of virulence and other properties in satellite RNA.

INTERACTIONS BETWEEN VIRULENT AND BENIGN SATELLITE RNAS

It has been shown previously that plants pre-infected with CMV containing a benign satellite RNA would resist the effects of a challenge infection with CMV containing virulent satellite RNA (16). As described above, however, it is possible that the challenge infection may prevail in transgenic plants, where the satellite RNA is not present initially at high levels. In order to assess the ability of satellite RNA in transgenic plants to cross protect, plants producing the $I_{17}N$ satellite RNA were challenged with CMV inocula containing the Y satellite RNA described above. Different results were observed in two types of experiment. In the first, the Y satellite RNA was combined with an isolate of CMV with which it is not naturally associated. On control plants which were not transformed this combination resulted in the production of the normal yellow chlorotic symptoms characteristic of a Y satellite infection. On the satellite-producing plants, however, the effect was a gradual amelioration of the chlorotic symptoms in the leaves which were invaded systemically at later times in the infection. RNA analysis showed that the Y satellite was gradually competed out of the virus culture.

In a second type of experiment the plants were infected with the Y satellite RNA with its natural helper strain of CMV. In this instance, no symptom attenuation was observed, although both the Y satellite and the $I_{17}N$ satellite were detected in the systemically infected leaves. This result suggests therefore that satellite RNAs vary in their affinities with different CMV strains and that this may be an important factor affecting the disease attenuation capability in satellite transformed plants exposed to infection with a CMV inoculum containing sat CMV.

THE BASIS OF SATELLITE RNA VIRULENCE

Different types of sat CMV induce different symptoms depending on the host plant. A summary of the symptoms induced by three satellite RNAs with which we work, is given in Table 1. Other known satellites of CMV may induce a white leaf symptom on tomato or may give no visible signs of their presence in the infected plant (9,17). How these effects arise is completely unknown. They may result from RNA interactions with the host, either directly or via the

TABLE 1
SYMPTOM INDUCTION BY THREE TYPES OF SAT CMV

Satellite	Tobacco symptoms	Tomato symptoms	Reference
$I_{17}N$	viral attenuation	lethal necrosis	14
Y	chlorosis	lethal necrosis	15
R	viral attenuation	viral attenuation	14

virus. Alternatively, short satellite encoded peptides may be implicated (6). In order to address these questions we are firstly attempting to identify the domains within the satellite RNA which are involved in the symptom induction. Our approach involves construction of recombinant satellite RNAs which incorporate elements of the 3 different satellite RNAs. This is achieved by manipulations of cDNAs which are inserted in derivatives of the vector pPM1 (18). This plasmid allows the production by transcription *in vitro* of satellite RNA which is highly infectious when inoculated onto plants together with CMV RNA. The conclusions from these experiments may be summarised as follows:

(1) Yellow chlorotic and necrotic symptom determinants are located in different regions of the satellite RNA. The yellow chlorotic domain is located centrally around a region where the sequence is unique to the Y satellite RNA. The necrotic domain is in the 3' part of the satellite RNA.

(2) It is unlikely that satellite encoded peptides are involved because the symptom domains are located away from the open reading frames at the extreme 5' end. Furthermore, for the necrotic domain it is not possible to identify a peptide in the 3' region which would be consistently encoded by different necrotic isolates of the satellite RNA (2,3).

The identification of these symptom forming domains now opens up the possibility of tracing the relevant interaction of the satellite RNA with other viral or host plant components. It may be possible also to remove or modify these domains so that rapid mutation to virulence would become unlikely.

THE EFFECT OF SATELLITE RNA PROCESSING

In a natural infection of CMV containing sat CMV it is likely that the satellite RNA and the CMV RNA compete for limiting amounts of replicase (19). As the infection progresses a point is reached in which the sat CMV has caused a reduction in the CMV RNA down to the minimum level necessary for continued replication of viral RNA in the plant. In contrast, in transgenic plants, production of satellite RNA is not coupled to viral RNA replication or replicase production. It was therefore expected that the relationship between viral and sat CMV synthesis would be altered so that viral RNA replication would be inhibited completely at, or close to, the site of inoculation.

In experiments with transgenic plants producing satellite RNA of tobacco ringspot virus (sat TobRSV) the challenge TobRSV infection was restricted to the inoculated leaves (20). However, with plants expressing sat CMV, the resistant plants still allowed CMV to spread systemically.

It is likely that two major reasons account for the difference between the results with sat CMV and sat TobRSV systems. Firstly, the symptom attenuation by sat CMV does not depend necessarily on a competition with the helper viral RNA. This was seen when CMV plants transformed with sat CMV were infected with TAV. Neither TAV production nor TAV RNA synthesis was reduced in systemically infected leaves, even when symptom production is almost completely inhibited (11).

Sat CMV causes inhibition of CMV accumulation in systemically infected leaves. It is quite possible therefore that sat CMV does interact competitively with CMV. However, the action in transgenic plants of sat CMV against CMV may be limited by a second factor, which is the form of sat CMV transcript in these plants.

It is now known that the sat CMV multimers, which were thought to mimic replication intermediates, will initiate replication of monomers only inefficiently. If they are replication intermediates it is probably only as part of a minor replication cycle. The inefficiency of multimer replication has been shown in experiments comparing the infectivity of _in vitro_ transcripts from multimeric and monomeric cDNA of sat CMV. The multimeric RNA was at least four orders of magnitude less infectious than monomeric cDNA and so its presence in the transgenic plants would have little effect on the final balance of sat CMV and CMV RNA.

In the plants transformed with sat TobRSV, the multimeric transcripts were processed autocatalytically into monomers so that there was a supply of active satellite RNA, even before the challenge inoculation with TobRSV (20). This active sat TobRSV could cause the inhibition of TobRSV in the inoculated leaves, as speculated above. If this interpretation is correct, the efficiency of resistance mediated by sat CMV would be improved if the constructions expressed in transgenic plants were engineered to contain the sequence elements active in autocatalysis, positioned such that active monomers would be produced (21).

FUTURE PROSPECTS

Only when a sat CMV has been disabled to prevent virulence and expressed in a highly active form in transgenic plants can it be used to engineer resistant plants. The modified sat CMV could be used also as a component of a mild strain inoculum to protect plants, as carried out already with natural benign sat CMV, in China (22).

An understanding of how sat CMV acts and is replicated may allow other satellites to be engineered from viruses which do not contain natural satellite RNAs. The studies on virulence and symptom attenuation by sat CMV may provide new information about the mechanisms of viral pathogenesis.

REFERENCES

1. Hidaka S, Ishikawa K, Takanami Y, Kubo S, Miura K (1984). Complete nucleotide sequence of RNA 5 from cucumber mosaic virus (strain Y). FEBS Letts 174:38-42.
2. Devic M, Jaegle M, Baulcombe DC (In preparation).
3. Richards KE, Jonard G, Jacquemond M, Lot H (1978). Nucleotide sequence of cucumber mosaic virus-associated RNA 5. Virology 89:395-408.
4. Gordon KHJ, Symons RH (1983). Satellite RNA of cucumber mosaic virus forms a secondary structure with partial 3'-terminal homology to genomal RNAs. Nucl Acids Res 11:947-960.

5. Collmer CW, Tousignant ME, Kaper JM (1983). Cucumber mosaic virus-associated RNA 5: X. The complete nucleotide sequence of a CARNA 5 incapable of inducing tomato necrosis. Virology 127:230-234.
6. Avila-Rincon MJ, Collmer CW, Kaper JM (1986). In vitro translation of cucumoviral satellites. I. Purification and nucleotide sequence of cucumber mosaic virus-associated RNA 5 from cucumber mosaic virus strain S. Virology 152:446-454.
7. Garcia-Arenal F, Zaitlin M, Palukaitis P (1987). Nucleotide sequence analysis of six satellite RNAs of cucumber mosaic virus: primary sequence and secondary structure alterations do not correlate with differences in pathogenicity. Virology 158:339-347.
8. Kaper JM, Waterworth HE (1981). Cucumoviruses. In Kurstak E (ed): "Handbook of Plant Virus Infections and Comparative Diagnosis," Elsevier/North Holland Biomedical press, p 258-322.
9. Mossop DW, Francki RIB (1979). Comparative studies on two satellite RNAs of cucumber mosaic virus. Virology 95:395-404.
10. Baulcombe DC, Saunders GR, Bevan MW, Mayo MA, Harrison BD (1986). Expression of biologically active viral satellite RNA from the nuclear genome of transformed plants. Nature 321:446-449.
11. Harrison BD, Mayo MA, Baulcombe DC (1987). Virus resistance in transgenic plants that express cucumber mosaic virus satellite RNA. Nature 328:799-802.
12. Bevan MW (1984). Binary Agrobacterium vectors for plant transformation. Nucl Acids Res 12:8711-8721.
13. Powell Abel P, Nelson RS, De B, Hoffman N, Rogers SG, Fraley RT, Beachy RN (1986). Delay of disease development in transgenic plants that express the tobacco mosaic virus coat protein gene. Science 232:738-743.
14. Jacquemond M, Lot, H (1981). L'ARN satellite du virus de la mosaique du concombre I. - Comparaison de l'aptitude a induire la necrose de la tomate d'ARN satellites isoles de plusieurs souches du virus. Agronomie 1:927-932.
15. Takanami Y (1981). A striking change in symptoms on cucumber mosaic virus-infected tobacco plants induced by satellite RNA. Virology 109:120-126.

16. Jacquemond M (1982). Phenomena of interferences between the two types of satellite RNA of cucumber mosaic virus. Protection of tomato plants against lethal necrosis. C R Acad Sc Paris, Serie III 294:991-994.
17. Gonsalves D, Provvidenti R, Edwards MC (1982). Tomato white leaf: the relation of an apparent satellite RNA and cucumber mosaic virus. Phytopathology 72:1533-1538.
18. Ahlquist P (1986). In vitro transcription of infectious viral RNA from cloned cDNA. Meth Enzymol 118:704-716.
19. Piazzolla P, Tousignant ME, Kaper JM (1982). Cucumber mosaic virus-associated RNA 5. IX. The overtaking of viral RNA synthesis by CARNA 5 and dsCARNA 5 in tobacco. Virology 122:147-157.
20. Gerlach WL, Llewellyn D, Haseloff J (1987). Construction of a disease resistance gene using the satellite RNA of tobacco ringspot virus. Nature 328:802-806.
21. Forster AC, Symons RH (1987). Self-cleavage of plus and minus RNAs of a virusoid and a structural model for the active sites. Cell 49:211-220.
22. Tien P, Zhang X, Qui B, Qin B, Wu G (1987). Satellite RNA for the control of plant diseases caused by cucumber mosaic virus. Ann appl Biol 111:143-152.

Molecular Biology of Plant–Pathogen Interactions, pages 269–281

GENETICALLY ENGINEERED CROSS PROTECTION AGAINST TMV INTERFERES WITH INITIAL INFECTION AND LONG DISTANCE SPREAD OF THE VIRUS

James C. Register, III, Patricia A. Powell, Richard S. Nelson, and Roger N. Beachy

Department of Biology, Washington University, St. Louis, MO 63130

ABSTRACT Experiments designed to elucidate the mechanism(s) of genetically engineered cross protection against tobacco mosaic virus (TMV) in transgenic plants are described. The TMV cDNA sequence which originally conferred protection in transgenic plants (Powell Abel, P, Nelson, RS, De, B, Hoffmann, N, Rogers, SG, Fraley, RT, Beachy, RN [1986] Science 232, 738) was specifically altered in order to compare the roles of the TMV coat protein (CP) and mRNA molecules in protection. The results of these experiments showed that CP, rather than the mRNA, was the "protecting molecule." Protoplasts from transgenic TMV CP-expressing (CP^+) plants were likewise protected against infection by TMV. Inoculation of transgenic protoplasts with TMV treated at pH 8.0 (a treatment which removes approximately one turn of CP subunits from the 5′ end of the virus) or TMV RNA overcame the protection, suggesting that initiation of virus uncoating was blocked in these cells. Two models for the mechanism of this blockage are presented. Analysis of virus spread has shown that although there is little or no inhibition of cell-to-cell spread of TMV in CP^+ plants, there is a block to long distance spread.

INTRODUCTION

The initial descriptions of a method for introducing foreign genes into higher plants (see ref. 1 for review) were accompanied by numerous predictions of a new "green revolution." While it is too early to assess the validity of these predictions, progress has been made in the use of genetic engineering in agriculture by producing virus-resistant plants. Two types of protection have successfully been demonstrated in the laboratory. The first type was originally obtained by introducing the coat (or capsid) protein (CP) gene from the common (U_1) strain of tobacco mosaic virus (TMV) into tobacco (2). These plants and their progeny were protected against infection by U_1 TMV. Because of similarities with cross protection, this protection has been termed genetically engineered cross protection (3). The second type of protection was generated when virus satellite RNAs were expressed in transgenic plants (4,5). These plants were resistant to disease caused by the virus associated with the satellite. Because protection by satellites is restricted to a limited number of viruses, genetically engineered cross protection appears to be the more generally applicable approach for producing virus resistant plants.

Genetic transformation has been used to generate plants that are protected against infection by alfalfa mosaic virus (AlMV; 6-8), potato virus X (PVX; 9), cucumber mosaic virus (CMV; 10), tobacco streak virus (11), and tobacco rattle virus (11), as well as TMV, in tobacco (2, 6-11) and tomato plants (6,12). Recently completed field tests of transgenic tomato plants expressing the TMV CP gene (CP^+) have shown that protection in the field is similar to or superior to that observed in the laboratory (12). In all examples of engineered cross protection, protection is characterized by a delay in or escape from systemic disease symptoms and virus spread following inoculation with the virus from which the protecting CP gene was isolated (2,3, 6-12). As described for classical cross protection (13), the protection against systemic disease development was reduced in plants expressing the TMV (2), AlMV (6), or PVX (9) CP genes when the concentration of virus inoculum was increased; this did not appear to be the case in CMV CP^+ plants (10). Genetically engineered cross protection is virus-specific: plants which express the AlMV CP gene are not protected against TMV infection (7), and TMV CP^+ plants show only a very low level of protection against infection by AlMV, PVX, potato virus Y, CMV, or the cowpea strain of TMV (TMV-Cc, also called sunn-hemp mosaic virus [SHMV]) (Anderson, EJ, Stark, D, Nelson, RS, Beachy, RN, manuscript in prep.). In contrast, tomato plants which expressed the TMV CP gene were protected against infection by tomato mosaic virus (12), a tobamovirus closely related to the U_1 strain of TMV (14).

Several types of studies have contributed to our understanding of the mechanism(s) of classical and engineered cross protection. Where appropriate virus-host combinations have been available, the effects of engineered cross protection on lesion development (both chlorotic and necrotic) have shown that there is a reduction in lesion numbers on the inoculated leaves of transgenic CP^+ plants. This indicates that at least part of the protection is due to inhibition of infection (3,6-9). An insight into the mechanism of classical cross protection was provided by the findings that inoculation with viral RNAs could overcome TMV- or CMV-mediated cross protection (15,16). However, Zinnen and Fulton (17) found that RNA from a severe strain of SHMV could not overcome the protection conferred by a mild strain. There are similar differences between examples of engineered cross protection. While TMV and AlMV RNAs can overcome protection in transgenic plants expressing the homologous CP gene (3,7,8), Hemenway et al. (9) reported that PVX RNA does not break down the protection in PVX CP^+ plants. The most straightforward interpretation of these results is that cross protection (classical as well as genetically engineered) is mediated by several mechanisms. Under this interpretation, protection results whenever a product or component of a virus (expressed in a plant following either virus infection or genetic transformation) inhibits infection by a second, homologous or closely related, strain. According to this definition, protection due to the accumulation of viral anti-sense RNA in transgenic plants (9,10, Powell, PA, Beachy, RN, manuscript in prep.) would be considered a type of cross protection.

Because it is difficult to address the mechanism(s) of engineered cross protection in whole plants, recent efforts in this laboratory have concentrated on analyzing TMV infection of transgenic TMV CP-expressing plants using techniques which allow the different stages of infection to be experimentally isolated.

RESULTS AND DISCUSSION

TMV Coat Protein Is Required For Protection

Because the experiments described above did not determine whether TMV CP or its mRNA was responsible for protection, experiments were designed to differentiate between these two possibilities. In addition, because the original plasmid construct contained untranslated viral sequence 3′ to the CP gene, experiments were conducted to determine if this region of the RNA (which contains a "tRNA-like" structure) was important in protection. To determine whether the mRNA function or the structural features of the transcript conferred protection, the TMV CP gene construct was modified in two ways. First, the translational capacity of the transcript was abolished by altering the sequence of the translation initiation codon using site-directed mutagenesis. Similarly, site-directed mutagenesis was used to generate a restriction site that permitted removal of over half of the 3′ untranslated region (including the sequences which encode the "tRNA-like" structure). Constructs containing either or both alteration(s) were expressed in transgenic tobacco plants, the progeny of which were tested for protection against TMV infection (Table I). No protection was observed unless CP was produced, and protection was not enhanced by the presence of the 3′ untranslated region. In addition,

TABLE 1
ROLE OF TMV COAT PROTEIN IN PROTECTION

Plant Line	CP	CP mRNA	tRNA	Protection
3011	+	+	+	+
3017	++	++	+	++
3012	+++	+++	+	+++
3030	+++	+	-	+++
3020	-	+	+	-
3051	-	+	-	-
306	-	-	-	-

Protection against systemic disease development caused by TMV infection was compared in seven transgenic tobacco plant lines. The presence or absence of the "tRNA-like" structure (+/-) as well as the relative levels of CP and CP mRNA (+, ++, +++) within these plants are shown. The criterion for infection was the appearance of vein clearing in upper canopy leaves, the first detectable visible symptom.

transgenic CP^+ lines were produced which synthesized CP at three different levels. In these lines, protection against systemic disease development increased as the CP level increased (Powell, PA and Beachy, RN, manuscript in prep.), in agreement with results previously reported for AlMV (6) and PVX (9), and confirming preliminary results obtained with the TMV CP gene under the control of different promoters (18). These results show that TMV CP is responsible for engineered cross protection against TMV.

Engineered Cross Protection In Protoplasts

Genetically engineered cross protection against both TMV and AlMV is expressed in protoplasts isolated from transgenic CP^+ plants (19,20; Fig 1A,B). To ascertain

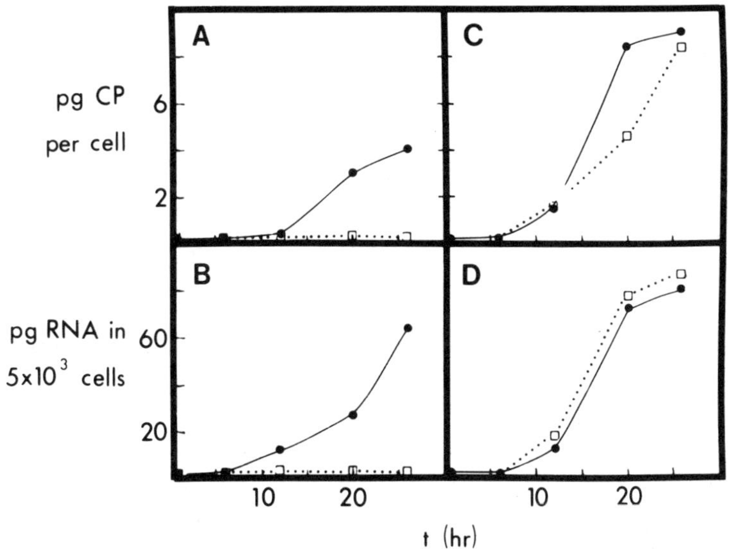

FIGURE 1. Accumulation of TMV CP and (+) strand RNA in protoplasts following inoculation with TMV or TMV RNA. Tobacco leaf mesophyll protoplasts from either transgenic CP^+ plant line 3404 (----□----) or CP^- plant line 306 (----•----) were inoculated with either 100 μg/ml of TMV (A,B) or 50 μg/ml of TMV RNA (C,D) using electroporation. Accumulation of TMV CP (A,C) or (+) strand RNA (B,D) was quantified as described (20).

whether the protection in protoplasts accurately reflects the situation in whole plants, this protection was characterized (20). Protection in protoplasts was not complete: a low percentage of CP^+ protoplasts became infected following inoculation with from 10 μg/ml to 1 mg/ml of TMV. As was the case for whole plants, protection in protoplasts could be overcome by inoculation with TMV RNA (Fig 1C,D). Finally, protection in protoplasts is virus-specific. As shown in Fig 2, inoculation of protoplasts from TMV CP^+ transgenic plants with either PVX or TMV-Cc resulted in infection, while inoculation with TMV did not.

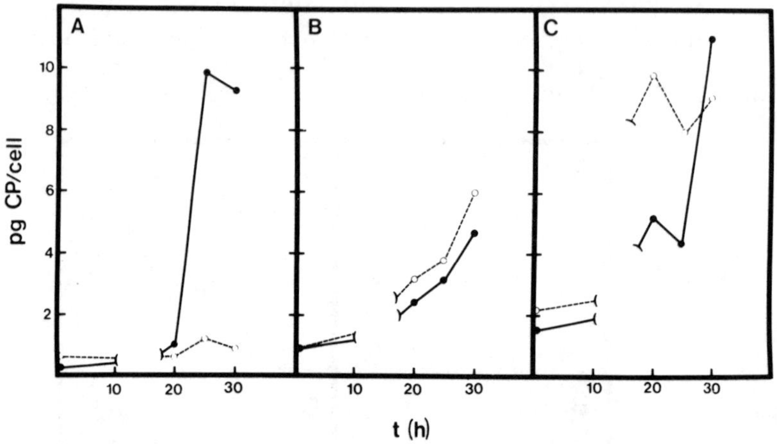

FIGURE 2. TMV CP expression in transgenic protoplasts does not confer protection against PVX or TMV-Cc infection. Leaf mesophyll protoplasts from transgenic CP^- tobacco lines 306 (——•——) or CP+ line 3646 (----o----) were inoculated with 50 μg/ml of TMV (A), PVX (B), or TMV-Cc (C) using polyethylene glycol (20). Virus replication was correlated with CP accumulation which was quantified using a dot immunobinding assay (3).

Unlike the situation in whole plants (2), protection in single cells is an all-or-none response; virus replication per infected cell (assayed by quantifying TMV CP accumulation) was similar in infected CP^+ and infected nonexpressor (CP^-) cells. In addition, protection was not overcome by high concentrations of virus inoculum as is the case in whole plants. We suggest that this result reflects the difference between protection in inoculated cells and a second type of protection, present in whole plants, which prevents systemic spread of the virus. The similarity of the protection in protoplasts and in the inoculated leaves of whole plants led us to use protoplasts for studying the mechanism of protection against TMV (20).

The finding that protection is expressed in protoplasts showed that a stage of infection prior to virus spread is blocked in CP^+ cells. This conclusion is supported by results with whole plants which showed that 100-fold more TMV was required to produce single sites of infection on CP^+ plants than on CP^- plants (Powell, PA, Nelson, RS, and Beachy, RN, manuscript in prep.). The finding that RNA replication was inhibited in protected cells (Fig 1B) showed that protection resulted from blockage of an event prior to RNA replication (20). Since viral RNA overcomes protection (Fig 1C,D) it can be argued that the blockage precedes release of viral RNA. To further define where the blockage occurs, we made use of the fact that as pH is increased, CP is progressively removed from TMV in a 5′ to 3′ direction (the same direction in which uncoating occurs *in vivo*; for review, see 21). The most subtle of these effects is observed at pH 8.0, where the *in vitro* translatability of the treated virus increases dramatically (22) in the absence of discernible alterations in virus structure (20,22). It has been proposed that pH 8.0 treatment removes the last turn of CP from the 5′ end of the virus rod (22). When pH 8.0-treated TMV was used to inoculate TMV CP^+ protoplasts, the protection was overcome as it was when the inoculum was TMV RNA (20). This suggests that the blockage of infection in TMV CP^+ cells is at or prior to initiation of uncoating. Treated virus also overcame protection in transgenic CP^+ local lesion host plants (20).

These results led us to propose two alternate explanations for how TMV CP could block TMV uncoating in transgenic plant cells (Fig 3). The first model proposes that there are specific sites in plant cells where TMV disassembly occurs. If these sites have an affinity for TMV CP (Fig 3, path a), the CP present in transgenic cells might physically block these sites and prevent TMV from binding and being disassembled (Fig 3B, path a, step 2). While this mechanism would require little endogenous CP (CP accumulates to relatively low levels in the transgenic protected plants; 2) it also proposes that specific "receptor-like" sites exist in plant cells - to date there is no evidence for the existence of such sites.

The second model proposes that CP-CP interactions are

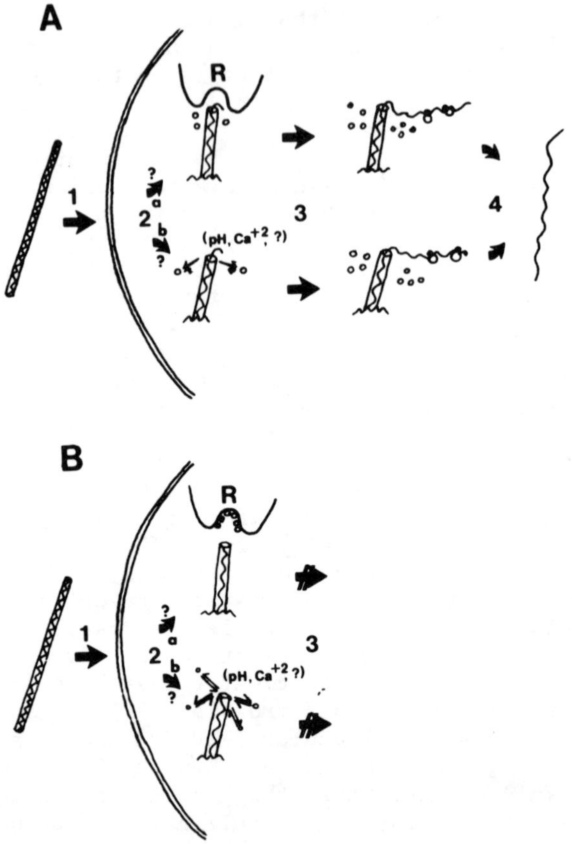

Figure 3. A model for the blockage of TMV uncoating in transgenic TMV CP^+ cells. Following entry (step 1) of TMV into either CP^- (A) or CP^+ (B) cells, virus uncoating initiates (step 2). Two ways in which this could occur are shown. In path a, interaction of TMV rods with an uncoating site (R) having a specific affinity for TMV CP initiates uncoating. In path b, local intracellular conditions favoring virus disassembly initiate uncoating. In CP^- cells, cotranslational disassembly ensues (step 3) and ultimitely a completely stripped viral RNA is released (step 4). In CP^+ cells, uncoating cannot initiate because of blockage of the uncoating site (path a) or because of a shifting of the disassembly kinetics such that virus disassembly is no longer favored (path b).

responsible for protection. If TMV uncoating occurs *in vivo* because of localized conditions which kinetically favor virus disassembly (for review, see 21), the presence of endogenous CP in transgenic cells could shift these kinetics, causing a fully assembled virus structure to be maintained (Fig 3, path b). It has been suggested that an extra turn of CP subunits exists on the ends of TMV rods, protecting the viral RNA ends from nucleolytic attack (23). This extra turn could potentially exist in equilibrium with free endogenous CP in transgenic cells, thereby preventing initiation of cotranslational disassembly. While both mechanisms are consistent with the observations about genetically engineered cross protection, including virus specificity, the latter mechanism does not require specific sites for virus uncoating.

Although no evidence exists to favor either mechanism, they appear to be experimentally testable. If the first mechanism is correct, a distinct threshold level of intracellular CP concentration should exist (correlating with the amount of CP required to saturate all uncoating sites) below which protection drops off markedly. Conversely, decreasing the intracellular CP concentration should gradually decrease protection if the second mechanism is valid. Determining the molecular details of the earliest manifestations of genetically engineered cross protection awaits completion of such experiments.

Engineered Cross Protection Inhibits Long Distance Spread

There are two types of virus spread in infected plants: local (or cell-to-cell) and long distance. It has been postulated that plasmodesmata provide the pathway for cell-to-cell-spread of virus and it is known that long distance spread occurs in the plant's vascular system (for review, see 24). Although TMV apparently spreads throughout a susceptible host as a nucleoprotein particle, the nature of this particle remains unknown. Because of these uncertainties and because it is a formidable task to experimentally isolate the process of virus spread, research in these areas has been slow to develop. Despite this, we are beginning to gain an understanding of the effects of genetically engineered cross protection on both processes.

The spread of TMV has been analyzed by inoculating TMV RNA onto small areas of leaves using tapered and polished ends of pasteur pipettes (the microinoculation procedure;

25,26). This technique allows for inoculation of small, yet reproducibly sized, leaf areas and provides a way to generate known numbers of infection sites. Inoculation of CP^+ and CP^- systemic host tobacco plants was carried out with TMV RNA such that equal numbers of infection sites were established on both plant genotypes. Cell-to-cell spread of virus was quantitated by removing several concentric rings of tissue surrounding the inoculation points and determining the amount of TMV within each sample by ELISA. Under these conditions, there was no difference in the rate of cell-to-cell spread of virus between the two plant types (Powell, PA, Nelson, RS, Beachy, RN, manuscript in prep.).

This approach was also used to examine the effects of genetically engineered cross protection on long distance spread. In such experiments, a delay in virus movement into the upper leaves of CP^+ plants and atypical symptom development on these leaves was observed compared to leaves from CP^- plants (Powell, PA, Nelson, RS, Beachy, RN, manuscript in prep.). Protection against systemic spread of TMV has also been examined by an independent experimental approach. When a leaf-bearing stem segment from a transgenic TMV CP^+ tobacco plant was grafted between lower and upper canopy sections from a CP^- tobacco plant, systemic movement of TMV into the upper canopy leaves was inhibited following infection of the lower nontransformed leaves (Wisniewski, LA, and Beachy, RN, manuscript in prep.). Although the role of the leaf in the CP^+ stem segment is not understood, we can conclude from these results that while genetically engineered cross protection against TMV has little or no effect on cell-to-cell virus spread it does interfere with long distance virus spread.

Taken together, these results demonstrate that genetically engineered cross protection can act by interfering with two events in virus infection and disease development. First, TMV CP produced in transgenic cells can block uncoating of the challenge virus. If a virus evades this block and sets up local sites of infection, systemic movement of the virus can subsequently be blocked. Although the mechanism responsible for protection in protoplasts and inoculated leaves is fairly well understood, the mechanism(s) responsible for inhibition of long-distance spread remains to be elucidated and may or may not be the same as that characterized in protoplasts. Finally, it appears that additional, or alternate, mechanisms are involved in genetically engineered cross protection against PVX (9) and perhaps CMV (1(. ; is possible that as viral CP-mediated engineered cross protection is extended to other classes of viruses additional mechanisms for protection will be identified.

ACKNOWLEDGEMENTS

The authors thank Dr. Milton Zaitlin for antibodies against TMV-Cc, Mike Dyer and Sally Leitner for greenhouse maintenance of plants, and Nancy Burkhart for expert secretarial assistance. This work was funded by a grant from the Monsanto Company. JCR III is a recipient of a Postdoctoral Fellowship in Plant Biology from the National Science Foundation awarded in 1986.

REFERENCES

1. Schell, JSt (1987) Transgenic plants as tools to study the molecular organization of plant genes. Science 237, 1176.
2. Powell Abel, P, Nelson, RS, De B, Hoffmann, N, Rogers, SG, Fraley, RT, Beachy, RN (1986) Delay of disease development in transgenic plants that express the tobacco mosaic virus coat protein gene. Science 232, 738.
3. Nelson, RS, Powell Abel, P, Beachy, RN (1987) Lesions and virus accumulation in inoculated transgenic tobacco plants expressing the coat protein gene of tobacco mosaic virus. Virology 158, 126.
4. Harrison, BD, Mayo, MA, Baulcombe, DC (1987) Virus resistance in transgenic plants that express cucumber mosaic virus satellite RNA. Nature 328, 799.
5. Gerlach, WL, Llewellyn, D, Haselhoff, J (1987) Construction of a plant disease resistance gene from the satellite RNA of tobacco ringspot virus. Nature 328, 802.
6. Tumer, NE, O'Connell, KM, Nelson, RS, Sanders, PR, Beachy, RN, Fraley, RT, Shah, DM (1987) Expression of alfalfa mosaic virus coat protein gene confers cross-protection in transgenic tobacco and tomato plants. EMBO J 6, 1181.
7. Loesch-Fries, LS, Merlo, D, Zinnen, T, Burhop, L, Hill, K, Krahn, K, Jarvis, N, Nelson, S, Halk, E (1987) Expression of alfalfa mosaic virus RNA4 in transgenic plants confers virus resistance. EMBO J 6, 1845.

8. Van Dun, CMP, Bol, JF, van Vloten-Doting, L (1987) Expression of alfalfa mosaic virus and tobacco rattle virus coat protein genes in transgenic tobacco plants. Virology 159, 299.
9. Hemenway, C, Fang, R-X, Kaniewski, WK, Chua, N-H, Tumer, NE (1988) Analysis of the mechanism of protection in transgenic plants expressing the potato virus X coat protein gene or its antisense RNA. EMBO J 7, 1273.
10. Cuozzo, M, O'Connell, KM, Kaniewski, WK, Fang, R-X, Chua, N-H, Tumer, NE (1988) Viral protection in transgenic plants expressing the cucumber mosaic virus coat protein or its antisense RNA. Bio/Technology 6, 549.
11. Van Dun, CMP, Overduin, B, van Vloten-Doting, L, Bol, J (1988) Expression of viral cDNA in transgenic plants and cross-protection. J Cellular Biochem Suppl. 12C, 298.
12. Nelson, RS, McCormick, SM, Delanney, X, Dube, P, Layton, J, Anderson, EJ, Kaniewski, M, Proksch, RK, Horsch, RB, Rogers, SG, Fraley, RT, Beachy, RN (1988) Virus tolerance, plant growth, and field performance of transgenic tomato plants expressing coat protein from tobacco mosaic virus. Bio/Technology 6, 403.
13. Cassells, AC, Herrick, CC (1977) Cross protection between severe and mild strains of tobacco mosaic virus in doubly infected tomato plants. Virology 78, 253.
14. Van Regenmortel, MHV (1986) Tobacco mosaic virus: antigenic structure. In Van Regenmortel, MHV, Fraenkel-Conrat, H, (eds.): "The Plant Viruses" Vol 2. New York:Plenum Press, p. 79.
15. Sherwood, JL, Fulton, RW (1982) The specific involvement of coat protein in tobacco mosaic virus cross protection. Virology 119, 150.
16. Dodds, JA, Lee, SQ, Tiffany, M (1985) Cross-protection between strains of cucumber mosaic virus: effect of host and type of inoculum on accumulation of virions and double-stranded RNA of the challenge strain. Virology, 144, 301.
17. Zinnen, TM, Fulton, RW (1986) Cross-protection between sunn-hemp mosaic and tobacco mosaic viruses. J Gen Virol 67,1679.
18. Beachy, RN, Powell Abel, P, Nelson, RS, Register III, JC, Tumer, N, Fraley, R. (1987) Genetic engineering of plants for protection against virus diseases. In "Plant Resistance to Viruses" CIBA Foundation Symp.

133. Chichester, Wiley, p. 151.
19. Loesch-Fries, LS, Halk, E, Merlo, D, Jarvis, N, Nelson, S, Krahn, K, Burhop, L (1987) Expression of alfalfa mosaic virus coat protein gene and antisense cDNA in transgenic tobacco tissue. In Arntzen, CJ, Ryan, C (eds.): "Molecular Strategies For Crop Protection," New York: Alan R. Liss, Inc., p. 221.
20. Register, III, JC, Beachy, RN Resistance to TMV in transgenic plants results from interference with an early event in infection. (manuscript submitted).
21. Wilson, TMA, Shaw, JG (1985) Does TMV uncoat cotranslationally in vivo? Trends in Biochemical Sciences 10, 57.
22. Wilson, TMA (1985) Cotranslational disassembly of tobacco mosaic virus in vitro. Virology 137, 255.
23. Butler, JG (1984) The current picture of the structure and assembly of tobacco mosaic virus. J Gen Virol 65, 253.
24. Atabekov, JG, Dorkhov, YuL (1984) Plant virus-specific transport function and resistance of plants to viruses. Adv Virus Res 29, 313.
25. Hooker, WJ, Benson, AP (1960) Time of symptom response in Datura tatula L. to potato virus X as a function of virus concentration. Virology 10, 245.
26. Konate, G, Fritig, B (1984) An efficient microinoculation procedure to study plant virus multiplication at predetermined individual infection sites on the leaves. Phytopathol Z 109, 131.

Molecular Biology of Plant-Pathogen Interactions, pages 283-296

RESISTANCE TO ALFALFA MOSAIC VIRUS IN TRANSGENIC TOBACCO AND ALFALFA

E.L. Halk, D.J. Merlo, L.W. Liao, N.P. Jarvis, S.E. Nelson, K.J. Krahn, K.K. Hill, K.E. Rashka, and L.S. Loesch-Fries

Agrigenetics Advanced Science Company
5649 E. Buckeye Road
Madison, Wisconsin 53716

ABSTRACT *Agrobacterium*-mediated gene transfer from a binary vector was used to produce transgenic tobacco plants that expressed the coat protein of alfalfa mosaic virus. Tobacco plants accumulating AMV coat protein under the direction of the cauliflower mosaic virus 19S or 35S promoters at 0.05% of soluble protein or higher were resistant to infection by AMV. The resistance or susceptibility of protoplasts from transgenic tobacco plants corresponded to that of the plant from which they were derived. Genotypes of five cultivars of alfalfa were also transformed using a binary vector carrying the AMV coat protein gene. Coat protein accumulation in the regenerated alfalfa transformants ranged from 5 to 493 ng per mg soluble protein. Protoplasts from four of these plants that expressed a high level of AMV coat protein were resistant to infection by AMV. Protoplasts from a low expresser were not resistant; therefore, there was a correlation between high levels of coat protein accumulation and resistance.

INTRODUCTION

Agrobacterium-mediated transformation of plants provides a means to investigate the role of individual genes or gene products in virus replication and disease development. Transgenic plants have been used to determine if the expression of specific viral genes in transgenic plants can confer resistance to infection by the virus. This approach is based on the phenomenon of cross-protection whereby a virus-infected plant becomes resistant to subsequent infection by related strains of the same virus. In a previous report (1), we have shown that expression of the alfalfa mosaic virus (AMV) coat protein gene under the direction of the cauliflower mosaic virus (CaMV) 19S promoter in tobacco conferred resistance to AMV infection. Our study showed that transgenic plants expressing a relatively high level of AMV coat protein (about 0.05% of soluble protein) were resistant to AMV, whereas plants expressing coat protein at one eighth this level were not resistant to infection. Resistance to AMV infection in transgenic plants mimicked the type of resistance observed by Sherwood and Fulton (2) and Dodds _et al_. (3) in cross-protection studies with tobacco mosaic virus and cucumber mosaic virus: _viz_., our transgenic plants were resistant to more than one strain of AMV but not resistant to an unrelated virus, and the transgenic plants were resistant to infection by AMV virions but not AMV RNA. The latter observation supports the hypothesis of Sherwood and Fulton (2) that coat protein plays a major role in cross-protection by inhibiting the uncoating of virus particles at an early stage of infection. Recently, the expression of other virus coat proteins in transgenic plants has been shown to confer resistance to infection by the viruses from which the coat proteins were derived (4-8).

We have regenerated transgenic tobacco and alfalfa plants that express the AMV coat protein gene under direction of the CaMV 35S promoter and tobacco plants that express a non-structural protein (P3) of AMV. In this report we present only the studies of the protein expression and disease resistance of transgenic tobacco and alfalfa plants that express the AMV coat protein gene; studies of P3 expression in tobacco will be presented elsewhere. Tobacco was used as a model plant; AMV does not cause an economically important disease in tobacco. Alfalfa, however, suffers significant yield depression when infected by AMV (9-15). Alfalfa cultivars exhibit a wide spectrum of susceptibility to AMV, ranging from susceptible to many strains through susceptible to a few strains to immune to many strains (16). Genetic resistance to one strain of AMV has been described in alfalfa; however, it was inherited as a recessive trait (17). We expect that expression of AMV coat protein in transgenic alfalfa plants will provide dominant resistance to multiple AMV strains. Transformation and regeneration of two species of alfalfa, *Medicago sativa* L. (18,19) and *Medicago varia* (20), have been reported, but only marker genes were inserted. This is the first report of alfalfa expressing a foreign gene of potentially economic importance.

METHODS

Vectors

Binary vectors were used to transform tobacco and alfalfa with the AMV coat protein gene. The pH400A4 vector contains the AMV coat protein gene under the direction of the CaMV 19S promoter (1). Figure 1 describes the vector pH575-35S-A4 which contains the coat protein gene under the direction of the CaMV 35S promoter (21).

Plant Transformation and Regeneration

Tobacco (*Nicotiana tabacum* L. cv. Xanthi-nc) was transformed and regenerated as previously described (1). Alfalfa (*Medicago sativa* L.) was transformed with *Agrobacterium tumefaciens* strain LBA4404 containing the vector pH575-35S-A4. Genotypes that could be regenerated from five cultivars of alfalfa were identified as described by Brown and Atanassov (22). Following co-cultivation, kanamycin-resistant alfalfa calli developed on the explants in six to eight weeks. Mature embryos were removed from calli as they appeared and were allowed to germinate on MS medium. Control plants were treated in the same manner but were neither incubated with *Agrobacterium* nor placed on kanamycin-containing medium. Regenerated plants were transplanted to soil mix and maintained in a growth chamber under a 16 hr photoperiod at 120 mE with temperatures of 22°C (day) and 20°C (night).

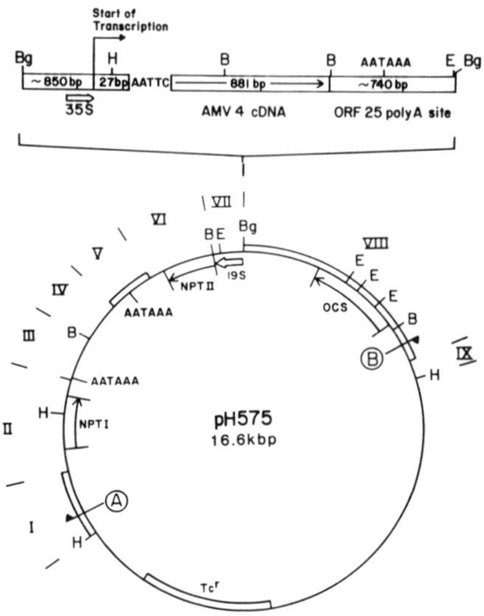

FIGURE 1. Map of the AMV binary vector, pH575-35S-A4. The vector carries a cDNA copy of AMV RNA 4 under control of the CaMV 35S promoter and is terminated by the T-DNA ORF 25 RNA polyadenylation signals. pH575 is a "micro Ti" binary vector described by Firoozabady et al. (24). Abbreviations are as follows: "AATAAA", RNA polyadenylation signal; 19S or 35S, CaMV 19S or 35S promoter sequence; OCS, octopine synthase sequence; NPT II, neomycin phosphotransferase II sequence; NPT I, prokaryotic neomycin phosphotransferase I sequence; Tc^r, tetracycline resistance sequence; B, Bg, E, and H, recognition sites for restriction endonucleases BamHI, BglII, EcoRI, and HindIII, respectively.

Analysis of Transformed Plants

Analyses of DNA and RNA, quantitation of coat protein and gene copy number, and assays of virus susceptibility were done as previously described (1). Protoplast isolation and inoculation methods have been previously described (23). Virions and RNA of AMV strain 425 were used for inoculation (1).

RESULTS

Transgenic Tobacco

The pH575-35S-A4 vector, containing the AMV coat protein gene under the direction of the CaMV 35S promoter and terminated by T-DNA Orf 25 poly(A) site, was used to transform tobacco. The level of AMV coat protein in 34 transformants ranged from 330 to 1300 ng coat protein per mg soluble protein (ng cp/mg p). Genetic analysis of the progeny was used to determine the copy number of the NPT II locus (the selectable marker) and presumably of the linked coat protein gene. Coat protein levels in transformants containing a single locus ranged from 330 to 760 ng cp/mg p; coat protein levels in transformants with two or more loci ranged from 340 to 1300 ng cp/mg p. In contrast, coat protein levels in the 33 regenerants from transformations with pH400A4, containing the AMV coat protein gene under the control of the CaMV 19S promoter and terminated by the CaMV poly(A) site, ranged from 25 to 560 ng cp/mg p. Only 4 of these 33 plants contained AMV coat protein at greater than 150 ng cp/mg p. Genetic analysis of the progeny of these four high expressers indicated that these plants had two loci of the AMV gene.

The pH575-35S-A4 transformant 105-2, which contains the coat protein gene at a single locus and expresses approximately 350 ng cp/mg p, and the pH400A4 transformant 14-1, which contains the coat protein gene at two loci and expresses approximately 540 ng cp/mg p, were compared in a further study. Two classes of 105-2 self-crossed progeny and 14-1 self-crossed progeny, those that expressed no detectable coat protein (non-expressers) and those that contained high levels of coat protein (expressers), were inoculated with AMV. The high level expressers developed significantly fewer lesions on inoculated leaves than their non-expressing counterparts, indicating resistance to primary (local) infection (Table 1). To analyze resistance to secondary (systemic) infection, young uninoculated leaves of inoculated progeny were assayed by ELISA for the presence of AMV. Non-expressers contained high concentrations of virus in young leaves. One of the six inoculated 105-2 high expressers contained a high concentration of virus in young uninoculated leaves 20

TABLE 1
RELATIVE SUSCEPTIBILITY OF TRANSGENIC TOBACCO PROGENY TO AMV INFECTION

Transformant	Average Number of Lesions per half leaf: Expressers	Average Number of Lesions per half leaf: Non-expressers	Relative Susceptibility[a]
105-2	0.16±0.05(6)[b]	36±16(6)	0.5%
14-1	3±5(9)[c]	22±9(8)[c]	14.0%[c]

[a]Relative susceptibility is defined as (number of lesions per half leaf on expressers ÷ number of lesions per half leaf on non-expressers) x 100.

[b]Numbers in parentheses denote the number of inoculated plants.

[c]Data from Experiment 1, Table III, ref. 1.

(Reprinted from EMBO J (1) with permission of IRL Press.)

days after inoculation, while the other 5 plants did not contain detectable levels of virus in uninoculated leaves. As reported previously, 14-1 high expressers showed a delay of systemic spread relative to control plants and some expressers did not develop systemic infection up to 16 days after inoculation (1). The results suggest that systemic virus infection was either delayed or prevented in these transgenic plants.

Protoplasts from transgenic and control plants were inoculated with AMV to determine if resistance to virus infection in protoplasts was similar to that of the whole plant. Only a small percentage of protoplasts from transformants 105-2 and 105-5, expressing coat protein under control of the CaMV 35S promoter, became infected following inoculation (Table 2). Similarly, inoculation of protoplasts from 14-1, expressing coat protein under control of the CaMV 19S promoter, also resulted in a low percentage of infection, whereas greater than half of the protoplasts from an untransformed Xanthi-nc became infected. This confirms and extends our previously reported results that demonstrated that transgenic protoplasts accumulating a relatively high level of virus coat protein are virus resistant (25).

TABLE 2
VIRUS SUSCEPTIBILITY OF TRANSGENIC TOBACCO PROTOPLASTS

Protoplast Source	Infected Protoplasts (%)
Experiment 1	
Xanthi- nc	54
14-1	9
105-2	2
Experiment 2	
Xanthi-nc	62
14-1	14
105-5	5

Inoculum for 10^5 protoplasts consisted of 1-5 μg of AMV virions. Protoplasts were assayed for infection by an immunofluorescent assay that discriminated between infected and uninfected protoplasts.

Transgenic Alfalfa

Following co-cultivation with Agrobacterium containing the pH575-35S-A4 vector, plants from five alfalfa cultivars were regenerated. Forty percent of the 240 regenerated plants expressed coat protein. The levels of AMV coat protein in some of these plants are shown in Table 3. Transformants of genotype K2H1 which were regenerated from a single callus were low expressers. Similar results were obtained for transformants from single calli of genotypes K2H4 and K2H5. The six transformants from a single callus of genotype K2H2 accumulated much higher levels of coat protein, up to 493 ng cp/mg p, while the transformants from a single callus of K2H3 exhibited a broad range of protein expression. DNA analyses were performed to identify plants carrying distinctive gene insertion patterns. The DNAs were digested with BamHI, and the fragments were separated by electrophoresis, blotted to

TABLE 3
EXPRESSION OF AMV COAT PROTEIN IN TRANSGENIC ALFALFA

Transformant[a]	Amount of Coat Protein (ng/mg soluble protein)
K2H1-10-1-1	13
K2H1-10-1-2	17
K2H1-10-1-3	6
K2H1-10-1-4	5
K2H1-10-1-6	26
K2H2-11-1	162
K2H2-11-2	477
K2H2-11-3	368
K2H2-11-5	423
K2H2-11-6	369
K2H2-11-7	493
K2H3-4-1-2	13
K2H3-4-1-3	24
K2H3-4-1-4	29
K2H3-4-1-9	236
K2H3-4-1-11	148
K2H4-28-2-1	27
K2H4-28-2-2	41
K2H4-28-2-3	43
K2H4-28-2-4	30
K2H5-4-2-1	15
K2H5-4-2-2	13

[a]Individual transformants listed arose from a single callus of genotype K2H1, K2H2, K2H3, K2H4, or K2H5. The genotypes are from five separate cultivars.

nylon membrane and hybridized to probes for NPT I, NPT II, AMV cDNA, or OCS. All K2H1 regenerants had an identical DNA pattern with the expected BamHI fragments of the T-DNA (Fig. 1). The DNA patterns of three of the regenerants of genotype K2H2 that were tested were also identical to each other but differed from genotype K2H1 regenerants; the left T-DNA was shorter than expected and did not contain NPT I. These data suggest that K2H1 regenerants are siblings, as are three K2H2 regenerants. The DNA patterns of the three low expressers of genotype K2H3 were different from each other, suggesting that they arose from independent transformation events. The DNA of the two high expressers from K2H3 and of the regenerants from K2H4 and K2H5 have not been analyzed.

The resistance of transgenic tobacco protoplasts to infection proved to be a reliable predictor of resistance of intact transgenic tobacco (Table 2). Therefore, we inoculated protoplasts from transformed alfalfa plants to ascertain their virus susceptibility. Inoculation of protoplasts from four high-level expressers of genotype K2H2 resulted in a significantly lower frequency of infection than in untransformed controls (Table 4). Protoplasts from a transgenic plant that accumulated a low level of coat protein, genotype K2H1, were as susceptible to AMV as were untransformed control protoplasts. These results suggest that high levels of coat protein accumulation are required for virus resistance in alfalfa, as was previously determined in tobacco (1). Experiments to determine the virus susceptibility of intact transgenic alfalfa plants are in progress.

While the amount of coat protein in the K2H1-10-1-4 low expresser was insufficient for protection from infection by AMV virions, it was possible that it would complement the infectivity of an AMV RNA preparation lacking coat protein or its mRNA. AMV RNA is not infectious unless RNA 4 or coat protein is present (26). Table 4 shows that only a small percentage of untransformed protoplasts of genotype K2H1 were infected when exposed to RNAs 1+2+3. This slight infectivity is probably due to residual RNA 4 in the RNA 1+2+3 preparation. In contrast, protoplasts from the K2H1-10-1-3 low expresser exhibited a five-fold higher level of infection, similar to that obtained when untransformed K2H1 protoplasts were exposed to AMV virions. Apparently, 6 ng cp/mg p is sufficient to promote infection but not enough to confer virus resistance.

TABLE 4
SUSCEPTIBILITY OF TRANSGENIC ALFALFA PROTOPLASTS TO INFECTION BY AMV

Protoplast Source	Inoculum[a]	Coat Protein Accumulation in Transgenic Plants (ng/mg protein)	Infected Protoplasts (%)
Experiment 1			
K2H2, untransformed	AMV	0	47.0
K2H2-11-6	AMV	369	2.4
K2H2-11-7	AMV	493	1.6
Experiment 2			
K2H2, untransformed	AMV	0	72.0
K2H2-11-2	AMV	477	1.6
K2H2-11-5	AMV	423	0.4
Experiment 3			
K2H1, untransformed	AMV	0	22.0
K2H1-10-1-4	AMV	5	27.0
Experiment 4			
K2H1, untransformed	AMV RNA1+2+3	0	5.4
K2H1-10-1-3	AMV RNA1+2+3	6	25.0

[a]Inoculum consisted of 5 μg/ml of AMV or 2 μg/ml AMV RNA 1+2+3.

DISCUSSION

We have examined the expression of the AMV coat protein gene in transgenic tobacco and alfalfa. Transgenic tobacco plants containing the AMV coat protein gene directed by the CaMV 35S promoter were compared to plants in which this gene was directed by the CaMV 19S promoter. The respective gene constructs also differed in the leader and polyadenylation sequences. A high level of expression of coat protein was achieved in plants containing a single gene copy under control of the 35S promoter, while two gene copies under control of the 19S promoter were needed to achieve similar expression levels. Therefore, the gene construct containing the 35S promoter is preferred because the transformants are genetically simplier. Analysis of virus susceptibility of progeny from transformant 105-2 showed that expression from a single locus gave excellent resistance at both primary (local) and secondary (systemic) levels.

This is the first report of transgenic alfalfa expressing a foreign gene other than ones from the T-DNA of Agrobacterium or a selectable marker, such as NPT II. The expression of the gene construct directed by the CaMV 35S promoter in transgenic alfalfa resulted in the accumulation of up to nearly 500 ng cp/mg p, whereas in transgenic tobacco, up to 1300 ng cp/mg p accumulated. This suggests that the plant species influenced relative expression levels (27).

Viral resistance was observed in protoplasts isolated from transgenic alfalfa plants expressing high levels of the AMV coat protein. Studies of whole plants are in progress; nonetheless, our studies of the viral resistance of protoplasts and whole plants of transgenic tobacco indicate that the protoplast system is valid for predicting resistance of the intact plant. Protoplasts from transgenic alfalfa expressing low levels of coat protein were not resistant to AMV infection. The expression of coat protein in these protoplasts complemented the infectivity of AMV RNAs 1+2+3 which are not infectious in the absence of coat protein or its mRNA, RNA 4. These results show that a small amount of coat protein is enough to complement non-infectious AMV RNA but is not enough to confer virus resistance. Therefore, it is likely that the capacity of transgenic plants to exhibit virus resistance will not be simply a consequence of their ability to produce biologically active coat protein, but also to accumulate a sufficient amount of the protein.

Alfalfa is the major forage legume in North America. AMV is the predominant virus infecting this crop and is often found in 1-3% of the seeds of commercial seed lots (28). Aphids, the virus vector, quickly spread the disease throughout a field. Disease control is largely ineffective; most of the plants in mature alfalfa stands are virus-infected (9,10,29). Incorporation of virus resistance into elite alfalfa cultivars has the potential to significantly improve yield and perhaps to increase the longevity of alfalfa stands.

This is Agrigenetics Advanced Science Company manuscript no. 88.

REFERENCES

1. Loesch-Fries LS, Merlo D, Zinnen T, Burhop L, Hill K, Krahn K, Jarvis N, Nelson S, Halk E (1987). Expression of alfalfa mosaic virus RNA 4 in transgenic plants confers virus resistance. EMBO J 6:1845.
2. Sherwood JL, Fulton RW (1982). The specific involvement of coat protein in tobacco mosaic virus cross protection. Virology 119:150.
3. Dodds JA, Lee SQ, Tiffany M (1985). Cross protection between strains of cucumber mosaic virus: effect of host and type of inoculum on accumulation of virions and double-stranded RNA of the challenge strain. Virology 144:301.
4. Abel PP, Nelson RS, De B, Hoffmann N, Rogers SG, Fraley RT, Beachy RN (1986). Delay of disease development in transgenic plants that express the tobacco mosaic virus coat protein gene. Science 232:738.
5. Tumer NE, O'Connell KM, Nelson RS, Sanders PR, Beachy RN, Fraley RT, Shah DM (1987). Expression of alfalfa mosaic virus coat protein gene confers cross-protection in transgenic tobacco and tomato plants. EMBO J 6:1181.
6. Van Dun CMP, Bol JF, and Van Vloten-Doting L (1987). Expression of alfalfa mosaic virus and tobacco rattle virus coat protein genes in transgenic tobacco plants. Virology 159:299.
7. Hemenway C, Fang R-X, Kaniewski WK, Chua N-H, Tumer NE (1988). Analysis of the mechanism of protection in transgenic plants expressing the PVX coat protein gene. J Cell Biochem Suppl 12C:281.
8. Cuozzo M, O'Connell KM, Kaniewski W, Fang R-X, Chua N-H, Tumer NE (1988). Viral protection in transgenic tobacco plants expressing the cucumber mosaic virus coat protein or its antisense RNA. Bio/technology 6:549.

9. Gibbs AJ (1962). Lucerne mosaic virus in British lucerne crops. Plant Pathol 10:61.
10. Crill P, Hagedorn DJ, Hanson EW (1970). Incidence and effect of alfalfa mosaic virus on alfalfa. Phytopathology 60:1432.
11. Hemmati K, McLean DL (1977). Gamete-seed transmission of alfalfa mosaic virus and its effect on seed germination and yield in alfalfa plants. Phytopathology 67:576.
12. Tu JC, Holmes TM (1980). Effect of alfalfa mosaic virus infection on nodulation, forage yield, forage protein, and overwintering of alfalfa. Phytopath Z 97:1.
13. Bailiss KW, Ollennu LAA (1986). Effect of alfalfa mosaic virus isolates on forage yield of lucerne (Medicago sativa) in Britain. Plant Pathol 35:162.
14. Miczynski KA, Hiruki C (1987). Effect of alfalfa mosaic virus infection on the yield and regeneration of alfalfa at different growth temperatures. Can J Plant Pathol 9:49.
15. Dall D, Randles J, Francki R (1987). Alfalfa mosaic virus - a novel pathogen in Australian pastures. In "VII International Congress of Virology, Abstracts," Ottawa: National Research Council Canada, p 259.
16. Frosheiser FI (1969). Variable influence of alfalfa mosaic virus strains on growth and survival of alfalfa and on mechanical and aphid transmission. Phytopathology 59:857.
17. Crill P, Hanson EW, Hagedorn DJ (1971). Resistance and tolerance to alfalfa mosaic virus in alfalfa. Phytopathology 61:369.
18. Shahin EA, Spielmann A, Sukhapinda K, Simpson RB, Yashar M (1986). Transformation of cultivated alfalfa using disarmed Agrobacterium tumefaciens. Crop Sci 26:1235.
19. Schreier PH, Kuntz M, Lipphardt S, Lörz H, Baker B, Simons A, de Bruijn F, Schell J, Bohnert HJ, Reiss B, Wasmann CC (1985). New developments in plant transformation technology: its application to cellular organelles, cereals, and dicotyledonous crop plants. In Zaitlin M, Day P, Hollaender A (eds): "Biotechnology in Plant Science: Relevance to Agriculture in the Eighties," Orlando: Academic Press, p. 237.

20. Deak M, Kiss GB, Koncz C, Dudits D (1986). Transformation of Medicago by Agrobacterium mediated gene transfer. Plant Cell Rep 5:97.
21. Odell JT, Nagy F, Chua N-H (1985). Identification of DNA sequences required for activity of the cauliflower mosaic virus 35S promoter. Nature 313:810.
22. Brown, DCW, Atanassov A (1985). Role of genetic background in somatic embryogenesis in Medicago. Plant Cell Tissue Organ Cult 4:111.
23. Loesch-Fries LS, Jarvis NP, Krahn K, Nelson SE, Hall TC (1985). Expression of alfalfa mosaic virus RNA 4 cDNA transcripts in vitro and in vivo. Virology 146:177.
24. Firoozabady E, DeBoer DL, Merlo DJ, Halk EL, Amerson LN, Rashka KE, Murray EE (1987). Transformation of cotton (Gossypium hirsutum L.) by Agrobacterium tumefaciens and regeneration of transgenic plants. Plant Mol Biol 10:105.
25. Loesch-Fries LS, Halk E, Merlo D, Jarvis N, Nelson S, Krahn K, Burhop L (1987). Expression of alfalfa mosaic virus coat protein gene and anti-sense cDNA in transformed tobacco tissue. In Arntzen CJ, Ryan C (eds): "Molecular Strategies for Crop Protecion," New York: Alan R Liss, Inc., p. 221.
26. Bol JF, Van Vloten-Doting L, Jaspars EMJ (1971). A functional equivalence of top component a RNA and coat protein in the initiation of infection by alfalfa mosaic virus. Virology 46:73.
27. Harpster MH, Townsend JA, Jones JDG, Bedbrook J, Dunsmuir P (1988). Relative strengths of the 35S cauliflower mosaic virus, 1′, 2′, and nopaline synthase promoters in transformed tobacco sugarbeet and oilseed rape callus tissue. Mol Gen Genet 212:182.
28. Graham JH, Frosheiser FI, Stuteville DL, Erwin DC (1979). "A Compendium of Alfalfa Diseases," St. Paul: The American Phytopathological Society, p. 46.
29. Frosheiser FI (1964). Prevalence of alfalfa mosaic virus in alfalfa in Minnesota. Plant Dis Rep 48:506.

Index